MW01428924

Study guide to accompany

Clinical pharmacology and nursing management

Fifth edition

Laurel Eisenhauer, R.N., Ph.D., F.A.A.N.
Professor of Nursing
Boston College School of Nursing
Chestnut Hill, Massachusetts

Lynn Wemett Nichols, R.N., M.S.N.
Doctoral Student
School of Nursing
University of Rochester
Rochester, New York

Associate Professor, Ret.
Department of Nursing
State University of New York College at Plattsburgh
Plattsburgh, New York

Roberta Todd Spencer, R.N., M.S.
Associate Professor, Ret.
Department of Nursing
State University of New York College at Plattsburgh
Plattsburgh, New York

Frances West Bergan, R.N., M.S.N.
Director, Hospital Administration
University Hospital
SUNY Health Sciences Center
Syracuse, New York

Lippincott
Philadelphia • New York

Ancillary Editor:	*Doris S. Wray*
Acquisition Editor:	*Margaret Zuccarini*
Editorial Assistant:	*Sara Lauber*
Production:	*Shepherd, Inc.*
Printer/Binder:	*Victor Graphics, Inc.*

ISBN: 0-7817-1721-3

Contents

Unit eight: Drugs affecting the gastrointestinal system 135

Unit nine: Drugs affecting the endocrine system 149

Unit ten: Drugs affecting the immune system 171

Unit eleven: Drugs affecting other body systems 179

Unit twelve: Drugs affecting inflammation and infection 191

Unit thirteen: Drugs affecting neoplastic disease 211

Unit fourteen: Miscellaneous drug families 215

Answer Section 231

Preface

The purpose of this study guide is to assist students in mastering the content of *Clinical Pharmacoogy and Nursing Management.* The study guide contains exercises that involve students with material from the text to develop further relationships between facts and to provide repetition conducive to learning. Completion of the study guide promotes a degree of overlearning favorable to the retention of essential content. Students are stimulated to relate pharmacology to their own life experiences by analyzing personal exposure to and attitudes toward chemicals used as drugs.

A variety of approaches to learning are used in this study guide. For the most part, each chapter stands alone. In a few instances, however, mainly relating to the student's self-study, an exercise may relate to previous work. With these exceptions, each study guide chapter can be completed without reference to previous chapters. Answers are provided in the back of the book.

It is our hope that this study guide will function as both an aid to learning and a means for measuring progress in the mastery of content in pharmacology relative to nursing practice.

—The Authors

UNIT ONE
Introduction to pharmacology

1 ▪ *Orientation to pharmacology*

Pharmacology is one of the oldest sciences known to humankind. It is the study of the effects of chemical substances on living tissue. An interdisciplinary study, pharmacology helps to find a balance between the use of drugs in preventing or ameliorating illness and danger of toxicity and user dependence.

Drug therapy has evolved from primitive cultures to modern times, reflecting the quest for knowledge about the world and its natural resources and desire to influence the outcome of natural events. Drug therapy has evolved from three major areas:

1. Development and transmission of oral tribal traditions in drug folklore (magical approach)
2. Experience, observation, and analysis of cultural traditions in the use of environmental elements (empirical proto pharmacologic approach)
3. Development of chemical and biological research methodologies (scientific rational approach)

The nurse must know the facts pertaining to any and all drugs a particular client is using. This requires a basic knowledge of pharmacology. Drugs used frequently can and should be memorized but it is not possible to memorize all drugs. No single source provides all the pertinent information needed. A sound scholarly approach and the use of a variety of sources promote the development of a solid knowledge in the discipline.

Sequences

Arrange the following in chronologic order by numbering each in sequence:

_______ Ebers Medical Papyrus (Egypt)
_______ Injection techniques
_______ Use of foxglove by William Withering
_______ Drug production as a major technical industry
_______ Chinese codification of mixtures for medicine
_______ Roman Materia Medica
_______ Sophisticated Arabian pharmacology

Matching

Match the substance in the left-hand column with the result in the right-hand column. Place your answer in the space provided. Common substances have been used historically for mood alteration and as laxatives. Match the following:

_______ 1. Alcohol
_______ 2. Coca
_______ 3. Senna
_______ 4. Tobacco
_______ 5. Opium
_______ 6. Rhubarb
_______ 7. Marijuana
_______ 8. Betel

a. Mood alteration
b. Laxative

Match the definition in the left-hand column with the approach in the right-hand column. Place your answer in the space provided.

_______ 9. Use of antibiotics to treat a sore throat without a throat culture

_______ 10. Development of designated methodologies to demonstrate cause and effect

_______ 11. Use of religious amulets

_______ 12. Development and communication of traditional cures

_______ 13. Experience, observation, and analysis of traditional drug uses

a. Rational approach
b. Empirical approach
c. Magical approach

Match each item in the left-hand column with the most appropriate reference in the right-hand column. Place your answer in the space provided.

_______ 14. Contains extensive material on adverse reactions

_______ 15. Is the best reference for determining the generic name for a new trade name drug

_______ 16. Contains extensive material on nursing implications

_______ 17. Is written primarily for practicing physicians

_______ 18. Is written primarily for medical students

_______ 19. Is written primarily for nursing students and practicing nurses

_______ 20. Contains pharmaceutical data but has few medical or nursing implications

a. USP
b. Goodman & Gilman's *The Pharmacological Basics of Therapeutics*
c. PDR
d. Eisenhauer et al., *Clinical Pharmacology and Nursing Management*

Completion exercises

Read each question carefully and place your answer in the space provided.

1. Reflect on your most recent use of medicinal agents. As accurately as possible, identify the following aspects of your selection and use of these drugs.

Substance Used

____

____

____

Who Prescribed

____

____

____

Reason for Use

____

____

____

Type of Approach Represented

____

____

____

2. Pure drugs were first available for scientific study in the _______________________.
3. The type of drugs used by homeopaths are _______________________.
4. One value of homeopathy was that it _______________________.

5. In the United States, the first official standards designated for drugs were the ______________ and ______________.

Personal exercise: History of pharmacologically active substances

As completely as possible, list in the table the pharmacologically active substances to which your body has been exposed over the past week; describe your response(s) to them and identify whether each response was desirable or undesirable.

Drug Name	**Response**	**Desirable**	**Undesirable**
Prescription Drug		*(Check one)*	
Patent Medicines			
Folk Remedies			
Herbs			
Foods			
Social Drugs			
Poisons			

Pollutants

____________ ____________ ____________ ____________

____________ ____________ ____________ ____________

(Save this list. You will be asked to refer to it in later exercises.)

Short answer questions

1. List six major characteristics of the 20th century, relative to pharmacology.

2. List five problems addressed by scientists using the rational approach for the evaluation of pharmacologic agents.
   a.
   b.
   c.
   d.
   e.

3. Whom or what can the nurse consult if printed information about a drug that is to be administered is not readily available?

Multiple choice questions

For each of the following, choose the one best answer:

1. One traditional use of alcohol is
   a. as an anesthetic
   b. as an antidiarrheal
   c. to relieve fatigue
   d. to relieve nausea
2. Saki is an example of a drug that was developed from
   a. grapes
   b. corn
   c. potatoes
   d. rice
3. When did the study of pharmacology begin?
   a. in the prehistoric times, through trial and error
   b. about 3000 B.C. in China
   c. about 2000 B.C. in Egypt
   d. during the Renaissance, when chemical reach began
4. In what century was aspirin discovered as a drug to treat pain and fever?
   a. 13th
   b. 16th
   c. 19th
   d. 20th
5. A drug applied to arrow tips as a poison is
   a. coca
   b. curare
   c. alcohol
   d. caffeine
6. During the 17th and 18th centuries the progress of pharmacology was characterized by
   a. wide distribution and use of drug information by physicians and laypersons
   b. reliance on scientific principles as a basis for knowledge
   c. reliance on herbal remedies for drug effects
   d. the tailoring of drugs for a specific effect through chemical manipulation of molecular structure

7. When were the stimulant properties of tea, coffee, and cocoa first recognized by European cultures?
   a. in prehistoric times
   b. during the Middle Ages
   c. in the Renaissance
   d. during the 17th century
8. In which century was foxglove first used as a heart stimulant?
   a. 13th
   b. 16th
   c. 18th
   d. 20th
9. The magical approach furthered the development of pharmacology because it
   a. involved clients in their own treatment
   b. fostered the experimental use of natural elements
   c. helped physicians realize some illnesses are caused by supernatural forces
   d. stimulated the growth of the material sciences
10. Which of the following had the most profound effect on the advancement of pharmacology during the 17th and 18th centuries?
    a. The scientific method was used to investigate drugs.
    b. The five major problems of pharmacology were recognized.
    c. The active ingredients of specific drugs were isolated.
    d. Toxicity and harmful effects were recognized.
11. Aspirin is still incompletely understood in relation to its
    a. mechanism of action
    b. safety margin
    c. allergenicity
    d. potency index
12. Localization of the site of drug action was a factor in the development of which approach to pharmacology?
    a. magical
    b. empiric
    c. scientific
13. Which of the following represents the empiric approach to drug use?
    a. prescribing antacids to relieve gastric distress after eating spicy foods
    b. prescribing penicillin to treat a sexually transmitted disease
    c. using garlic to ward off a cold
    d. none of the above
14. *The United States Pharmacopeia and National Formulary* is written for
    a. laypersons
    b. nurses
    c. pharmacists
    d. physicians
15. A drug that causes sedation in most people causes a coma in one person. This example best reflects
    a. an adverse reaction
    b. an allergic reaction
    c. a side effect
    d. a toxic effect
16. When a client is admitted to the hospital, she shows the nurse a blue tablet that she describes as a "nerve pill." She thinks the pill is Valium but doesn't know the dosage. To find a colored picture of Valium in varying dosage forms, the best action for the nurse to pursue initially is to
    a. ask the pharmacist to provide a drug package insert
    b. call a pharmaceutical manufacturer
    c. consult the *Physician's Desk Reference*
    d. telephone the client's physician

Essay question

List and briefly describe the types of required information needed about a drug preparation to give safe care to the client receiving it.

Personal exercise

Write a 100-to-150-word description of your own attitude toward "drugs." On a scale of 10, with 1 equaling extreme permissiveness toward medication use and 10 extreme avoidance of use, what value would you assign to your viewpoint.

Learning experience 1-1

1. Interview a friend or family member to explore his or her beliefs about the use of medications and personal drug habits related to taking prescribed medicines. Explore the following questions in your interview:
   a. What was the subjects presenting problem?
   b. What interventions, if any, did the individual try before seeking medical advice?
   c. How did he or she approach the healthcare provider to resolve a problem?
   d. How did he or she comply with the recommended regimen for taking the medication?
   e. What approaches to using mycologic agents are you able to identify in this interview?
2. Interview friends and peers to solicit information regarding health-seeking practices that reflect an empirical orientation.
3. Explore the availability of folk remedies or herbal products in a health food store and identify the rationale for using these specific products.
4. Prepare an outline of essential information for a drug ordered for a client or acquaintance. Use at least five references, including (if possible) Drug Information, Facts and Comparisons, or Compendium of Pharmaceutical and Specialities; a nursing textbook on pharmacology; a medical textbook on pharmacology; and the Physicians's Desk Reference.

Enrichment experience 1-1

Interview an older relative or friend to explore the experiences he or she has had with drug use throughout the life span. Ask questions about traditional family remedies, patent medicines, prescription drugs, and nonmedicinal drugs (alcohol, nicotine, caffeine, and so forth.) If the person remembers anything about life in the 1960's, find out how he or she felt about drug use in this period. How does this attitude compare with the person's opinion on decriminalizing the use of marijuana?

Compare your findings with those of your classmates. What cultural contexts are reflected in the drug practices reported? Are the attitudes expressed similar or dissimilar? Do the data offer any clues to factors influencing these attitudes? How do the attitudes of older adults compare with those of young people today?

2 ▪ *Drug preparations, controls, and standards*

The drugs produced by pharmaceutical firms today are ready-to-use products that have been purified, modified, formulated, named, and packaged to appeal to physicians, other healthcare providers and consumers. Their manufacture, marketing, and use are regulated by controls ranging from formal laws to cultural mores and family values. Some basic knowledge of these preparations and controls is essential for safe drug use by nurses and clients alike.

Matching

For each item in the left-hand column, select the most appropriate item from the right-hand column.

_______ 1. Binders
_______ 2. Disintegrators
_______ 3. Dyes
_______ 4. Fillers
_______ 5. Preservatives
_______ 6. Vehicles
_______ 7. Flavoring

a. Aid in identifying unlabeled drugs
b. Prevent microbial growth in injectable solutions
c. Decrease the risk of tablets crumbling
d. Give form and substance to a drug
e. Enable a manufacturer to adjust dosage of a preparation
f. Make drugs more palatable
g. Promote dissolution of a tablet

Match the drug in the left-hand column with its classification in the right-hand column according to the standards presented in the Controlled Substance Act of 1970.

_______ 8. diazepam (Valium)
_______ 9. peyote
_______ 10. heroin
_______ 11. cough syrups containing codeine
_______ 12. meprobamate (Miltown)
_______ 13. methadone
_______ 14. secobarbital ("reds")
_______ 15. amphetamines ("speed")
_______ 16. LSD
_______ 17. nalorphine

a. Schedule I
b. Schedule II
c. Schedule III
d. Schedule IV
e. Schedule V

True and false

In the space in front of each statement, place a T if the statement is true; place an F if the statement is false.

_______ 1. The generic name of a drug is usually the same as its official name.

_______ 2. In the United States, official names are printed in *Drug Information,* published by the United States Pharmacopeia Association.

_______ 3. A drug may have many proprietary names.

_______ 4. *The United States Pharmacopeia and National Formulary* publishes a list of approved abbreviations for drug names.

_______ 5. Nurses should not reveal to the client the names of prescribed drugs unless the physician has asked that the name be listed on the prescription label.

_______ 6. Enteric-coated tablets are designed to delay the release of their ingredients until they reach the intestinal mucosa.

_______ 7. Drug experience reports submitted to the Food and Drug Administration (FDA) must originate with a physician or dentist.

_______ 8. Drugs classified under Schedule I of the Controlled Substance Act of 1970 are medicinal agents with the greatest potential for causing dependence.

_______ 9. At present there is no legally sanctioned medicinal use for heroin in the United States.

_______ 10. In the United States, prescriptions for narcotics such as morphine may be refilled only once before renewal.

_______ 11. According to federal FDA regulations, medicinal drugs sold in the United States must be 100 percent pure.

_______ 12. At present there is no legally sanctioned medicinal use for thalidomide in Canada.

Multiple choice questions

For each of the following, choose the one best answer:

1. Aspirin is usually manufactured
   a. from a plant source
   b. from a mineral source
   c. from animal tissues
   d. by synthesis in a laboratory
2. Insulin is an example of a drug derived from
   a. animals
   b. chemicals
   c. minerals
   d. plants
3. Which of the following drugs is least likely to be prescribed for oral administration?
   a. polypeptides
   b. steroids
   c. glycosides
   d. salts
4. Which of the following drugs is least likely to be compatible with morphine sulfate?
   a. atropine sulfate
   b. sodium pentobarbital
   c. meperidine hydrochloride
   d. magnesium chloride
5. Which of the following drug families contains substances whose pharmacologic action is attributed to the formation of charged ions upon dissolution?
   a. polypeptides
   b. steroids
   c. glycosides
   d. salts
6. Which of the following substances is not a steroid?
   a. cholesterol
   b. estrogen
   c. digitalis
   d. glycerin
7. Atropine, codeine, and morphine belong to which major class of drugs?
   a. alkaloids
   b. glycosides
   c. polypeptides
   d. steroids
8. Which class of drugs are protein in nature, tend to be high molecular weight compounds, and must be given parenterally?
   a. alkaloids
   b. glycosides
   c. polypeptides
   d. salts
9. Which class of drugs are organic compounds containing nitrogen with a basic pH and found in seeds, roots, leaves, and bark?
   a. alkaloids
   b. glycosides
   c. polypeptides
   d. steroids
10. An example of a glycoside is
    a. insulin
    b. morphine sulfate
    c. digitalis
    d. testosterone
11. Powders added to a drug to delay the dissolution of the medication for a timed-release effect would be an example of which type of drug additive?
    a. binders
    b. diluents
    c. fillers
    d. vehicles

12. Substances added to a drug that increase bulk and reduce the concentration of the active ingredient are called
   a. binders
   b. diluents
   c. disintegrators
   d. vehicles
13. Drugs most likely to act as ions (electrically charged particles) are
   a. salts
   b. steroids
   c. alkaloids
   d. polypeptides
14. Which of the following is most likely to taste sweet?
   a. an extract
   b. a fluid extract
   c. an elixir
   d. an aromatic water
15. Asthmatic clients are most likely to experience allergic reactions to dyes that color tablets
   a. red
   b. blue
   c. green
   d. yellow
16. Tartrazine is added to drug formulations for the purpose of
   a. making pills taste better
   b. making tablets look more attractive
   c. preventing tablets from crumbling
   d. increasing the bulk of a tablet without increasing the dose
17. An example of a generic name for a drug is
   a. acetylsalicylic acid
   b. Ascriptin
   c. aspirin
   d. Bufferin
18. If a drug label is difficult to read, the nurse should
   a. ask a colleague to verify the name
   b. contact the physician to verify the order
   c. return the drug and container to the pharmacist
   d. rewrite the label clearly
19. If successive prescriptions for a drug use different names, the client is most likely to
   a. refuse to take the second prescription
   b. skip doses of the drug
   c. take a double dose of the drug
   d. alternate doses
20. If the drug name is capitalized, it is most likely to be a/an
   a. chemical name
   b. generic name
   c. official name
   d. trade name
21. Which method would most likely be used to determine potency of a drug?
   a. blood sampling
   b. chemical analysis
   c. double-blind studies
   d. tissue concentration analysis
22. In comparing the various testing procedures available for drugs, the major disadvantage of chemical assay is that this method
   a. involves risks to human subjects
   b. is expensive
   c. is not always available
   d. is time consuming
23. The incidence and severity of adverse reactions attributable to the use of a drug determines which property of that drug?
   a. efficacy
   b. potency
   c. purity
   d. safety/toxicity
24. Which property of drugs is determined by the degree that a drug can be absorbed and transported by the body to its active site?
   a. bioavailability
   b. efficacy
   c. purity
   d. safety/toxicity
25. Of the following choices, which method would be the most appropriate to measure efficacy of a drug?
   a. analyzing chemically the ingredients of the drug for impurities
   b. asking clients if their symptoms were relieved after taking the drug
   c. observing clients for harmful side effects while being treated with the drug
   d. testing blood samples for concentration of the drug after the drug has been given
26. The first narcotic control act passed by any nation was
   a. the Food, Drug, and Cosmetic Act of 1906
   b. the Harrison Act of 1914
   c. the Food, Drug, and Cosmetic Act of 1938
   d. the Durham-Humphrey Amendment of 1952

27. Under Canadian law, examples of "designated" drugs would include
    a. opiates
    b. amphetamines
    c. tranquilizers
    d. antibiotics
28. The cheapest and most valid test for drug evaluation is usually through
    a. chemical assay
    b. bioassay
    c. bioimmunoassay
    d. animal trials
    e. clinical trials on humans
29. Legislative guidelines for drug controls are largely at which level?
    a. local
    b. state
    c. national
    d. international
30. The main purpose of the Food, Drug, and Cosmetic Act of 1938 was to
    a. prevent consumers from taking drugs with poisonous properties
    b. prohibit fraudulent therapeutic claims by drug manufacturers
    c. provide for certification of certain drugs through testing by the FDA
    d. regulate the importation, manufacture, sale, and use of habit-forming drugs
31. The tragic birth defects from the drug thalidomide were a major factor that led to the passage of which law?
    a. Canadian Narcotic Control Act
    b. Controlled Substance Act
    c. Durham-Humphrey Amendment
    d. Kefauver-Harris Amendment
32. In describing the relationship between federal drug laws and state laws, which of the following is the most accurate? State laws must be
    a. compatible with federal laws
    b. identical to federal laws
    c. less stringent than federal laws
    d. more specific than federal laws
33. At which level are restrictions on the sale or use of alcohol or tobacco usually enacted?
    a. local
    b. state
    c. national
    d. international
34. At which level would restrictions on the use of drugs vary the most?
    a. institutional
    b. local
    c. state (provincial)
    d. national
35. When transferring to a new state, to obtain accurate and complete information about current drug regulations, the nurse should
    a. ask the manager in charge of the nursing unit on which he or she works
    b. contact a pharmacy for institutional and state regulations
    c. request the state drug laws from the governor's office
    d. write to the Federal Drug Administration
36. Which of the following actions is within the role of the nurse administering medications?
    a. giving an aspirin to a client without a physician's order
    b. leaving the medication at the bedside for a client to take when she finishes eating
    c. insisting the client take the prescribed medication when he refuses
    d. recording each dose of opiates administered to clients
37. The Ames test measures
    a. carcinogenicity of chemicals in animals
    b. bioavailability of chemicals in humans
    c. potency of chemicals
    d. mutagenicity of chemicals in bacteria
38. Refill of prescription drugs in Canada is limited to a period of
    a. 2 weeks
    b. 1 month
    c. 3 months
    d. 6 months
39. An important nursing responsibility related to clinical trials of experimental drugs on humans is
    a. recording data identifying subjects as members of either the experimental or the control group
    b. testing blood samples to determine the drug level in the serum
    c. assessing subjects' responses to treatment
    d. all of the above

Selection of options

For each drug in the left-hand column, select from the right-hand column the type of constraint(s) that currently exist in the United States

_______ 1. Alcohol
_______ 2. Caffeine (tea, coffee, cola)
_______ 3. Marijuana
_______ 4. Heroin

a. Legal control (federal, state, local)
b. Institutional policies in, for example, hospitals and nursing homes
c. Religious proscriptions
d. Cultural mores
e. Family values

For each name in the left-hand column, select all appropriate items in the right-hand column.

_______ 5. Abbreviation
_______ 6. Trade name
_______ 7. Official name
_______ 8. Chemical name
_______ 9. Generic name
_______ 10. Proprietary name
_______ 11. Brand name

a. Tends to be long and cumbersome
b. In the *United States Pharmacopeia and National Formulary*
c. In the United States, is chosen by the United States Adopted Name Council
d. Is protected by copyright
e. Is usually an acronym
f. Is capitalized when written
g. Denotes molecular structure of a drug
h. Often has no written standard

For each of the following, select all appropriate responses:

12. Techniques frequently employed in the laboratory production of drugs include
    a. maintaining a natural drug in its crude form to preserve all active principles
    b. modifying natural drugs to increase specificity
    c. building complex molecules from pure chemical elements
    d. altering genes of microorganisms to induce production of drugs in short supply
    e. altering drug molecules to reduce toxicity
13. Data appropriate to a drug history include
    a. chemical names of drugs used by the client
    b. generic names of drugs used by the client
    c. trade names of drugs used by the client
    d. allergic reactions to drugs
    e. allergic reactions to foods
14. Why are enteric coatings applied to tablets?
    a. to make them easier to swallow
    b. to make them taste better
    c. to delay their absorption
    d. to protect the drug from stomach secretions
15. The term *lozenge* is synonymous with
    a. tablet
    b. pill
    c. capsule
    d. troche

Rank-order question

Arrange the following in rank order according to their viscosities, starting with the most viscous.

_______ a. Magma
_______ b. Solution
_______ c. Suppository
_______ d. Cream
_______ e. Ointment
_______ f. Paste

Correct the false statement

Indicate whether the following statements are true or false; correct the underlined words or phrases.

_______ 1. A single drug may have multiple generic names.

_______ 2. The proprietary name identifies the manufacturer of the drug.

_______ 3. Individual drugs may be members of more than one drug family.

_______ 4. Acids and salts are among the drugs derived from mineral sources.

_______ 5. In most cases, synthetic drugs are not as effective as are natural drugs.

_______ 6. The purpose of adding lubricants to tablets is to make them easier to swallow.

_______ 7. Fixed oils evaporate easily, leaving no greasy residue.

_______ 8. A foam is a homogeneous mixture of two liquids that do not dissolve in each other.

_______ 9. The federal agency charged with the task of controlling the smuggling of heroin or cocaine into the United States is the Food and Drug Administration.

_______ 10. According to the text, penalties for drug infractions in many countries are more lenient than in the United States.

_______ 11. In the United States, the first federal legislation that dealt with drug controls was the Food, Drug, and Cosmetic Act of 1906.

_______ 12. The Shirley Amendment of 1912 was effective in requiring that efficacy of drug remedies be proven.

_______ 13. The first federal controls on habit-forming drugs were established by the Controlled Substance Act of 1970.

_______ 14. The Food, Drug, and Cosmetic Act of 1938 placed specific controls on the labeling of drugs.

_______ 15. A legend drug may be sold without a prescription.

_______ 16. Only physicians can file adverse drug reaction reports with the Food and Drug Administration.

_______ 17. In Canada nurses may receive sample drugs from pharmaceutical firms.

Short answer questions

Define the following terms relating to drug preparations:

1. Purity

2. Potency

3. Bioavailability

4. Efficacy

Define and give an example of each of the following terms:

5. Generic name

6. Official name

7. Active ingredient

8. Additive

9. Alkaloid

10. Glycosides

11. Polypeptides

12. Steroids

13. Vehicles

14. Fillers

15. Diluents

16. Binders

17. Disintegrators

18. Lubricants

19. Flavorings

20. Dyes

Name the type of drug preparation described by the following:

21. Mixtures of oils, water, and drug ingredients

22. Compressed powders or granulated ingredients

23. Molded mixtures of a drug's ingredients in a firm base with a low melting point

24. Drug ingredients mixed with alcohol, oil, soap, or water

25. Saturated solutions of water and volatile substances

26. High concentration of alcohol solution of vegetable drugs

27. Mixtures of alcohol, volatile oils, and sweeteners

28. Generic names ending in "ine"

Answer the following questions:

29. For what is the Ames text used?

30. List the attitudes and practices in your family that exert control over drug use, for example, the use of social drugs and illegal drugs, adherence to physicians' orders for prescription drugs, and preferred patent medicines. Include avoidance of drugs known to cause adverse reactions, such as those causing allergies or idiosyncratic reactions.

Identify the drug property described in the following:

31. The relative strength of drug action: ____________________

32. The magnitude of the difference between safe and toxic doses: ____________________

33. Ability to produce desired therapeutic responses: ____________________

34. Freedom from contaminating substances: ____________________

35. Degree to which a drug is absorbed and transported to target tissues: ____________________

Answer the following questions:

36. According to the provisions of the Controlled Substances Act of 1970, how does drug dependence differ from drug addition?

37. List one or more examples of legal drug controls in the United States that have been more strict than the customs or mores of the population at large or of a substantial subculture. What happened as a consequence?

38. List at least eight provisions of the Canadian Food and Drugs Act. Identify one drug forbidden by Canadian law. Define the legal meaning of *controlled, designated,* and the abbreviation *Pr.*

Completion exercise

Read each question carefully and place your answer in the space provided.

1. A drug that causes congenital absence or severe deformity of the limbs in children exposed to it *in utero* is ____________________.
2. Inadequate control of production in the manufacture of the drug ____________ caused permanent paralysis in some recipients.
3. A drug for which there is substantial evidence of effectiveness would be rated according to the rating scale adopted by the National Research Council of the National Academy of Science as ____________________
4. The law requiring that effectiveness of drugs must be established by substantial evidence is the ____________________.
5. The factor most important in determining a person's drug use is ____________________.

Learning experience

Examine the policy and procedure manuals at a hospital or nursing home to determine drug controls in effect in that healthcare setting. Compare these requirements with those imposed by the state or provincial government. Which policies represent controls that are stricter than state or provincial requirements? Are any of them required by county or town ordinance? Pay particular attention to policies regarding automatic expiration of drug orders, security measures for controlled drugs, and recording of the disposition of narcotics.

Enrichment experiences

1. Write a letter to the drug manufacturer that advertises "candylike" medicines for children. As a professional nurse and consumer, explain your concerns and the potential dangers associated with this type of drug promotion.
2. List drug abbreviations noted on clients' charts and Kardexes or medication administration records in a medical unit within a healthcare facility. Compare this list with those abbreviations noted in two other specialty units (e.g., pediatrics, maternity, or psychiatric unit). Fill in the correct generic or brand name for each abbreviation. Ask a colleague to do the same; then compare responses. Consider the professional and legal implications if you were unable to identify a drug correctly.

3 ▪ *Nursing process: Management of clients with drug-related problems*

The nursing process provides the framework for logical scientific problem solving in nursing care. The process includes the following: assessment, diagnosis, planning, intervention, and outcome evaluation. The nurse uses the nursing process to promote optimal response to chemicals, to decrease the risk of adverse reactions, and to assist clients to achieve optimal health through the proper use of drugs.

Personal exercise: Nursing care plan

Select one medicinal substance that you use regularly or sporadically. Using the nursing process, develop a nursing care plan tailored to your own personal needs. Identify interventions in the care plan of which you had not previously been aware that will enhance the effectiveness of the medication and minimize adverse reactions to the drug.

Correct the false statement

Indicate in the blanks whether the following statements are true or false; if false, correct the underlined words or phrases.

_______ 1. Nursing responsibilities for clients receiving therapeutic drugs <u>are limited primarily to the dependent function of administering drugs prescribed by the physician.</u>

_______ 2. The nursing care plan should include consideration <u>of potential as well as actual problems</u> arising from drug use.

_______ 3. Detailed teaching regarding drug properties is particularly important for <u>institutionalized clients</u> receiving drugs for <u>treatment of acute health problems.</u>

_______ 4. Nurses should <u>teach clients to avoid the use of drugs whenever possible.</u>

_______ 5. Criteria for outcome evaluation should be formulated <u>at the time evaluation data are collected.</u>

Short answer questions

1. Name three general objectives of nursing care related to the proper use of drugs.

2. Name the steps in the nursing process.

3. Identify four categories of data required for assessing drug use.

4. Identify five types of goals that are appropriate in the care of clients receiving therapeutic drugs.

5. Identify five types of reactions that should be investigated while taking a drug history.

6. Why are data about unusual drug reactions in family members important?

7. What elements are desirable in a measurable criterion for evaluating nursing care?

Multiple choice questions

For each of the following, choose the one best answer:

1. The first step in the nursing process is
   a. assessment
   b. diagnosis
   c. intervention
   d. planning
2. The nurse is asking a client if he has any allergies. The nurse is using which step of the nursing process?
   a. assessment
   b. evaluation
   c. intervention
   d. planning
3. Which of the following best describes the planning step of the nursing process?
   a. arranging for the social services department to assist the client with finances so he can afford to buy his medication
   b. documenting that the client's blood pressure has increased since he started taking a medication
   c. reporting to the physician that the client has developed a goal that the client will report any dizziness he may have from a medication
4. Of the following, which best describes what occurs in the outcome evaluation step of the nursing process?
   a. carrying out nursing actions to enhance the effectiveness of the medication regimen
   b. collecting data from the client that might indicate his response to medications
   c. reporting to the physician that the client developed a rash after he started taking a new medication
   d. setting a goal that the client will report any dizziness he may have from a medication
5. Of the following, which best describes what occurs in the outcome evaluation step of the nursing process?
   a. carrying out nursing actions to enhance the effectiveness of the medication regimen
   b. collecting data from the client that might indicate his response to medications
   c. comparing what actually happened during medication therapy with the preestablished goal
   d. identifying potential problems the client may experience from his or her medications
6. The identification of contraindications for a drug to be used is the primary responsibility
   a. of the nurse
   b. of the physician
   c. of the pharmacist
   d. equally of all of the above
7. Consultation with a pharmacist is likely to be required when clients
   a. cannot metabolize or eliminate normal dosages of the drug
   b. experience severe adverse reactions to drugs
   c. receive many drugs concurrently
   d. all of the above
8. Factors such as poverty, confusion, lack of education, emotional nonacceptance of a disease, stiffness in the hands from arthritis, and poor vision would have the greatest impact on which aspect of drug therapy for the client?
   a. reactions
   b. compliance
   c. contraindications
   d. tolerance

9. Which of the following would best apply to the term, *drug interactions* (as opposed to *contraindications, precautions,* and *adverse reactions*)?
   a. Every drug has some side effects that many clients may experience when taking the drug.
   b. One drug may counteract or enhance the effect of another drug the client is taking.
   c. Specific drugs should not be used under certain conditions, such as when a client is pregnant.
   d. The risk of complications is increased if the drug is given to a client with an organ impairment, such as kidney

Selection of options

For each of the following, select all appropriate responses. Circle the correct answers.

1. The part(s) of the nursing diagnosis that must be amenable to nursing interventions is (are) the
   a. problem
   b. cause of the problem
   c. underlying factors that contribute to the cause of the problem
2. Clients who are most likely to need a drug dosage smaller than the usual range for their age and body size are clients with
   a. malabsorption
   b. impaired circulation
   c. renal impairment
   d. hepatic impairment
3. Inherited factors affecting response to drugs include
   a. ability to absorb oral doses
   b. microsomal enzymes in the liver
   c. kidney function
   d. allergic tendencies

Using a drug history form

Using the form that follows, select a client, friend, or family member and obtain a drug history.

Enrichment experience

Observe a nurse caring for clients for 4–8 hours to determine how pharmacologic aspects of care are integrated into the nursing care plan.

DRUG HISTORY FORM FOR HOME USE   Today's Date ______

Client's Name ______   Date of Birth ______
Address ______   Telephone ______
______

Occupation ______
Present Concern ______
Physician's Name ______   Telephone ______
Referral Source ______   Telephone ______
______
______

Informant (if other than client) ______
______

I. Medications

What drugs are you now taking?

Prescription ______
______

Over-the-counter ______
______

Home remedies ______
______

For what reasons do you take these drugs? ______
______

Do they work as intended? ______
______

What drugs have you taken in the last 2 weeks? ______
______
______
______

What drugs have you taken in the past year? ______
______
______
______

Have you experienced any problems when taking drugs?

Skin rash ______   Blurred vision ______
Nausea/vomiting ______   Ringing in the ear ______
Drowsiness ______   Loss of hair ______
Constipation ______   Tremors ______
Diarrhea ______   Other ______
Dry mouth ______

What do you use for the following conditions?

Dry skin ______
Rashes ______
Deodorant ______
Diaper ______
Athlete's foot ______
Poison ivy ______
Insect bites ______
What kind of soap do you use? ______
What kind of detergent/fabric softener? ______
What kind of perfume/cologne/after-shave? ______

(Continued)

DRUG HISTORY FORM FOR HOME USE (*Continued*)

Dandruff ____________________
Hair color treatments/special shampoos and rinses ____________________
Toothache ____________________
Do you wear dentures? ____________________
If yes, how do you care for them? ____________________
Ear problems (excessive wax, itching, discharge) ____________________
____
Eye problems (too little or too much water, redness, discharge, irritation) ____________________
____
Do you wear glasses or contact lenses? ____________________
If yes, how do you care for them? ____________________
Headaches ____________________
Cold and virus ____________________
Wheezing ____________________
Chest pain ____________________
Allergies ____________________
Sinus condition/runny nose ____________________
Sore throat ____________________
Stomach ache/indigestion ____________________
Nausea and vomiting ____________________
Constipation ____________________
Diarrhea ____________________
Gas pains/cramps ____________________
Hemorrhoids/rectal bleeding ____________________
Menstrual cramps ____________________
Vaginal or penile discharge ____________________
Contraception ____________________
Muscle ache/back ache ____________________
Burns ____________________
Cuts ____________________
Hangover ____________________
Nervous anxiety/tension ____________________
Feelings of depression or loss ____________________
Sleep disturbances ____________________
Fatigue ____________________
Sexual difficulties ____________________
Feeling overweight ____________________
Feeling underweight ____________________

II. *Drug Storage*

Where do you store your medicines? (Describe)
Medicine cabinet ____________________
Shelf ____________________
Table ____________________
Purse ____________________ Where is purse kept? ____________________
Refrigerator ____________________
Other ____________________
____
Are any medicine storage areas locked? ____________________ Which? ____________________
____
____

(Continued)

DRUG HISTORY FORM FOR HOME USE (*Continued*)

Where do you store your household and other chemicals? (Describe)

Kitchen cupboard ________

Closet ________

Garage ________

Shed ________

Cellar ________

Other ________

Are any of these storage areas locked? ________ Which? ________

____

____

III. *Environment*

What household chemicals do you use regularly? ________

Is your water fluoridated? ________ Is it hard or soft? ________

Does it have a particular taste? ________

Do you have a deodorizer in use in your home? ________

What type of heating do you have in your home? ________

Is your street a heavily traveled bus/truck route? ________

What kind of paint was used on the floors, walls, and woodwork in your home? ________

If you have a garden, do you use any pesticides, herbicides, or fertilizers? ________

What kinds of house plants do you have? ________

Would you consider this climate a healthy one for you and your family (e.g., smog, industrial pollutants)? ________

____

Do you wash fruits and vegetables before you use them? ________

Do you do your own home canning of foods? ________

IV. *Habits*

How much of the following do you consume per day? Per week?

Soda (diet, regular, decaffeinated) ________

Tea (herbal, regular) ________

Coffee (decaffeinated, regular) ________

Alcohol (beer, wine, liquor) ________

Candy (chocolates, licorice, diet candy) ________

Vitamins ________ Minerals ________ Herbal preparations ________

Do you smoke any of the following? If yes, how often?

Cigarettes ________

Cigars ________

Pipe ________

Marijuana ________

Other ________

Do you use any inhalants? If yes, how much? What kind? How often? ________

____

Do you use any artificial sweeteners? If yes, how much? What kinds? How often? ________

____

Do you use any salt or salt tablets? If yes, how much? How often? ________

Do you regularly use cosmetics? If yes, which ones? ________

What do you use for skin care? ________

Do you take vitamins or minerals? If so, what kind? How many? How often? ________

Do you regularly use laxatives, antacids? If yes, what kind? How many? How often? ________

Do you use, or have you used, food for medical purposes? If so, what have you taken and for what? ________

________ How often? ________

Do you use any recreational drugs? If yes, specify. ________

(*Continued*)

DRUG HISTORY FORM FOR HOME USE (*Continued*)

V. *Specific Problems and Concerns*

Do you have any allergies?

To drugs? ______

To foods? ______

To animals? ______

To the environment? ______

Have you ever experienced any difficulty taking drugs? ______

The pills are difficult to swallow ______

The pills or liquid do not taste right (e.g. bitter) ______

The dose is too complicated to take as prescribed ______

You forgot to take drugs at different times of the day ______

Do you ever give your medicines to others—a family member or friends? ______

Have you ever taken anyone else's medicine? ______

Have you ever experienced any ill effects from medicines (e.g., dizziness, loss of consciousness, tremors, rash, upset stomach)? ______

Have you had any allergic reaction to drugs? ______

Has anyone in your family experienced an allergic reaction? ______

How do you measure your liquid medicine (e.g., teaspoon)? ______

Have you ever stopped taking a prescribed medicine before it was finished, If yes, for what reason? ______

How are you affected when you forgot to take your medication? ______

______

What do you do about missed doses of medication? ______

What happens when you forget to take your medication? ______

How do you pay for your medicines? ______

How do you obtain medications? Yourself? Home delivery? Friend or family member? ______

How do you dispose of unused, unknown, or out-of-date medications? ______

How would you contact the local poison control center? ______

Do you use an identification bracelet or carry a drug information card? ______

Have you ever purchased drugs outside the United States? If so, which ones? Do you continue to take them? ______

Do you use any self-testing products (e.g., Clintest, Diastix, or pregnancy testing products)? ______

Do you use or have you used illegal drugs? (specify)? ______

Who are your current physician(s)? ______

______ Telephone ______

______ Telephone ______

______ Telephone ______

______ Telephone ______

Nurse(s)? ______ Telephone ______

______ Telephone ______

Pharmacist(s)? ______ Telephone ______

______ Telephone ______

Dentist(s)? ______ Telephone ______

______ Telephone ______

Podiatrist(s)? ______ Telephone ______

______ Telephone ______

Ophthalmologist(s)? ______ Telephone ______

______ Telephone ______

(Continued)

DRUG HISTORY FORM FOR HOME USE (*Continued*)

Other health care providers? (Please be specific)

_______________________________________ Telephone ______________
_______________________________________ Telephone ______________
_______________________________________ Telephone ______________
_______________________________________ Telephone ______________

This drug history should be adapted as applicable for each client interview and situation. Because of specialization, a client may have more than one dentist, doctor, and so forth. Moreover, those who have more than one home may have health care professionals in each location. Be sure to note these situations. (Form developed by Martha Fortune, R.N., M.S., Consultant)

UNIT TWO
Therapy with drugs

4 ▪ *Pharmacodynamics and pharmacokinetics*

Individual response to drugs is determined in large part by inherited processes affecting the absorption, distribution, storage, receptor interaction, and excretion of active chemicals. The following exercises relate to these processes of pharmacokinetics and pharmacodynamics.

Matching

A. Match the term in the left-hand column with the most appropriate item in the right-hand column. Place your answer in the space provided.

_______ 1. Urinary acidifier
_______ 2. Osmotic diuretic
_______ 3. Lubricant
_______ 4. Agonist
_______ 5. Saline cathartic
_______ 6. Antacid
_______ 7. Antagonist
_______ 8. Endorphin

a. Alteration of the physical environment of the cell
b. Alteration of the chemical environment of the cell
c. Interaction with a cell receptor

B. Match the tissue in the left-hand column with the most appropriate item in the right-hand column. Place your answer in the space provided.

_______ 1. Tissue that tends to store metallic ions
_______ 2. Tissue that tends to store acidic drugs
_______ 3. Tissue that tends to store hydrocarbons
_______ 4. Tissue that most actively breaks down drugs

a. Fat
b. Bone
c. Liver
d. Plasma proteins
e. Brain

C. Match the phrase in the left-hand column with the terms in the right-hand column. Place your answer(s) in the space provided. (More than one answer may be correct.)

_______ 1. Movement across a membrane requiring dissolution in the lipid portion of the membrane
_______ 2. Transport mechanism(s) that require(s) energy expenditure
_______ 3. Transport mechanism that is most specific (i.e., is highly selective of the type of molecule transported)

a. Active transport
b. Diffusion
c. Pinocytosis
d. Osmosis

_______ 4. Movement of water across a membrane that is impervious to some or all of the chemicals in the solution

_______ 5. Movement across a membrane by means of encapsulation in an envelope of membranous material

_______ 6. Movement across a membrane against a pressure gradient

_______ 7. Mechanism whose maximum capacity is limited only by the area of the membrane

_______ 8. Mechanism that allows free movement of polar compounds

a. Active transport
b. Diffusion
c. Pinocytosis
d. Osmosis

Checklist

Using a check mark, indicate the administration routes involving absorption by mucous membranes.

_______ 1. Subcutaneous
_______ 2. Sublingual
_______ 3. Intrathecal
_______ 4. Intramuscular
_______ 5. Rectal
_______ 6. Buccal
_______ 7. Nasal
_______ 8. Intra-arterial
_______ 9. Vaginal

Correct the false statement

Indicate in the blanks whether the following statements are true or false; if false, correct the underlined words or phrases.

_______ 1. Desensitization may involve an increase in the number of cell receptors.

_______ 2. Refractoriness may involve a decrease in the number of cell receptors.

_______ 3. The greater the specificity of a drug, the narrower the margin of safety.

_______ 4. The wider the margin of safety of a drug, the lower its therapeutic index.

_______ 5. A drug with a therapeutic index of 1.0 would have a wide margin of safety.

_______ 6. Water-soluble drugs are absorbed most readily by the skin.

_______ 7. Inflamed tissue such as meninges and skin tend to absorb drugs more readily than normal tissue.

_______ 8. Drugs are applied to the skin only for a local effect.

_______ 9. Salts in solution ionize more readily than nonelectrolytes.

_______ 10. Drugs that are basic in nature are absorbed rapidly by the gastric mucosa.

_______ 11. The administration of large doses of antacids with oral acidic drugs facilitates the absorption of the drug.

_______ 12. The absorption of basic drugs is retarded in persons with low levels of or no hydrochloric acid in gastric secretions.

_______ 13. Enteric-coated tablets are designed to disintegrate rapidly in the stomach.

_______ 14. Oral administration of medications is desirable because it is convenient and provides for rapid absorption.

_______ 15. A given dose of drug (corrected for body weight) is likely to exert a greater effect in normal young adults than in an infant or an elderly person.

_______ 16. Starvation is likely to make a person more sensitive to drug effects.

_______ 17. Induction of liver enzymes is likely to increase a person's response to a given dose of drug.

_______ 18. Loading doses are recommended when beginning therapy with most drugs.

_______ 19. Clients in shock caused by trauma are likely to receive medication by inhalation and by intravenous injection.

_______ 20. The organ that is most active in metabolizing drugs is the brain.

_______ 21. The organ that is most active in excreting drugs is the kidney.

_______ 22. The metabolism of drugs is not affected by the sex of the recipient.

_______ 23. The results of pharmaceutical research involving animals are not always applicable to humans.

Completion exercise

Read each question carefully and place your answer in the space provided.

1. Two routes of administration that provide higher concentrations of drug at the target tissues than in the systemic circulation are ______________ and ______________.
2. A drug used to facilitate absorption of subcutaneous medication is ______________.
3. A drug used to delay absorption of local anesthetics is ______________.
4. Water-soluble compounds with a molecular weight of ______________ are usually eliminated by the kidneys.
5. Large molecules are usually excreted by the ______________.
6. A steady state blood level of drug is usually best achieved by means of the ______________ method of administration.

Draw a drug map

Using standard pharmacologic references, determine the usual pharmacokinetic processes involved when each of the following drugs is administered (penicillin G procaine, prednisone, insulin, milk of magnesia, morphine sulfate, and methotrexate sodium). Complete the diagrams* by drawing arrows to delineate the pathways the drug takes and by identifying the specific organs and tissues involved in the process. Note any special characteristics (e.g., protein binding in the blood, active secretion in the kidneys).

Learning experience

1. Investigate the pharmacokinetic processes involved in glucose administered intravenously, halothane administered by inhalation, sulfamethoxazole administered by mouth, and chlorpromazine administered intramuscularly. What can you deduce about risk factors for toxicity, nursing measures to prevent adverse reactions, and emergency treatment for harmful reactions from this information?

2. Select one of the following drugs to study: atropine, secobarbital, or warfarin. Look up the drug you select to determine the specific mechanism of action. Can you explain how the drug's action determines therapeutic effect? Side effects? Toxic manifestations? Compare the action of the drug with that of antidotes and/or corrective treatment of toxicity.

*Supp. 30–32.

1. penicillin G procaine

Sites of Absorption	Sites of Biotransformation
Vascular Compartment	**Sites of Inactive Storage**
Target Tissues	**Sites of Excretion**

2. prednisone

Sites of Absorption	Sites of Biotransformation
Vascular Compartment	**Sites of Inactive Storage**
Target Tissues	**Sites of Excretion**

3. insulin

Sites of Absorption	Sites of Biotransformation
______	______
______	______

Vascular Compartment	Sites of Inactive Storage
______	______
______	______

Target Tissues	Sites of Excretion
______	______
______	______

4. milk of magnesia

Sites of Absorption	Sites of Biotransformation
______	______
______	______

Vascular Compartment	Sites of Inactive Storage
______	______
______	______

Target Tissues	Sites of Excretion
______	______
______	______

5. morphine sulfate

Sites of Absorption	Sites of Biotransformation
______________________	______________________
______________________	______________________

Vascular Compartment	Sites of Inactive Storage
______________________	______________________
______________________	______________________

Target Tissues	Sites of Excretion
______________________	______________________
______________________	______________________

6. methotrexate sodium

Sites of Absorption	Sites of Biotransformation
______________________	______________________
______________________	______________________

Vascular Compartment	Sites of Inactive Storage
______________________	______________________
______________________	______________________

Target Tissues	Sites of Excretion
______________________	______________________
______________________	______________________

5 ▪ *Adverse drug reactions*

Every physiologically active drug has the potential to cause an undesirable reaction that may induce illness in the recipient. Such conditions are termed *iatrogenic.*

Adverse reactions include side effects, toxic reactions, allergic and immunologic reactions, carcinogenic reactions, chain reactions, cumulative reactions, idiosyncratic reactions, teratogenic reactions, and tolerance and dependence.

Matching

Read the section in the text about commonly abused substances (in Chapter 14). Study the description of the opiate withdrawal syndrome. Match the signs and symptoms of the syndrome in the left-hand column with the phase of the syndrome in the right-hand column. Place your answers in the space provided.

_______ 1. Abdominal cramps
_______ 2. Diaphoresis
_______ 3. Diarrhea
_______ 4. Extreme restlessness
_______ 5. Yawning
_______ 6. Mydriasis
_______ 7. Nausea and vomiting
_______ 8. Insistent drug-demanding behavior
_______ 9. Muscle twitching
_______ 10. Hyperglycemia
_______ 11. Elevated vital signs
_______ 12. Rhinorrhea

a. First phase
b. Second phase
c. Third phase
d. Fourth phase

Short answer questions

1. Define the following terms:
   a. Iatrogenic

   b. Adverse drug reaction

   c. Side effect

   d. Toxic effect

   e. Allergic reaction

   f. Carcinogenic

g. Chain reaction

h. Cumulative reaction

i. Idiosyncratic reaction

j. Teratogenic

k. Tolerance

l. Dependence

2. Look up *penicillin* in the text. Describe the allergic reactions seen with this drug.
   a. Most frequent reaction

   b. Most serious reaction

3. List some factors that might be elicited through taking a detailed client history that would indicate to the nurse that the client may well be a candidate for an adverse drug reaction.

4. List appropriate nursing approaches to ameliorate the following problems:
   a. Cardiovascular reactions

   b. Cutaneous reactions

   c. Gastrointestinal reactions

Enrichment experience

In clinical laboratory, select a client receiving multiple therapeutic drugs on a regular basis (suggestion: six or more).

***Before* investigating these drugs, assess the client's condition. During the physical examination, list subjective complaints and objective evidence that seem outside of normal ranges.**

Look up the drugs included in the client's medication regimen, studying particularly the adverse reactions they can cause.

1. **What are the most common adverse reactions for each medication?**
2. **What are the life-threatening adverse reactions for each medication?**
3. **How many of your client's subjective complaints could be caused by medication? Which one(s)?**
4. **What findings from objective evidence that you gathered could be caused by medication?**
5. **List possible nursing diagnoses that relate to adverse drug reactions.**
6. **What interventions would you perform to assist the client to prevent adverse drug reactions?**
7. **What interventions would you perform to assist the client to eliminate or alleviate any actual adverse drug reactions?**
8. **What questions might you raise about the medication regimen?**

Completion exercise

Study this diagram, which illustrates a chain reaction to cortisone. Fill in the blanks.

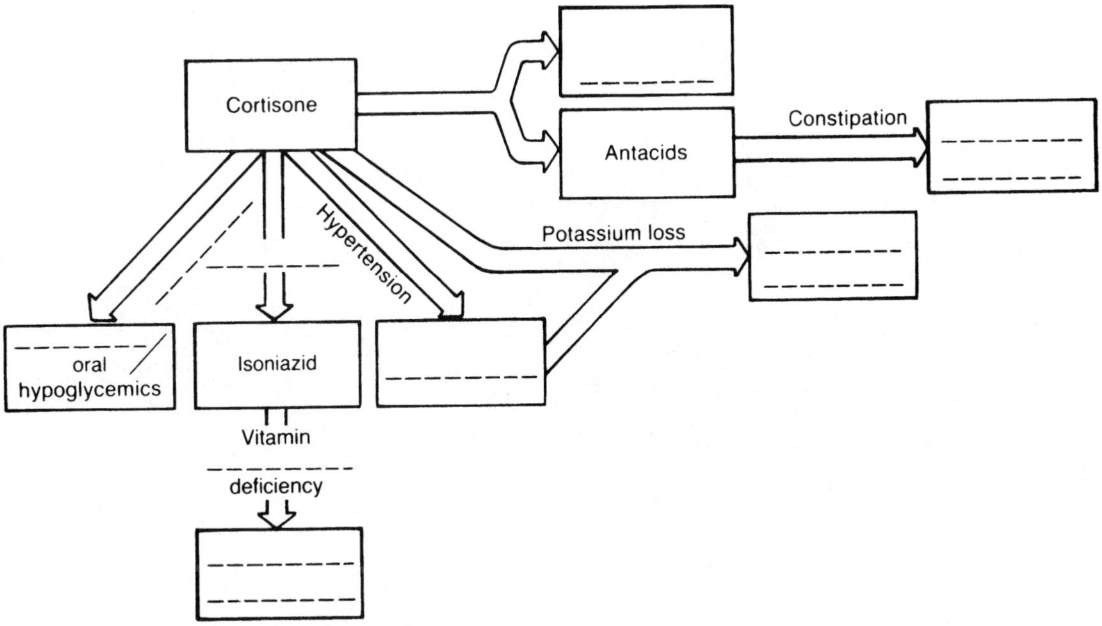

6 ▪ *Drug interactions*

Foods contain nutrients and natural and artificial toxins. These components can produce therapeutic effects or adverse reactions and are capable of producing drug-food interactions.

Drug-drug interactions are varied and may affect the absorption, distribution, biotransformation, or excretion of drugs. They may be beneficial or hazardous and may differ from person to person. The following exercises relate to this textbook material.

Matching

A. Match the medications listed in the left-hand column with their physiologic antagonists from the list of nutrients in the right-hand column.

_______ 1. Coumarin anticoagulants	a. Calcium
_______ 2. Digoxin	b. Potassium
_______ 3. Hydrochlorothiazide	c. Sodium
	d. Zinc
	e. Vitamin A
	f. Vitamin C
	g. Vitamin D
	h. Vitamin K

B. Match each nutrient listed in the left-hand column with all the signs and symptoms of its deficiency syndrome.

_______ 4. Vitamin A	a. Anemia
_______ 5. Vitamin B_6	b. Leg pains
_______ 6. Vitamin B_{12}	c. Dermatitis
_______ 7. Niacin	d. Abnormal gastrointestinal bleeding
_______ 8. Riboflavin	e. Loss of night vision
_______ 9. Vitamin C	f. Hypotension
_______ 10. Vitamin K	g. Petechiae
_______ 11. Sodium	h. Sore tongue

C. Match the mechanism of drug interaction in the left-hand column with its pharmacokinetic phase in the right-hand column.

_______ 12. Competition for carrier mechanism for secretion	a. Absorption
	b. Distribution
_______ 13. Acceleration of metabolism	c. Biotransformation
_______ 14. Dissolution rate change	d. Excretion
_______ 15. Insufficient ingestion of solvent	
_______ 16. Displacement	
_______ 17. Change in pH of urine	
_______ 18. Inhibition of metabolism	
_______ 19. Direct interaction	

D. Drug excretion may be affected by drug-drug interaction. The secretion of digoxin, penicillin, and acetohexamide (hydroxyhexamide) will be decreased by certain other drugs. Match these drugs in the left-hand column with their interactant drug in the right-hand column.

_______ 20. Digoxin
_______ 21. Penicillin
_______ 22. Acetohexamide (hydroxyhexamide)

a. Acetylsalicylic acid
b. Indomethacin
c. Phenylbutazone
d. Spironolactone
e. Lithium
f. Probenecid

Correct the false statement

Indicate in the blanks whether the following statements are true or false; if false, correct the underlined words or phrases.

_______ 1. A client known to have food allergies should avoid eating <u>foods known to act frequently as allergens</u>.

_______ 2. Charcoal-broiled foods are known to <u>facilitate absorption of tetracycline</u>.

_______ 3. Dissolution of most drugs is promoted by the ingestion of <u>warm liquids</u>.

_______ 4. Enteric-coated tablets should be administered with <u>milk to facilitate absorption</u>.

Selection of options

For each of the following, select *all* appropriate responses. Circle the correct answers.

1. Foods rich in potassium include
   a. apples
   b. apricots
   c. bananas
   d. cranberries
   e. orange juice
   f. soup
2. Minerals that exert a direct effect on cardiac function include
   a. aluminum
   b. copper
   c. calcium
   d. iron
   e. potassium
   f. phosphorus
   g. zinc
3. Sulfites are used as preservatives in
   a. baked goods
   b. fresh salads
   c. meats
   d. wines
4. Additives likely to cause allergic reactions in asthmatic individuals include
   a. vinegar
   b. BHT
   c. caffeine
   d. sulfites
   e. tartrazine
5. Medications likely to impair intestinal absorption include
   a. broad-spectrum antibiotics
   b. digestants
   c. diuretics
   d. laxatives
6. Diuretics that conserve body potassium include
   a. ethacrynic acid
   b. furosemide
   c. hydrochlorothiazide
   d. spironolactone
   e. triamterene

Learning experiences

1. Investigate through library research and/or discussion with nutritionists, chemists, or other knowledgeable professionals, some issue related to drug-food interaction. Examples of such issues include the listing of ingredients on food labels and the use of additives. Write a letter to your senator or representative expressing your concerns regarding this issue.

2. Select two drugs from any of the drug chapters in this book. Study the material in the chapter on the drugs for potential drug-drug interactions. Identify the mechanisms of drug interaction that are operating. Determine what the nurse should do when such interactions can be predicted. Write up a teaching plan for a client who will receive one of these drugs, emphasizing how to avoid harmful interactions. Repeat the exercise with drugs from other chapters of the book.

Short answer questions

1. List at least six types of food additives.

2. List at least four foods that should not be ingested by individuals receiving monoamine oxidase (MAO) inhibitors.

3. List at least six factors predisposing to drug-induced nutritional deficiency.

4. Define the following terms:
   a. Detrimental drug interaction

   b. Clinically desirable interaction

5. List some factors that might be elicited through taking a detailed client history that would indicate to the nurse that the client may well be a candidate for a drug-food or drug-drug interaction or both.

6. List six drugs whose absorption will be decreased by concurrent administration of another drug, and list the interactant drug responsible for the decreased absorption.

   Drug with Decreased Absorption

   ____
   ____
   ____
   ____
   ____
   ____

   Interactant Drug

   ____
   ____
   ____
   ____
   ____
   ____

7. Explain how drug interactions during the absorptive phase can be avoided. Give one specific example.

8. Drugs do compete with other drugs for drug-binding sites on albumin but often the drug-drug interaction is really a result of a second mechanism. List three examples of drugs that interact as a result of displacement and of another mechanism.
   a.

   b.

   c.

9. Define the terms *drug inhibitor* and *drug inducer.* Give three examples of each type of drug.
   a. Drug inhibitor

   b. Drug inducer

10. Identify two drugs involved in both inhibition and acceleration reactions.

11. Look up *allopurinol* in the text. Describe how metabolic inhibition occurs when allopurinol is used.

12. Look up *cimetidine* in the text. Identify drugs and classes of drugs that may interact with cimetidine.

13. Explain how tyramine could cause an accentuated hypertensive effect.

14. Smoking (nicotine) appears to be a drug inducer. How would you explain to a heavy smoker the effects of smoking on an interactant drug?

15. List seven routes by which drugs may be excreted.

16. How could you increase the rate of excretion of salicylates?

UNIT THREE
Administration of medications

7 ▪ Principles of medication

Many people are involved in the various processes required for the manufacture, distribution, prescription, administration, and monitoring of drugs used to treat human diseases, but it is vital that the nurse be aware of all drugs taken by the client, that the client be evaluated regularly and comprehensively for therapeutic response and adverse reactions, and that intervention be initiated when necessary to ensure optimal effects of drug therapy.

Effective drug therapy depends on the delivery of accurate doses of active chemicals to the body tissues at the proper site of action for the drug involved. To complete this process successfully, the practitioner must master certain technical skills: proper storage and handling of drugs; command of the language used in drug therapy; accurate computation of drug doses; and techniques used in delivering drugs by specific routes to specific sites. The following exercises will help you to develop knowledge related to drug therapy.

Matching

A. Match each measure of weight in the left-hand column with the letter designating the equivalent volume(s) (of water) in the right-hand column. Place your answer(s) in the space provided.

______	1. Dram	a. Milliliter
______	2. Ounce	b. Pint
______	3. Gram	c. Fluidounce
______	4. Grain	d. Cubic centimeter
______	5. Pound	e. Tablespoon
______	6. Kilogram	f. Minim
		g. Fluidram
		h. Liter

B. Match the healthcare personnel in the left-hand column with their legal rights in the right hand column. Place your answer in the space provided.

______	1. Physicians	a. May compound drugs
______	2. Physician's assistants	b. May dispense drugs
______	3. Pharmacists	c. May administer drugs to clients
______	4. Nurses	
______	5. Dentists	

Correct the false statement

Indicate whether the following statements are true or false; if false, change the underlined words or phrases.

______ 1. Insulin should be stored in the refrigerator <u>at all times</u>.

______ 2. The best way to warm a medication to body temperature is <u>to place the container in warm water</u>.

_______ 3. The best place to store most drugs in the home is in the bathroom medicine cabinet.

_______ 4. In healthcare institutions, narcotics are usually stored in areas secured by at least two locks.

_______ 5. A bottle of elixir of phenobarbital used to pour medication for all clients receiving the drug is an example of unit dosage.

_______ 6. When a medication order does not specify the route to be used, the drug is administered by mouth.

_______ 7. Once a physician has verified a drug order that the nurse has feared may harm the client, the nurse may administer the dose.

_______ 8. After a telephone order is written by the nurse on the physician's order sheet, it must be countersigned as soon as possible by the physician.

_______ 9. The nurse who administers a drug in accordance with a verbal order can be charged with practicing medicine without a license if the physician later repudiates the order.

_______ 10. The substance used as a standard for equating measures of weight and volume in both the apothecary and metric systems is wine.

_______ 11. When the route is not specified in a medication order, the drug is administered by hypo.

_______ 12. In hospital situations, only physicians and nurses commonly administer drugs to clients.

_______ 13. In administering drugs, the nurse must adhere to the order as written by the physician.

_______ 14. For many drugs, the time required for elimination of residues from the body in a normally healthy adult is about 2 weeks.

Multiple choice questions

For each of the following, choose the one best answer:

1. Your client is to receive digoxin 0.375 mg PO. In the drug supply you find that all the digoxin tablets are scored and that each contains 0.25 mg. There are three whole tablets and one half-tablet. You would
   a. give the half-tablet and one whole tablet to the client
   b. break another tablet; give the half-tablet and a whole one to your client and leave the original half-tablet for the nurse who broke it to administer
   c. call the pharmacy for a tablet containing 0.125 mg digoxin to administer with one 0.25-mg tablet
   d. call the physician to request an order consistent with the drug preparations available
2. The most critical nursing responsibility related to medication is
   a. preparing and administering the dose with 100 percent accuracy
   b. explaining the purposes of therapy to the client
   c. warning the client of the risk of drug use
   d. assessing client response to drugs
3. In which of the following settings is the nurse likely to have the greatest latitude in the administration of medications and the greatest influence on drug regimens?
   a. care of clients in the home (community nursing)
   b. skilled nursing care (nursing home)
   c. acute care facility (hospital)
   d. primary practice (private office for independent nursing)
4. In hospital settings, professional nurses are responsible for the accuracy of medications administered to clients by them and also for those administered by
   a. vocational-technical nurses
   b. respiratory therapists
   c. physicians
   d. a and b above
   e. all of the above
5. If the required dose of a drug is half of a tablet, the drug can be administered provided that
   a. the tablets furnished are scored
   b. the tablets furnished are enteric-coated
   c. the tablets furnished are water-soluble
   d. none of the above; fractional parts of a tablet should not be given
6. The label on a container of liquid medication has become soiled from spilled medication. The nurse should
   a. relabel the container clearly, verifying the accuracy of the new label by checking three times
   b. return the container to the pharmacy for relabeling

c. discard the container and medication and secure a new supply
d. ask the nursing supervisor to assist in relabeling the container to ensure against error

7. Child-protective packaging should be used for all medications
a. without exception
b. except topical ointments, eye drops, and nose drops
c. except for drugs used by clients with impaired manual dexterity
d. except for drugs given by injection

8. The best organization for storage of stock drug supplies is
a. separation of injectable preparations from topical and oral drugs
b. separation of injectable drugs from preparations for external use
c. arrangement in alphabetical order
d. separation of light-sensitive from light-stable drugs

9. When the medication nurse leaves a unit for lunch, what should be done with the key to the medication cart (closet)? The key is
a. kept in the possession of the medication nurse
b. left with the charge nurse
c. left with the ward secretary or manager
d. hidden in a place known only to members of the nursing staff

Selection of options

For each of the following, select all appropriate responses. Circle the correct answers.

1. A nurse working in a physician's office could appropriately advise a client to
a. inform the physician if improvement does not occur as expected
b. discontinue drug therapy when symptoms subside
c. adjust the dosage in accordance with severity of the symptoms
d. report adverse reactions associated with taking the medication

2. To measure accurately an 18-ml dose of liquid medication, you could use a
a. medicine glass
b. measuring teaspoon
c. fluted paper cup
d. 6-ml syringe

3. What should the nurse do when a medication order specifies a dose that is more than the usual dosage range?
a. give the dose as ordered; physicians are responsible for their actions
b. consult with the physician to clarify the accuracy of the order
c. refuse to give the drug if the dose is likely to harm the client

4. To assess client response to drug therapy, the nurse must have knowledge of
a. therapeutic effects expected of the drug
b. side effects of the drug
c. signs and symptoms of drug toxicity
d. the specific dose administered to the client

5. In which of the following situations are medications commonly used without the involvement of healthcare professionals?
a. use of legend drugs
b. use of over-the-counter drugs
c. use of folk remedies
d. medicinal use of narcotics
e. therapy by an herbalist

6. Most drugs maintain their safety, potency, and stability longest when stored in environments that are
a. light
b. airy
c. cool
d. moist
e. dark
f. dry
g. warm
h. clean

7. Drugs likely to require refrigeration include
a. elixirs
b. suppositories
c. vaccines
d. parenteral fluids
e. liquid antibiotics
f. oral liquids with a bitter taste
g. eye and ear drops

Sequences

A nurse caring for a hospital client notes that the signs and symptoms of infection remain unabated 3 days after an oral antibiotic has been ordered. (Acute signs and symptoms of infection usually subside about 24 hours after effective antibiotic treatment is begun.) Arrange the following steps in the order in which the actions should be taken.

_______ Notify the physician of the client's failure to improve.

_______ Check the chart to see how many doses of antibiotic the client has received.

_______ Interview the client to determine whether the oral antibiotic has been retained.

Completion exercises

Read each question carefully and place your answer in the space provided.

1. Protocols are defined as ______________________________.
2. The three essential parts of a prescription are ______________________________.
3. Name the three systems used to measure drugs: ______________________________.
4. Which system is preferred for medication? ______________________________.
5. Distribution of a drug supply is termed ______________________________.
6. When a physician or dentist recommends a medicinal substance and specifies the way it is to be used, this is known as ______________________________.
7. Preparation of medicinal substances from raw ingredients is termed ______________________________.

Short answer questions

1. Identify the five "rights" of medications.

2. How many serum half-lives ($t_{1/2}$) elapse before drug residues in the blood are reduced to less than 1 percent?

3. If a drug has a half-life of 24 hours, how long would it take for 99 percent of a given dose to be eliminated from the body of a normally healthy adult? (Ignore the factor of storage in tissue depots.)

Define the following abbreviations:

4. IV

5. OD

6. od

7. ac

8. hs

9. gtt I

10. ℥ i

11. ʒ i

12. mg

13. g

14. ml

15. SOS

16. pc

17. qd

18. qlh

19. STAT

20. IM

21. H

22. v

23. ss

24. SSKI

25. SSE

26. ms

27. MOM

28. MO

29. TWE

30. g

31. mcg

32. kg

33. cc

34. l

35. ASA

Situational exercises

What would you do in the following situations? Write your answers on a separate sheet of paper.

1. A physician with a heavy accent gives you a telephone order to give one of his patients "one Eva Coogan." You know he means to order a medication, but you do not recognize this drug name.

2. When you offer your client his daily dose of allopurinol at 10 A.M. he asks you to leave it on the bedside table, saying that he doesn't want to take it until his dinner tray arrives because he experiences stomach distress when taking it on an empty stomach.

Personal exercise: Drug history

Pretend that you are acutely ill with abdominal pain and are admitted to the hospital. What information should you give the nurse who is taking your drug history? Write your answer on a separate sheet of paper, using the form on page 3 of the Study Guide.

Learning experiences

Visit a healthcare or health-related facility to explore drug practices in the setting. Consider questions such as the following:

Is a member of the staff responsible for administering drugs?
What education and training in pharmacology has this person had?
If the individual is not a nurse, by what legal authority have these functions been assigned to him or her?
Has the institution provided an opportunity for the individual to acquire adequate knowledge and skills to administer drugs safely?
What is the nature of this training?
If residents administer their own drugs, what precautions are taken to prevent errors of dosage, detect untoward response, or prevent abuse of drugs?

Share your findings with those of your classmates. Discuss the legal factors contributing to the practices you observed. What changes would you recommend to improve the safety and therapeutic efficacy of drug regimens in these institutions?

Learning experiences

1. Observe a nurse caring for clients for a period of 4 to 8 hours to determine how pharmacologic aspects of care are integrated into the nursing care plan.
2. While caring for clients in the clinical laboratory, integrate pharmacologic aspects into your care plan at every step in the process.
3. Discuss medication practices you have observed in healthcare settings. What method of assignment has been utilized for patient care (functional, team, primary)? Was the same method used for the administration of drugs? How many people, on average, use the medication area during a given shift? Do the facilities for preparing drug doses appear adequate? Describe the procedures used for administering drug doses. What are their strengths and weaknesses?
Are you aware of any medication errors that have occurred? Were these reported? Discuss measures that might be taken to improve the safety and therapeutic efficacy of the drug regimens of clients in these settings.
In a hospital or nursing home, explore the medication area of a nursing unit. Is the area well ventilated or air conditioned? Well lighted? Locked?
How many people have access to the area? Is the area neat and clean? Does it contain adequate work space for drug preparation? If there is a sink in the room, wash your hands and observe whether this procedure poses risks of contaminating equipment or materials used for preparing medication (e.g., from splashing).
Examine packaged drugs. Which have light-resistant containers? Air-tight seals? Which are refrigerated? Are all labels clearly legible? What precautions are taken to secure drugs, including controlled drugs like narcotics? Examine the sheets used for monitoring use of controlled substances.
4. Assess drug storage practices in the home of a client or acquaintance. Are the drugs kept in locked storage areas? Are conditions of storage appropriate for the substances in use?
Examine the tools available in the hospital or nursing home for measuring drugs. Are these adequate for accurate preparation of doses?
What additional tools would you recommend?
In the library investigate attempts to promote the use of the metric system in the United States. List situations in daily living in which you use the metric, apothecary, and household systems of measurement. Do you think the metric system should be adopted by the United States for all purposes? Why or why not?

8 ▪ *Strategies to promote therapeutic alliance*

A person's physiologic response to a particular drug is affected by the psychological response to drugs, as is the reverse. Each person's response is unique. An understanding of these factors helps the nurse to obtain a more effective response from the client when administering drug therapy.

Short answer questions

1. Drug effectiveness is influenced by psychological response and pharmacodynamic actions. Identify the three resulting degrees of effectiveness and define each term.
   a.

   b.

   c.

2. List various emotional responses a person may have to drug therapy.

3. Give several instances in which placebos are used.

4. Ways in which the angry client might respond to drug therapy include the following:

5. Ways in which the "good" client might respond to drug therapy include the following:

Matching

Match the behavioral response in the right-hand column with the supporting statement in the left-hand column. Place your answer in the space provided.

_______ 1. Hidden beliefs unconsciously affecting the emotional state and responsiveness to drug therapy

_______ 2. A positive or negative attitude affecting the therapeutic value of a drug

_______ 3. State of mind, or opinions, that influence behavior

_______ 4. Behavior arising from attitudes held toward people, drugs, drug therapy, health care, and self

a. Attitude
b. Motivation
c. Meaning attached to drugs
d. Power of suggestion
e. Type of illness
f. Nurses' behavioral response

_______ 5. Acuteness or chronicity of illness, leading to positive or negative responsiveness

_______ 6. Causative factors activating behavior for need satisfaction

Multiple choice questions

For each of the following, choose the one best answer:

1. Placebos are thought to be effective because of the
   a. production of endorphins in the brain
   b. pharmacologic action of the active drug in the placebo
   c. nurturing attitude of healthcare providers
2. Mrs. Brown has continued to take her digitoxin regularly, as prescribed by her physician, although she has experienced extreme nausea and vomiting, headaches, and drowsiness for the last 5 days. Mrs. Brown could be
   a. exhibiting anger and resentment about her condition
   b. gaining a feeling of security from taking the digitoxin
   c. manifesting fear over her drug dependency
   d. exhibiting physical symptoms of psychological origin
3. In this instance, an appropriate nursing diagnosis for Mrs. Brown would be
   a. ineffective individual coping (displaced anger) related to feelings of helplessness
   b. overcompliance related to knowledge deficit and the need for security
   c. fear related to knowledge deficit
   d. anxiety related to chronic physical illness
4. An important nursing intervention for Mrs. Brown would be
   a. encourage verbalization of anger
   b. provide information on digitoxin toxicity and her responsibilities
   c. explore with Mrs. Brown her fears about drug dependency
   d. discuss with Mrs. Brown the relationship between her physical symptom and her anxiety
5. When assessing a client for drug therapy, one of the first areas to be assessed is
   a. length of time of therapy
   b. family support of drug therapy
   c. types of drugs available
   d. client attitude toward drugs and drug taking
6. Successful drug therapy is most apt to be accomplished when
   a. both client and healthcare providers strive toward the same goal
   b. the nurse is knowledgeable about the drugs administered
   c. the right drug in the right dosage is given at the right time
   d. the client substitutes drugs for the sick role

Learning experiences

1. Identify a time during childhood when you were ill and received medication.
- **Who administered the drug?**
- **What were the behaviors of this person, both verbal and nonverbal?**
- **How did family members respond to you? Was this response similar to or different from other members when they were ill?**
- **How were drugs administered? Were they disguised, given with something else, given alone, or was bribery used?**

2. Identify your attitude now toward drug taking.
- **Are there similarities between present and childhood experiences, between you and the family member who administered the drug?**
- **Identify your verbal and nonverbal behaviors when administering drugs. Which might have a positive effect? Which might have a negative effect on a client?**
- **Do different kinds of drugs elicit different responses? What values are affecting your responses?**

The ability to establish a therapeutic alliance between a client and the healthcare provider is a key factor contributing to overall client compliance with a plan of care and medication regimen. There

are a variety of psychological factors that impact upon the unique physiological responses of each individual to drug therapy. An understanding of these factors, including the values and beliefs the nurse/provider brings to the relationship, helps the nurse to identify potential or actual barriers to compliance and to work with the client to overcome them.

Multiple choice questions

For each of the following, choose the one best answer.

1. When a client lacks commitment to a strict regimen, it is likely that:
   a. the family's influence is unimportant
   b. the client cannot find the incentive to achieve the goals of satisfying a basic need
   c. there is little significance attached to drug taking
   d. the client's symptoms are not significant
2. Placebos are thought to be effective because of the
   a. production of endorphins in the brain
   b. pharmacologic action of the active drug in the placebo
   c. nurturing attitude of health care providers
3. Mrs. Brown has continued to take her digitoxin regularly, as prescribed by her physician, although she has experienced extreme nausea and vomiting, headaches, and drowsiness for the last 5 days. Mrs. Brown could be
   a. exhibiting anger and resentment about her condition
   b. gaining a feeling of security from taking the digitoxin
   c. manifesting fear over her drug dependency
   d. exhibiting physical symptoms of psychological origin
4. In this instance, an appropriate nursing diagnosis for Mrs. Brown would be
   a. ineffective individual coping (displaced anger) related to feelings of helplessness
   b. overcompliance related to knowledge deficit and the need for security
   c. fear related to knowledge deficit
   d. anxiety related to chronic physical illness
5. An important nursing intervention for Mrs. Brown would be
   a. encourage verbalization of anger
   b. provide information on digitoxin toxicity and her responsibilities
   c. explore with Mrs. Brown her fears about drug dependency
   d. discuss with Mrs. Brown her physical symptom and her anxiety
6. When assessing a client for drug therapy, one of the first areas to be assessed is
   a. length of time of therapy
   b. family support of drug therapy
   c. types of drugs available
   d. client attitude toward drugs and drug taking
7. Successful drug therapy is most apt to be accomplished when
   a. both client and healthcare providers strive toward the same goal
   b. the nurse is knowledgeable about the drugs administered
   c. the right drug in the right dosage is given at the right time
   d. the client substitutes drugs for the sick role

9 ▪ *Cultural aspects of drug therapy*

Understanding health beliefs and traditional practices is fundamental to the development of care plans which are culturally sensitive and responsive to the needs of the client. Of equal importance is the ability to incorporate effective self-treatments and use of natural substances when these folk practices and medicinal plants are known to be effective for maintaining health and treating common illnesses.

Personal exercise

Make a list of interventions you take when treating your own illnesses. Consider what you do at the first sign of a cold, sore throat, earache, headache, sore muscles, or cold sore to relieve the symptoms. Evaluate each intervention and consider whether your actions are based on family traditions, home remedies, medicinal herbs, prescribed medications, or a combination. Take a family history by asking parents and grandparents what remedies they choose for the same conditions. Consider the degree of influence these family practices have had on your own behavior.

Matching

A. Match the term in the right-hand column with the definition in the left-hand column.

_______ 1. The observation, description, and experimental study of indigenous drugs and their biological activities

_______ 2. Method used to prepare a tisane when the active ingredients of the medicinal plant are found in the mucilage

_______ 3. Any plant-containing substances that can be used for therapeutic purposes

_______ 4. Holistic approach to illness that takes into consideration folk beliefs and psychosocial, cultural, physiologic, and spiritual forces

_______ 5. Most common way to used dried plants for medicinal purposes; requires a basic remedy, adjuvant, complement, and correctors

_______ 6. Use of roots, stem, or bark of a vegetable drug to form a medicinal liquid by soaking the parts in cold water and boiling

a. Tisane
b. Ethnomedicine
c. Decoction
d. Medicinal plant
e. Maceration
f. Ethnopharmacology

B. Match the ethnic group in the right-hand column with the list of common characteristics defining health beliefs of that group.

_______ 1. Universal balance is dependent on harmony between elemental forces of fire, water, wood, earth, and metal.

_______ 2. God is responsible for allowing health or illness; fatalism is dominant; maintaining a balance between hot and cold forces promotes wellness.

_______ 3. Health denotes harmony with nature and the body, mind, spirit; restoring harmony restores sense of self.

_______ 4. Human body is one with the universe; respect for the body; belief that the body and universe are interdependent; belief in cause and effect; illness is purposeful and is related to past or future events.

a. African American
b. Hispanic American
c. Native American
d. Asian American

Short answer questions

1. Define the terms *Doctrine of Signatures* and *moxibustion.*

2. Identify several factors that may affect the potency and usefulness of an herbal plant.

3. Identify at least four factors that generally determine the health and illness beliefs and practices of different ethnic groups.

4. List examples of several biologic variations among different racial groups in response to the use of chemical substances.

Completion exercises

Read each question carefully and place your answers in the spaces provided.

1. For each cultural group listed, identify folk remedies used in treating common illnesses.

Group	Common Illness	Remedy
African Americans	open wound	_______________
	congestion/cold	_______________
	boil	_______________
Hispanic Americans	menstrual disturbances	_______________
	stomach aches	_______________
	whooping cough	_______________
Native Americans	headache	_______________
	constipation	_______________
European Americans	sore throat	_______________
	burns	_______________

2. Complete the table, giving potential body effects caused by the following common chemical components of plants.

Chemical Component	Effect on the Body
Vitamins	________________
Alkaloids	________________
Antibiotics	________________
Heterosides (sugars)	________________
Acids	________________
Minerals	________________

3. Listed below are several medicinal plants. Identify the active ingredients and their therapeutic uses.

Medicinal Plant	Active Ingredient(s)	Medicinal Use
American hellebore *(Veratrum viride)*	________________	________________
Periwinkle *(Catharanthus roseus)*	________________	________________
American mandrake *(Atropa mandragora)*	________________	________________
Rauwolfia *(Rauwolfia serpentina)*	________________	________________
Purple foxglove *(Digitalis purpurea)*	________________	________________
Cocaine *(Erythroxylon coca)*	________________	________________
Opium poppy *(Papaver somniferum)*	________________	________________

Checklist

Using a check mark, indicate the category of the body fluids listed according to traditional Hispanic practices.

1. Blood
   ________ a. hot, wet
   ________ b. hot, dry
   ________ c. cold, wet
   ________ d. cold, dry
2. Yellow bile
   ________ a. hot, wet
   ________ b. hot, dry
   ________ c. cold, wet
   ________ d. cold, dry
3. Black bile
   ________ a. hot, wet
   ________ b. hot, dry
   ________ c. cold, wet
   ________ d. cold, dry
4. Phlegm
   ________ a. hot, wet
   ________ b. hot, dry
   ________ c. cold, wet
   ________ d. cold, dry

UNIT FOUR
Developmental considerations in drug therapy

10 ▪ *Drug therapy in maternal care*

Anything that is eaten, inhaled, injected, or used topically by a pregnant woman has the potential to harm or help the fetus. The same is true of the breast-feeding mother and her infant. Nurses must be aware of the need for maternal education to protect the fetus and infant from adverse effects of medication, as well as from pollutants found in the environment.

Labor should occur about 280 days after conception (9 calendar months, or 10 lunar months). If it starts much before the expected date of delivery, the infant may be too immature to live outside the uterus. If it occurs too long after the expected date, the fetal life may not be sustained properly *in utero,* and to lessen maternal pain during labor and delivery. In some instances, labor may have to be induced or made more forceful, or may take place after the baby has died *in utero.* Regardless of the circumstances, nurses attending the mother must understand the rationale and effects of any drugs that are used.

Matching

A. Mrs. T. has been admitted to the hospital for induction of labor because of gestational diabetes. She has completed all the necessary testing. Match each procedure in the left-hand column with its rationale in the right-hand column. Place your answer in the space provided.

_______	1. Amniocentesis	a. Helps to ripen cervix
_______	2. Sonogram	b. Establishes L/S ratio
_______	3. PGE_2 given in gel	c. Establishes fetal age
_______	4. Oxytocic drug administration	d. Stimulates contractions

B. Match the causative agent in the left-hand column with the resulting condition in the right-hand column.

_______	1. Maternal alcoholism	a. Small for gestational age infant
_______	2. Anesthetic gases	b. Abruptio placentae
_______	3. Cigarette smoking	c. Spontaneous abortion
_______	4. Gestational DM	d. FAS
_______	5. Cocaine snorting	e. Large for gestational age infant

C. Match the medication in the left-hand column with the reason for which it is given to the pregnant client in the right-hand column.

_______	1. Steroids	a. Prevention of isoimmunization
_______	2. Erythromycin	b. Relief of stress during asthma
_______	3. Sulfa	c. Treatment of *Chlamydia trachomatis* infection
_______	4. Rh (D) immune globulin (RPIG)	d. Treatment of toxoplasmosis
_______	5. Ampicillin with probenecid	e. Treatment of gonorrhea
_______	6. Benzathine penicillin	f. Treatment of syphilis

Correct the false statement

Indicate whether the following statements are true or false; if false, correct the underlined words or phrases and place your answer in the space provided.

_______ 1. Proper maternal weight gain during pregnancy should be 25 pounds or more for most women.

_______ 2. Antiemetic drugs taken early in the day are a safe way to control nausea and vomiting associated with pregnancy.

_______ 3. Fat-soluble substances penetrate the placental barrier more easily than nonfat-soluble substances.

_______ 4. Overweight women should be encouraged to lose weight during pregnancy.

_______ 5. Immediate intervention to prevent further labor should be undertaken when premature labor is diagnosed.

_______ 6. Ultrasound can distinguish uterine contractions producing changes in the cervix from those that do not.

_______ 7. Possible maternal overhydration is a complication of ritodrine combined with corticosteroids.

_______ 8. Patients receiving ritodrine should be evaluated for dyspnea, chest pain, pulse over 120 beats/min, and blood pressure below 90/60 mm Hg.

_______ 9. Patients receiving ritodrine should have fluid intake limited to 300 ml/hr.

_______ 10. Drugs used for pain relief can be given at any time during labor if dose is low.

Short answer questions

1. Pregnancy affects the speed with which drugs pass through the placenta. Indicate in the space provided whether the reaction is slower or faster because of body changes.
   a. No increase in hepatic blood flow: _______________
   b. Increased renal perfusion: _______________
   c. Changes in placenta in third trimester: _______________
2. Treatment of pregnancy-induced hypertension (PIH) includes dietary advice. Fill in the recommended daily allowances for the following:
   a. Protein: _______________
   b. Sodium, if no edema present: _______________
   c. Fluids: _______________
3. Name four classes of tocolytic agents:
4. Ritodrine should never be used in the presence of:
5. The half-life of IV oxytocic drugs is _______ to _______ minutes.
6. Discuss briefly why the following drugs are not recommended for pregnant patients with cardiac problems:
   a. Propranolol:
   b. Procainamide:

c. Warfarin:

d. Diuretics:

Completion exercises

Read each question carefully and place your answer in the space provided.

1. Following delivery of the neonate and placenta, ____________________ is administered to promote uterine contraction.
2. An oral drug used postpartum to contract the uterus is ____________________.
3. The newborn's eyes are treated immediately after birth with ____________________ or ____________________ because both drugs are effective against gonorrhea and *Chlamydia trachomatis.*
4. Fill in the possible side effects for the following drugs, which are frequently used for pain relief during labor.

Drug	Possible Maternal Side Effects	Possible Fetal Side Effects
Meperidine	____________________	____________________
Hydroxyzine	____________________	____________________
Valium	____________________	____________________

Situational exercises

What would you do in the following situations? Write your answer in the space provided.

A. Mrs. J. arrives at the hospital stating that she thinks she is in labor, and that her due date is 6 weeks from now. Her physician is expected to arrive shortly, and wants certain information available at the time.

1. Provide three appropriate comments for the following procedures that have been ordered.
   a. Constant fetal monitoring:

   b. Ultrasonography:

   c. Maternal history and physical examination:

   d. Preparation for administration of ritodrine hydrochloride:

2. Nursing actions during administration of ritodrine hydrochloride for premature labor include the following:

3. Patient education following discharge with orders for taking ritodrine hydrochloride PO at home include these instructions:

B. Infants of diabetic mothers are usually large for their gestational age, and may develop hypoglycemia after birth. Explain the reasons for each of these and place your answer in the space provided.

C. A group of young women are discussing their use of alcohol and cigarettes. They turn to you for information about the effects of these substances on the fetus. What would you tell them?

D. Analyze a 1-week intake of a pregnant woman in her 6th week of gestation. Develop a nutrition counseling plan which will assist the mother to increase her caloric and nutritive intake appropriately.

11 ▪ *Drug therapy in pediatric nursing*

Pediatric clients are members of a unique population in their response to pharmacologic agents. The child requires special consideration in the calculation of medication doses. Knowledge of physiology, psychology, and cultural beliefs, as well as the child's age, health state, development, and genetic endowment will assist the nurse in the safe administration of therapeutic agents to this population.

Matching

A. Match the appropriate form of oral medication listed in the left-hand column to the correct age group listed in the right-hand column. Assume that the child is at the normal level of physical development.

_______ 1. Capsules	a. School-age children
_______ 2. Chewable tablets or liquid medication	b. Infants and toddlers
_______ 3. Liquid medication	c. Preschoolers

B. Match the appropriate site for an intramuscular injection listed in the left-hand column with the age group or groups in the right-hand column. (You may have more than one answer.)

_______ 1. Dorsogluteal	a. Infants
_______ 2. Vastus lateralis	b. School-age children
_______ 3. Deltoid	c. Adolescents

Short answer questions

1. List two safety measures that would be used prior to the administration of medication to the child.

2. Discuss how knowledge of pediatric growth and development will assist the nurse in administering medication to a preschooler.

3. List two ways that play could be used to assist a school-age child prior to and following the administration of an intramuscular injection.

4. List eight factors that may influence a child's response to pharmacologic therapy.

5. List three aspects of an immature renal system and the effect these may have on response to medications.

6. Discuss the rationale for avoiding the use of intravenous solutions with preservatives in premature infants and neonates.

7. Which formula provides the greatest accuracy to determine a safe, therapeutic pediatric dosage for a child who is extremely obese for his age?

8. When administering intramuscular injections to infants, what is the preferred volume in milliliters that can safely be injected at each site?

9. A child weighing 13.5 pounds is to receive amoxicillin 55 mg q8h for bilateral otitis media. The recommended dose is 40 mg/kg/day in 3 divided doses every 8 hours.
   a. How much is the total daily dose?

   b. How many milligrams would be administered every 8 hours?

   c. Is amoxicillin 55 mg/dose a safe, therapeutic dose?

10. A child weighing 68 pounds experienced a witnessed seizure and is to receive phenytoin (Dilantin) orally. The recommended dose of phenytoin is 5 to 7 mg/kg/day.
    a. What is the safe high and low dose range for this child?

    b. What would the daily dose be if the pediatrician orders 6 mg/kg/day?

Computations

1. The usual dose of an antibiotic is 20 mg/kg/24 hours. The child weighs 48 pounds. Determine the maximum individual dose if the child was to receive the medication every 8 hours.

2. The usual dose for an antibiotic is 100–200 mg/kg/24 hours. The child weighs 18 kg. Determine the low and high safe dose range for 24 hours. Determine the maximum individual dose range if the child was to receive the medication every 8 hours.

Calculation exercises

Pediatrician order:

Ceftazidime 300 mg IV q8h for a 16.5-pound 3½-year-old with a bacterial respiratory infection. The child has no known allergies but does have a history of renal failure and is at risk for edema. Calculate the safe dosage range based on the child's weight to determine whether the individual dose is safe and effective. Then determine the correct volume of IV diluent for this medication and calculate the IV infusion pump rate.

Step 1: Convert the child's weight to kilograms.
a. 16.5 pounds equals _____ kg (2.2 kg equals 1 pound)
Step 2: Consult a drug reference for a standard safe pediatric dose. For example, the *Children's Hospital of Boston Formulary* recommends: ceftazidime 100–150 mg/kg/day in 3 divided doses. Total daily dose not to exceed 6 g/day.
Step 3: Calculate the low and high safe dose range for 24 hours using the recommendation.
b. Safe low dose range _____ mg/24 hr hours
c. Safe high dose range _____ mg/24 hr hours
Step 4: Calculate safe dose for each individual dose and determine whether this falls within the safe, effective range.
d. Safe low individual dose _____ mg/dose
e. Safe high individual dose _____ mg/dose
f. Safe dose? Yes or No

If yes, proceed to calculation of IV diluent and IV rate.
Step 1: Refer to unit recommendations for dilution of drug or contact pharmacist. In this example, the recommendation for ceftazidime is to dilute 10–20 mg of drug with 1 ml of solution and infuse over 30 minutes.
Step 2: Calculate the safe low and high dilution range.
g. Minimum dilution range at 20 mg/1 ml equals ____ ml
h. Maximum dilution range at 10 mg/ml equals ____ ml
Step 3: Consider the child's medical history. Evaluate renal status, cardiac status, presence of edema, number of medications administered and dilutions required, type and size of IV catheter, and daily maintenance fluid requirements/fluid balance before arriving at a decision.
Factors to consider with this child:
i. ______________________________

____

j. Dilution decision: ____ mg/ml.
k. Dilute in ____ ml.
Step 4: Calculate the IV rate if infusing through a burette on an infusion pump (drop factor [gtt] = 60). Medication would be delivered in 3 ml adding volume to total 18 ml over 30 minutes.
l. Pump rate equals ____

Case example

The client is a 7-year-old child admitted last evening with a diagnosis of a ruptured appendix. Surgery was successfully performed, and intravenous antibiotics are ordered. Vital signs are assessed every 4 hours and are as follows: T-39.5C, P-100, R-20, BP 100/60. A nasogastric tube is in place and is connected to a suction machine set on low. The child is to be ambulated this afternoon. Intramuscular analgesics are ordered.

Because this is the client's first hospital admission, the parents are anxious and concerned. They are reluctant to encourage respiratory exercises or ambulation. They state that the child is fearful of needles.

Devise a care plan stating assessment data, diagnosis, goal, interventions, and outcome criteria for evaluation.

Enrichment experiences

1. As a pediatric nurse in a primary care ambulatory clinic or on a busy inpatient pediatric unit, you will both administer and teach parents and guardians to administer medications to children. Consider the methods used to provide safe medication administration to children. What safety measures should be taught to families for home administration of medications?

2. Chronically ill children receive medications on a long-term basis. What strategies will encourage compliance in a 14-year-old with a seizure disorder? Consider approaches to assist a newly diagnosed diabetic 8-year-old in coping with injections. Determine supportive nursing care for the families of these children.

12 ▪ *Drug therapy in gerontological nursing*

There are many factors to consider when assessing drug use among elderly clients. Chapter 12 does not give you a "cookbook" approach to assessment but rather attempts to facilitate your ability to view your elderly clients as people. General guidelines are presented to enable you to check for signs of developing toxicity, to assess the effects of drugs your elderly clients are taking, and to be an advocate and teacher for an effective and safe medication regimen for your elderly clients.

Short answer questions

You may need to refer to other chapters for information regarding specific drugs.

1. Name several factors that contribute to drug toxicity among elderly clients.

2. Identify some changing resources of the elderly that may affect their drug use. How can the nurse help the client?

3. Give examples of how the pharmacist may be used as a resource person.

4. What could be the adverse effects of the following drugs in an elderly client?
   a. Sedatives in a client with chronic respiratory disease:

   b. Thyroid supplements in a patient with coronary artery disease:

   c. Antihypertensive drugs in a client with arteriosclerosis or cerebrovascular insufficiency:

5. Briefly list cognitive changes that elderly clients may exhibit as a result of drug toxicity.

6. Why is it important to know the level of kidney function in clients taking drugs, and what are some assessments you should make to evaluate kidney function?

Correct the false statement

Indicate whether the following statements are true or false; if false, correct the underlined words or phrases.

_______ 1. Polypharmacy occurs among elderly clients because <u>they frequently visit their physicians with complaints of aches and pains</u>.

_______ 2. Common signs of drug toxicity among the elderly include <u>mental status changes</u>.

_______ 3. Elderly clients who have difficulty getting childproof caps off their medication bottles should be encouraged to leave the caps off.

_______ 4. The elderly are more prone to drug toxicity because drugs are tested primarily on healthy young adults.

_______ 5. A major problem among elderly clients is compliance to their drug regimen.

_______ 6. Signs and symptoms of drug toxicity in the elderly client may mimic those of medical or psychiatric illness.

Matching

Match the term in the left-hand column with its definition in the right-hand column. Place your answer in the space provided.

_______ 1. Toxicity
_______ 2. Intramuscular injection
_______ 3. Absorption
_______ 4. Distribution
_______ 5. Metabolism
_______ 6. Excretion
_______ 7. Calendar
_______ 8. Pharmacokinetics

a. Process affected by increased gastric pH
b. Process influenced by liver function
c. Tool that may be used to facilitate the medication regimen
d. Reaction that may first manifest as acute confusion
e. Process that may be altered by changes in body mass
f. Process influenced by kidney function
g. Procedure that should be preceded by an evaluation of muscle mass
h. Dynamic factors that influence the effectiveness of a drug in the body

Personal exercise

Write your answers on a separate sheet of paper.

1. Devise the most optimal scheduling pattern for Mrs. M. at home. Her meals are usually 8 A.M., 12:30 P.M., and 5 P.M. She goes to bed at 9 P.M. and gets up at 7 A.M. She leaves for physical therapy every day at 9:30 A.M. and returns at 12 noon. Consider drug interactions and side effects, meals, and her lifestyle.

   Her medications are:

   multivitamin 1 qd
   digoxin 0.125 mg qd
   ranitidine (Zantac) 150 mg b.i.d.
   warfarin (Coumadin) 5 mg qd
   hydrochlorothiazide (HYDRODIURIL) 50 mg qd
   KCL tab qd
   docusate sodium (Colace) 100 mg qd
   milk of magnesia 1 tsp q 4 h prn
2. Mrs. X. is 79 years old and has been taking a tricyclic antidepressant for several years. She also takes diphenhydramine (Benadryl) as an antihistamine for her “allergies” in the summer. What signs and symptoms would you look for to see if she was experiencing anticholinergic side effects?
3. Go to your own or to your family’s medicine cabinet and make a list of all the medicines there. Be sure to include over-the-counter drugs. Also note expiration dates, prescription dates, or both.
4. Develop various creative aids that may be used by elderly clients for the facilitation of their medication regimen.
5. Your elderly client has a history of arteriosclerosis, hypertension, emphysema, and arthritis. Her medications include digoxin, furosemide, and aspirin. You find that she also occasionally takes the following: diazepam when she feels upset; multivitamins and mineral supplement; laxatives at least once a week; and an over-the-counter antihistamine when she gets a cold. This client lives with her husband, who is in good health. She frequently gets confused over how many “little white pills” to take each day. Briefly outline a teaching program you would initiate for this client.

UNIT FIVE
Pharmacology in community-based nursing

13 ▪ Drug therapy in the home and community

This chapter has two major areas of emphasis: nonprescription drugs and drug therapy in the home and community.

Section I: Nonprescription drugs

Hundreds of over-the-counter (OTC) drug products are available to the general public. These products are sold without prescription and may be obtained in many locations including drugstores, supermarkets, department stores, discount stores, and vending machines located in many areas. OTC preparations are used to relieve symptoms of minor, self-limiting conditions and control nonprogressive chronic conditions. As healthcare professionals, nurses are resources to consumers and have a responsibility for educating them about appropriate use of OTC preparations and other alternative or nonconventional therapies.

Matching

Match the legislative act in the right-hand column with the provisions affecting nonprescription drugs in the left-hand column.

_______ 1. Defined prescription and nonprescription drugs
_______ 2. Prohibited fraudulent claims of efficacy of drugs
_______ 3. Required reporting of adverse reactions to the government
_______ 4. First federal law to regulate drugs
_______ 5. Established panels to review OTC drugs

a. 1962 Kefauver-Harris Amendment
b. 1972 OTC Drug Review
c. 1952 Durham-Humphrey Amendment
d. 1912 Shirley Amendment
e. 1906 Federal Food and Drug Act

Multiple choice questions

Choose the one best answer for each of the following questions. Circle the letter of the appropriate response.

1. Regulation of OTC preparations is concerned with
   a. effectiveness of products
   b. safety of products
   c. truth in labeling
   d. all of the above

2. A common characteristic of OTC preparations is
   a. low dose of inactive ingredients
   b. low dose of active ingredients
   c. no risk of adverse reactions
   d. high risk of adverse reactions
3. A benefit of using OTC drugs is that
   a. OTC drugs cost less than prescription drugs but contain the same dose
   b. OTC drugs can be used safely to treat symptoms of minor illness
   c. OTC drugs never require supervision of their use by a healthcare professional
4. Federal Food and Drug Administration (FDA) regulations require that terminology on labels
   a. be stated as warnings to users
   b. be stated in precise terms that can be interpreted easily by a healthcare provider
   c. be clear and basic enough for ordinary individuals to understand directions for use, warnings, and contraindications
   d. be concise and list only possible allergic reactions as warnings
5. Since the FDA OTC Drug Review began in 1972, some products have been reclassified from OTC status to prescription status because
   a. they were determined to be safe for animals but not for humans
   b. clinical trials revealed serious side effects
   c. they were determined to be safe at any dose
   d. there were not enough data to warrant classification
6. The use of OTC drugs by consumers decreases the burden on the healthcare system by
   a. empowering consumers to manage minor conditions without the need for professional health care
   b. decreasing the variety of products used
   c. eliminating adverse reactions to drugs, thus eliminating the need for professional intervention
   d. all of the above
7. When eliciting a drug history from a client, the nurse should obtain information about the use of prescription and nonprescription products, including
   a. name of product, reason for use, where product was purchased, and cost
   b. name of product and any allergic reactions
   c. name of product, reason for use, frequency of use, response to product, and any adverse reactions
   d. name of product and frequency of use
8. Because dosages of OTC drugs are calculated for individuals in a specific age group who are of average height and weight,
   a. adverse reactions are likely to occur in overweight individuals
   b. use of these products may produce adverse reactions in the elderly
   c. adverse reactions are less common than with prescription drugs
   d. use of the products decreases the occurrence of adverse reactions in the elderly
9. The nurse needs to caution clients who use OTC products regularly that
   a. preparations with multiple active ingredients are more likely to cause adverse reactions than those with one or two active ingredients
   b. preparations that are long-acting have few adverse reactions
   c. preparations with multiple ingredients cost more than those with only one active ingredient
   d. preparations with one ingredient are less effective than those with multiple ingredients
10. The purpose of a tamperproof seal is
    a. to deny children access to medications
    b. to prevent accidental overdosage of a medication
    c. to prevent adulteration of a product
    d. to ensure compliance with federal legislation

Short answer questions

1. List three advantages of using OTC preparations.

2. List three disadvantages of using OTC preparations.

3. State three cautions that the nurse should give clients when discussing self-medication with nonprescription products.

4. Identify at least three active or inactive ingredients used in OTC drug preparations that are contraindicated for certain groups of consumers; for each ingredient, identify the consumer(s) at risk.

Completion exercise

Complete the following table, which compares the advantages and disadvantages of using prescription and nonprescription drugs. Use a separate sheet of paper to write your response.

Type of Drug	Advantages	Disadvantages
Prescription	______________	______________
Nonprescription	______________	______________

Learning experience

Study the list of product name and product category indexes of the current edition of *Physicians' Desk Reference for Nonprescription Drugs*. Note the variety and number of available products.

Enrichment experiences

1. Select an OTC product and analyze it using the following nurses' guide for evaluating nonprescription drugs:

a. Read the label carefully for inclusion of the following:

Description of tamper-resistant feature
Name of product
Active ingredients
Inactive ingredients
Quantity of contents
Name and address of manufacturer, packer, or distributor
Indications for use
Instructions for use
Warnings, contraindications, and interactions
Expiration date and lot or batch code

b. Compare brand-name products with generic products, noting:

Active and inactive ingredients
Amount of active ingredients
Warnings, contraindications, and interactions
Cost

c. Compare several products recommended for the same use, noting:

Active and inactive ingredients
Instructions for use
Warnings, contraindications, and interactions
Cost

d. Using a pharmacologic data source for reference, evaluate OTC preparations:

How does the OTC preparation compare with the recommended dosage range?
Does the pharmacologic source recommend the active ingredient for the purpose for which it is used in the OTC preparation?
What risks are involved in using the preparation?
Would use of the OTC preparation be likely to result in undue delay in seeking needed care from a healthcare professional?
Is the preparation safe for adults?
Is the preparation safe for the frail elderly?
Is the preparation safe for children?

2. Explore the sleep aid section at a local supermarket or drugstore. Note which products contain the same active ingredient. Compare amount of the active ingredient and price of the product.

3. Explore a community pharmacy for homeopathic remedies. How do labels differ from conventional drugs?

4. Analyze advertisements for nonprescription drugs that appear in the general media. What claim is being made? What indirect message is conveyed by pictures or graphics?

Personal exercise: OTC drug history

Make a list of the OTC products that you have used during the past month. Include drugs that have been taken for specific symptoms (e.g., headache, indigestion), cosmetics, sugar substitutes, weight loss products, and soaps. Identify active ingredients for each product. Evaluate each product in terms of safety for habitual use, efficacy, risk of adverse reaction, and risk of interaction with prescription drugs. List other nonprescription products that you are likely to use and the reasons for their use. List actions that enhance the safety of self-medication with OTC preparations. Write your answer on a separate sheet of paper.

Section II: Drug therapy in the home

This section attempts to achieve two broad goals: (1) to integrate your previous knowledge about pharmacology as it relates to various client variables, including beliefs, attitudes, and previous experiences with drugs; and (2) to enhance your perceptions about how you view drugs, and about how those views affect your nursing ability. Given these expected outcomes, the following questions are offered to provide you with an opportunity to test your knowledge of the chapter content, and also to assist you in applying the nursing process to at-home client situations.

Correct the false statement

Indicate whether the following statements are true or false; if false, correct the underlined words or phrases.

_______ 1. A thorough drug history <u>at home</u> is best achieved over several visits.

_______ 2. Clients will usually comply with drugs if they understand <u>their effects and actions</u>.

_______ 3. How <u>drugs are stored in the home</u> reflects a level of safety of their use.

_______ 4. The major goal of taking a drug history is to ensure that the client takes every prescribed <u>and over-the-counter drug</u>.

Short answer questions

1. List five client variables that reflect the client's knowledge of the drugs being taken.

2. Name four ways by which a prescription label is identified.

3. Explain why the following items are dangerous to the client and/or difficult for the community health nurse to assess:
   a. Multiple drug products:

   b. Sustained-release products vs. tablets and capsule preparations:

4. Using knowledge acquired from other chapters in this text, name three foods that have pharmacologic effects (e.g., salt–fluid retention):

5. Identify a problem relating to drug use in the home; state the problem in measurable terms.

Learning experience

1. Take a drug history from one or more of the following persons:
   a. Person over 70 years of age
   b. Mother of small children
   c. Teenager or young adult
   d. Someone of a different culture from you
2. List all the drugs in the household, noting expiration dates and where they are stored.

Enrichment experience

1. List the resources available in your community for determining the contents of OTC drugs.
2. Interview a member of the staff at the poison control center in your area regarding how drug problems are handled (e.g., OTC, overdose of medications, rising incidence of drug abuse).
3. Search your community for the sale of homeopathic remedies and literature or the open practice of homeopathy by community residents.
4. Assess the drug-taking characteristics of a group of high school students by giving them a pretest of their knowledge, attitudes, and behaviors about drugs. Prepare and deliver a lecture to them based on this assessment and, if possible, administer a post-test to detect any changes in the group's knowledge and behavior.
5. Learn what laws in your state pertain to
   a. Generic drugs
   b. Expiration dates on over-the-counter drugs
   c. Inclusion of patient information packets for both OTC and prescription drugs
   d. Controlled substance prescribing
   e. Disposal of toxic substances and infectious substances in the home

Situational exercises

What would you do in the following situations?

Mr. S., a 68-year-old widower and retired prison warden, was diagnosed 10 years ago with emphysema. He recently moved to this town to live with his daughter and grandchildren. His physician has sent you a referral after diagnosing metastatic cancer to ensure that he follows his medication regimen, especially during a 6-week course of outpatient chemotherapy.

1. Before your first home visit, what further information should you obtain to prepare for a thorough drug use assessment?
   a. past and present diagnoses
   b. other prescribed medications
   c. his prognosis
   d. the goals of chemotherapy
   e. all of the above

2. What client variable would be of greatest importance to ascertain on the first home visit?
   a. knowledge of drugs
   b. names of other physicians
   c. source of income
   d. attitude about drugs

3. Mr. S. becomes nauseated, and states that he doesn't want to continue chemotherapy. Which of the following measures would you undertake to augment his compliance?
   a. explain how cancer cells proliferate
   b. teach him a bland diet
   c. ascertain his goal of chemotherapy
   d. inform his physician of this decision

Jumbled words

For the following jumble, rearrange the three words in bold print to obtain the missing letters that form the word below it. Then rearrange all letters in boxes to form the last word.

This is what a client needs to take drugs safely:

D E L W O K G N E

_ _ ☐ _ ☐ _ _ _ ☐

+

T I N A M I V T O O

☐ _ _ _ _ ☐ _ _ _ ☐

+

L A C I T A P I Y B

☐ _ ☐ _ _ _ _ ☐ _ _ = **C** _ _ _ _ _ _ _ _ _ _

14 ▪ *Substance abuse*

The illicit use of chemical substances has become a recognized health problem in the general population. The ability to identify and intervene in the abuse cycle will provide positive strategies for the healthcare team to use in directing intervention plans. The following exercises will facilitate the development of knowledge in the area of substance abuse, and provide an understanding of the complexities of abuse cycles.

Matching

For each drug in the first column, select the appropriate street term from the second column:

_______ 1. Phencyclidine (PCP)
_______ 2. Amphetamine
_______ 3. Methaqualone
_______ 4. Heroin
_______ 5. Cocaine

a. DOA
b. Smack
c. Angel dust
d. Black beauty
e. Nose candy
f. Soaper

Correct the false statement

For each of the following items, mark T if the statement is true. If the statement is false, correct it by changing the underlined word(s):

_______ 1. The abuse of central nervous system depressants is more likely to be associated with homicidal and suicidal tendencies than is the use of central nervous system stimulants.

_______ 2. Hallucinogenic drugs appear to act as antagonists on nerve cell receptors that normally respond to endogenous neurotransmitters.

_______ 3. Xanthines can enhance the performance of motor skills that have been incompletely mastered.

Multiple choice questions

For each of the following, choose the one best answer:

1. Which of the following is true about the nature of drug dependence?
   a. Addictive behavior is dependent on the original motivating force.
   b. During the initial period of drug abuse, the user cannot control consumption.
   c. The more potent a chemical agent, the more rapidly addiction develops.
   d. A negative relationship exists between potency and dependency.

2. According to Bejerot's classification of addiction, therapeutic addiction
   a. may be a consequence of medical treatment
   b. is frequently contagious
   c. is the most common type in the Western world
   d. occurs rarely among health personnel

3. Which type of addiction occurs when a psychoactive substance is accepted and socially tolerated by the general population?
   a. endemic
   b. epidemic
   c. iatrogenic
   d. therapeutic
4. Nembutal and Seconal belong to which drug classification?
   a. CNS sympathomimetics
   b. general CNS depressants
   c. opioid analgesics
   d. hallucinogens
5. Heroin, morphine, codeine, and Demerol belong to which drug classification?
   a. CNS sympathomimetics
   b. general CNS depressants
   c. opioid analgesics
   d. hallucinogens
6. Which drug group causes the following symptoms: short-lived euphoria, drowsiness, lethargy, decreased physical activities, pinpoint pupils, decreased vision, and constipation?
   a. CNS sympathomimetics
   b. general CNS depressants
   c. opioid analgesics
   d. psychedelics
7. The common effects of CNS depressants include
   a. anxiety
   b. drowsiness
   c. insomnia
   d. irritability
8. In the treatment of heroin addiction,
   a. physical dependence is more difficult to eliminate than psychologic dependence
   b. treatment of dependence usually requires many months
   c. withdrawal is more dangerous than that from any other CNS depressant
   d. psychologic dependence resolves once physical dependence ends
9. Methadone is used
   a. as an antidote to opioids
   b. in the treatment of opioid overdose
   c. to minimize nausea from opioids
   d. for weaning a client from opioids
10. Acute alcohol toxicity that is life-threatening may require heroic measures to reduce alcohol concentration. The most likely treatment is
    a. mechanical ventilation
    b. rapidly flowing intravenous fluids
    c. bowel cleansing with purgatives
    d. hemodialysis
11. Acute alcohol withdrawal is typically treated with IV fluids and
    a. antiarrhythmics
    b. corticosteroids
    c. narcotic analgesics
    d. benzodiazepines
12. A person with little or no tolerance to alcohol is likely to die if the blood alcohol concentration exceeds
    a. 0.15 percent
    b. 0.5 percent
    c. 1.5 percent
    d. 5 percent
13. When an alcohol-addicted client is admitted to the hospital, observation for delirium tremens (DTs) would be most important during which time period? The first
    a. week only
    b. two weeks
    c. three weeks
    d. four weeks
14. Which group of drugs have these street names: *speed, uppers, crank,* and *truck drivers*?
    a. amphetamines
    b. barbiturates
    c. benzodiazepines
    d. hallucinogens
15. Disulfiram (Antabuse) is used medicinally in the treatment of alcoholism for the purpose of
    a. ameliorating the signs and symptoms of acute alcohol intoxication
    b. monitoring the sobriety of those under treatment for chronic alcoholism
    c. preventing habitual drinking
    d. preventing impulse drinking
16. Amphetamines act as stimulants to
    a. the central nervous system
    b. α-adrenergic receptors
    c. β-adrenergic receptors
    d. all of the above

17. Elimination of amphetamines is enhanced by
   a. stimulation of bile secretion
   b. lowering the pH of the urine
   c. raising the pH of the urine
   d. changes in the glomerular filtration rate
18. In chronic or heavy users, withdrawal of amphetamines is followed by physical and emotional symptoms. Are amphetamines considered to cause dependence?
   a. Yes, they are believed to cause psychologic dependence but not physical dependence.
   b. Yes, they are believed to cause physical dependence but not psychologic dependence.
   c. Yes, they are known to cause both psychologic and physical dependence.
   d. The extent to which the withdrawal syndrome is caused by psychologic or physical dependence is unknown.
19. During emergency treatment of victims of amphetamine overdose, the nurse should focus on interventions to treat
   a. hypotension
   b. hypothermia
   c. muscle stiffness
   d. seizures
20. How do the amphetamines affect sleep?
   a. They delay or inhibit onset of sleep by increasing mental alertness.
   b. They suppress REM sleep.
   c. neither of the above
   d. both a and b above
21. One drug that can promote elimination of amphetamines, in cases of acute toxicity, is
   a. sodium bicarbonate
   b. ammonium chloride
   c. 5 percent dextrose in water
   d. phentolamine
22. Cocaine is a derivative of
   a. the opium poppy
   b. the cocoa bean
   c. the coca leaves
   d. catecholamines
23. Persons who "snort" cocaine regularly are likely to develop
   a. hepatitis B
   b. lethargy and stupor
   c. needle "tracks" on the extremities
   d. perforation of the nasal septum
24. A hallucinogen approved for medicinal use is
   a. lysergic acid diethylamide
   b. psilocybin
   c. mescaline
   d. drombinol
25. Caffeine withdrawal is likely to be accompanied by
   a. lethargy
   b. headache
   c. convulsions
   d. hallucinations
26. A common adverse effect of caffeine is
   a. ataxia
   b. constipation
   c. insomnia
   d. vomiting
27. Which is an example of a hallucination (as opposed to an illusion)?
   a. answering the door when the phone rings
   b. misinterpreting a stick for a knife
   c. perceiving a red balloon as orange
   d. seeing a person that isn't there
28. Which drug group causes appetite suppression, mood elevation, insomnia, and hyperactivity?
   a. CNS sympathomimetics
   b. general CNS depressants
   c. opioid analgesics
   d. hallucinogens
29. What drug typically produces euphoria, total relaxation, and altered sensory and time perception, and is called *Acapulco gold, hay,* and *hemp*?
   a. cocaine
   b. LSD
   c. marijuana
   d. PCP
30. General CNS depressants are used medically to
   a. alleviate muscle spasms
   b. relieve pain
   c. suppress appetite
   d. treat glaucoma
31. Ritalin, a CNS sympathomimetic drug, is used medically to
   a. detoxify heroin addicts
   b. prevent insomnia
   c. relieve surgical pain
   d. treat hyperactive children

32. What drug is referred to by these street names: *snow, rock, white, crack, nose candy?*
    a. cocaine
    b. LSD
    c. marijuana
    d. PCP

Selection of options

For each of the following, select *all* appropriate responses. Circle the correct answers.

1. Clients recovering from amphetamine overdose are likely to experience
    a. prolongation of REM sleep
    b. fatigue and lethargy
    c. episodic hyperactivity
    d. emotional depression
2. Which of the following foods contain xanthine stimulants?
    a. coffee
    b. ginger ale
    c. chocolate candy
    d. licorice candy
    e. tea
    f. cola beverages
    g. wine
3. Use of which of the following combinations of drugs is likely to produce a life-threatening adverse reaction?
    a. alcohol and caffeine
    b. alcohol and tranquilizers
    c. hypnotics and tranquilizers
    d. alcohol and hypnotics
    e. opiates and alcohol
    f. hypnotics and opiates
4. Opioid dependence during pregnancy is likely to cause
    a. congenital defects in the baby
    b. prolonged labor during parturition
    c. opioid dependence in the newborn
    d. apnea in the newborn
5. In combination with certain drugs, opiates greatly increase the risk of toxicity. Some drugs that exhibit this synergism are
    a. alcohol
    b. analeptics
    c. hypnotics
    d. tranquilizers
6. What are the most likely effects when naloxone is administered to a person dependent on high doses of opiates?
    a. any "high" persisting after the last opioid dose will be decreased or abolished
    b. any "high" persisting after the last opioid dose will be enhanced
    c. nausea, vomiting, diarrhea
    d. miosis
7. Withdrawal of opiates from a dependent person is characterized by
    a. rhinorrhea
    b. midriasis
    c. nausea and vomiting
    d. diarrhea
8. Physiologic effects of opioid analgesics include
    a. a decrease in anxiety, fear, and pain
    b. depression of mood and dysphoria
    c. inhibition of sensory perception, especially that of pain
9. Gastrointestinal effects of opiates include
    a. nausea
    b. vomiting
    c. diarrhea
    d. biliary colic
10. What physiologic changes are most likely to occur during acute alcohol intoxication?
    a. dehydration
    b. hypoglycemia
    c. water retention
    d. depletion of B vitamins
11. By what routes may alcohol be absorbed by the body?
    a. PO
    b. SC
    c. IV
    d. inhalation
    e. topical
12. Chronic use of alcohol markedly increases the risk of serious health problems. These include
    a. teratogenic damage to a developing fetus
    b. cancer
    c. progressive liver deterioration
    d. peptic ulcers
    e. loss of control of epilepsy and diabetes
    f. brain degeneration
    g. peripheral neuritis

h. pancreatitis
i. skeletal and cardiac muscle degeneration
j. hypertension

13. Health problems most likely to be associated with chronic alcoholism are
a. muscle weakness
b. malnutrition
c. vitamin A toxicity
d. frequent or serious infections
e. cirrhosis of the liver

14. Lay terms for alcohol withdrawal include
a. the "shakes"
b. "DTs"
c. "clap"
d. being "bombed"

15. Examples of hallucinogens are
a. heroin
b. barbiturates
c. LSD
d. peyote

Short answer questions

1. Define the following terms:
a. Abuse:

b. Addiction:

c. Tolerance:

d. Dependence:

2. Describe the cycles of dependence reflected in each of the following:
a. Pharmacologic circle:

b. Cerebral circle:

c. Social circle:

d. Psychologic circle:

3. Give examples of street slang for these commonly abused drugs:
a. Barbiturates:

b. Heroin:

c. Cocaine:

d. Marijuana:

e. Hashish:

f. LSD:

g. Morphine:

h. Methaqualone:

i. Phencyclidine:

4. List at least three adverse effects of long-term use of cocaine.

5. By what route is medicinal cocaine administered?

6. What is a flashback?

7. Name two nursing measures helpful in the treatment of someone experiencing a "bad trip" following use of a hallucinogen.

Enrichment experiences

1. **Explore public health efforts to provide community education regarding the hazards of drug and alcohol abuse through health education curricula in schools, and public education through social organizations, national programs, and healthcare facilities.**
2. **Survey local middle schools (junior high schools), high schools, and emergency room nurses to explore the substances abused most frequently in your area. Identify high-risk populations based on this information.**
3. **Request an information and education seminar for your class with a narcotics agent from your local law enforcement agency.**
4. **Assess the type, availability, and efficacy of drug-related rehabilitation programs in your community.**
5. **Contact your regional office of the Drug Enforcement Administration to obtain information about current rates of substance abuse in your community.**

Learning experience

Review your personal experiences with alcoholic beverages. How does your use of alcohol compare with the "norm" for your peers? Have you ever become intoxicated? "Hung over"? What factors influenced your early decisions regarding acceptance or rejection of alcoholic beverages? In light of the information on alcohol previously presented, how would you evaluate the drinking habits of yourself and your peers?

15 ▪ *Toxicology*

The study of toxicology enables the student to develop an awareness about the differences between the therapeutic use of pharmacologic agents and their poisonous potential in lethal doses. The following exercises will provide a broad base of information related to poison intervention and control.

Multiple choice questions

For each of the following, choose the one best answer:

1. The three branches of the science of toxicology include
   a. adverse reactions to medications, economic toxicology, and environmental toxicology
   b. adverse reactions to medications, economic toxicology, and forensic toxicology
   c. adverse reactions to medications, environmental toxicology, and forensic toxicology
   d. economic toxicology, environmental toxicology, and forensic toxicology
2. The percutaneous route refers to the mode of entry when substances cross
   a. mucous membranes
   b. skin
   c. GI mucosa
   d. alveolar membranes
3. The gastrointestinal route designates the point of entry of substances crossing
   a. the gastric mucosa
   b. the intestinal mucosa
   c. the sublingual mucosa
   d. all of the above
4. Drugs that enter the body parenterally are
   a. ingested
   b. inhaled
   c. injected
   d. rubbed on the skin
5. By which route are substances most likely to be degraded before reaching the general circulation?
   a. percutaneous
   b. GI
   c. parenteral
   d. inhalation
6. By which route are chemicals likely to reach the circulation most quickly?
   a. percutaneous
   b. GI
   c. intravenous
   d. inhalation
7. Which route of entry provides the *least* opportunity to decrease or delay absorption of a poison?
   a. percutaneous
   b. GI
   c. subcutaneous
   d. intravenous
8. Children are most likely to be poisoned by
   a. household cleansers
   b. poisonous plants
   c. insect bites
   d. medicines
9. The environmental pollutant most likely to cause poisoning in children is
   a. dioxin
   b. lead
   c. mercury
   d. sulfites
10. The most likely cause of lead poisoning in small children is
    a. breathing fumes from vehicular traffic
    b. chewing the dark filler from lead pencils
    c. breathing fumes from pottery glazes containing lead
    d. chewing on items coated with lead-containing paints
11. Poisondex is
    a. a test for toxic potential of a substance
    b. a test for toxic levels of poison in the blood

c. a printed volume of information about toxic materials
d. a computerized system of information about toxic materials

12. A form of poisoning that can cause delayed pathology is that caused by
   a. acetaminophen
   b. insecticides
   c. diazepam (Valium)
   d. chlorine bleach
13. Which of the following chemicals has no known positive effects on the body?
   a. acetaminophen
   b. alcohol
   c. arsenic
   d. lead
14. The most feared effect of lead poisoning in children is
   a. anemia
   b. lead deposits in the bone
   c. mood swings
   d. neuropathy
15. How is lead poisoning diagnosed?
   a. by examination of the teeth
   b. by x-ray films of the bones
   c. by testing the blood
   d. only by the signs and symptoms of poisoning
16. Mercury concentrations in sea water are most likely to result from
   a. massive deaths of contaminated fish
   b. acid fresh water draining from rivers-heds
   c. emission of lead from underwater volcanic vents
   d. industrial pollution
17. The safest way of discarding poisonous materials is usually by
   a. flushing the material down a toilet
   b. burial in a landfill waste disposal site
   c. burning in an incinerator
   d. encasing them in concrete
18. Vapors most likely to cause poisoning in the hospital setting are
   a. alcohol and formaldehyde
   b. ethylene oxide and methylmethacrylate
   c. ether and halogens
   d. oxygen and helium
19. The *first* piece of information to secure when answering the telephone in a poison control center is
   a. the condition of the victim
   b. the identity of the poison affecting the victim
   c. whether or not emergency medical personnel are needed
   d. the telephone number and address of the caller
20. The first treatment given a poison victim should be
   a. support of vital functions
   b. removing or eliminating the poison
   c. administering an antidote
   d. emotional support of the victim and family
21. For how many poisons are antidotes available?
   a. virtually 100 percent
   b. about half (50 percent)
   c. about one fourth (25 percent)
   d. less than one-fiftieth (2 percent)
22. In regard to medications, the nurse should teach parents to
   a. discard old or expired medications in the trash
   b. keep all medications out of reach of children
   c. combine two partial bottles of aspirin so as not to confuse them
   d. tell the child taking a pill is as easy as eating an M&M

Selection of options

For the following question, select *all* appropriate responses. Circle the correct answers:

1. Which of the following are contraindications for inducing emesis in a poison victim?
   a. absence of gag reflex
   b. ingestion of aspirin
   c. ingestion of lye
   d. ingestion of kerosene

Short answer questions

1. Define the following terms:
   a. Antidote:

   b. Toxicology:

   c. FEP:

   d. Chelate:

2. Give the route of entry of a toxin and provide an example of each.

Toxin Route	Example

3. Briefly describe first-aid steps to be taken when intervening in a poison emergency under the following conditions:
   a. Ingestion in a conscious victim

   b. Inhaled poison

   c. Skin contamination

   d. Eye contamination

4. List five methods used to prevent absorption of poisons.

5. List five methods used to enhance excretion of a poison.

6. Identify the four criteria needed to diagnose plumbism positively.
   a.

   b.

   c.

   d.

Personal exercise: Poisons in the home

Survey your home environment for the storage of potentially toxic substances. Identify measures that could poison-proof your home.

Learning experience

Contact local emergency room departments to survey recent trends in accidental poisonings, or interview an emergency room nurse to explore the methods used for meeting the needs of acute poisoning victims.

Enrichment experience

Investigate the incidence of lead poisoning in your community. What populations are at risk of being in contact with toxic levels of lead? What other heavy metal toxins are present in your locality? How are hazardous waste materials disposed of in your community?

UNIT SIX
Drugs that affect the nervous system

16 ▪ *Drugs that affect the autonomic nervous system*

The autonomic nervous system controls vital functions of the body and the physiologic balance of the total organism. Autonomic drugs are those chemicals that change this balance, either by altering the function of the autonomic nervous system or by augmenting or counteracting its effects. Nurses must understand autonomic functions, therefore, to understand the actions and effects of autonomic drugs.

Matching

A. Match the drug or condition in the left-hand column with the appropriate antidote from the right-hand column. Place your answer in the space provided.

______	1. Parathion	a. Norepinephrine
______	2. Norepinephrine	b. Atropine
______	3. Mushroom poisoning	c. Epinephrine
______	4. Nerve gas	d. Phentolamine
______	5. Phentolamine	
______	6. Malathion	
______	7. Insect sting allergy	

B. Match the physiologic response in the left-hand column with its mode of autonomic activity in the right-hand column.

______	1. Miosis	a. Sympathetic
______	2. Bradycardia	b. Parasympathetic
______	3. Bronchodilation	
______	4. Increased respiratory secretion	
______	5. Constriction of gastrointestinal sphincters	
______	6. Increased contractility of the urinary bladder	
______	7. Secretion of epinephrine and norepinephrine	
______	8. Increased blood glucose concentration	

C. Match the drug in the left-hand column with its class(es) or use(s) in the right-hand column.

_______ 1. Epinephrine
_______ 2. Atropine
_______ 3. Ambenonium
_______ 4. Norepinephrine
_______ 5. Isoproterenol
_______ 6. Phenylephrine

a. Cholinergic
b. Adrenergic
c. Anticholinergic
d. Sympathetic blocking agent
e. Hyperglycemic
f. Used to control life-threatening vasogenic shock
g. Nasal decongestant
h. First choice for treating anaphylaxis
i. Administered preoperatively to inhibit respiratory secretions
j. Used to alleviate bronchospasm
k. Used in treating myasthenia gravis

Find the hidden words

Hidden within the following letter grid are words and phrases from Chapter 16. They may be vertical, horizontal, or diagonal. Circle the letters as you find the hidden words.

List of words and phrases

adrenalin
adrenergic
amnesia
anticholinergic
atropine
belladonna
cholinergic
epinephrine
ergot
ganglia
levophed
midriasis
miosis
muscarine
neostigmine
nerve gas
nicotine
norepinephrine
parasympathomimetic
phentolamine
sarin
scopolamine
sympathetic

d a r d r s c o p b u t a n t i a a d m p h e t n

t d a d a e i o a n t i p a r a i c g r a n t i i

a h a m u s c a r i n e h y p s s y m p a m i n c

e r a t r o p n a a d r e n e p i a s i s m b a t

d x c o p o r e s e r p i n e f n a g r e n e n a

c i g a r a p p y s o i m i o s i a d e n o m p b

n e p h r i r a m m e a n i t n n a r e v o l a p

d a i t l e v o p h e d d n l g i d n e a r d a h

n e d e d o n i a n t i a r l e a i e d e p e n i

s a r i n u b a t a c i g r e n i l o h c i t n a

i i a a b o s a h i s n p n i n e r s s t i t d u

i m m a d s u m o y d e i i i p e o t n c i g r t

p n s n i i d i m n e r p p i n b r i c a i c a o

n e i t m s a p i c h e c e o p e c g d c i b c a

s y m c h a a t m p p h e n t o l a m i n e s i u

e l h c o t e p e c o t i i t o i i i e c y c b t

i n e p h t o n t l v i n p t i a n n h m c m e o

a l i e p i i n i e e e h o g a d r e n a l i n n

p e t p e p h n e r l a g r n r o g i c a t d i o

n i a h e p e d e p h r n t e c n u s a n t r i m

c r n r a r p h r i e p i a i c n t i i t a i s i

t a o e g a n g l i a d e n a m a a i o s i a h c

t n a i s c o p o l a m i n e p n b n a m o s o m

n t e w p h e d r i a s i s i t a t d r e n i m a

a i i h a p p r i o d l n i i p i r i a s i s m n

n c t p o p h i a s r d e s p a e p i n e p i n e

i c i g r e n i l o h c i t n a p h e d r e i s t

Correct the false statement

Indicate whether the following statements are true or false; if false, correct the underlined words or phrases.

________ 1. Ephedrine has a shorter duration of action than does epinephrine.

________ 2. A serious adverse effect of adrenergic hormones and drugs is an increased risk of cardiac arrhythmias.

________ 3. The action of dobutamide is dependent on release of endogenous norepinephrine.

________ 4. It is important that the use of adrenergic vasoconstrictors to treat hypotensive shock be preceded by fluid volume replacement.

________ 5. When surgery is contemplated for persons who have been receiving adrenergic blocking agents, it is important that the dosage of the medication be increased on the day of the surgery.

________ 6. The active ingredients in many insecticides and nerve gas are anti-adrenergics.

________ 7. Cholinergic or anticholinesterase eye drops are often used in treating chronic glaucoma.

________ 8. The principal toxins in mushrooms are nicotinic compounds.

Completion exercises

On the drawing at right, identify and label the following:

1. The nerve terminal of the presynaptic nerve cell
2. The postsynaptic receptor cell
3. The synaptic contact zone
4. The postsynaptic receptor area
5. Organelles and enzymes that synthesize, store, release, and actively reuptake transmitter chemicals
6. Organelles that respond to receptor triggers

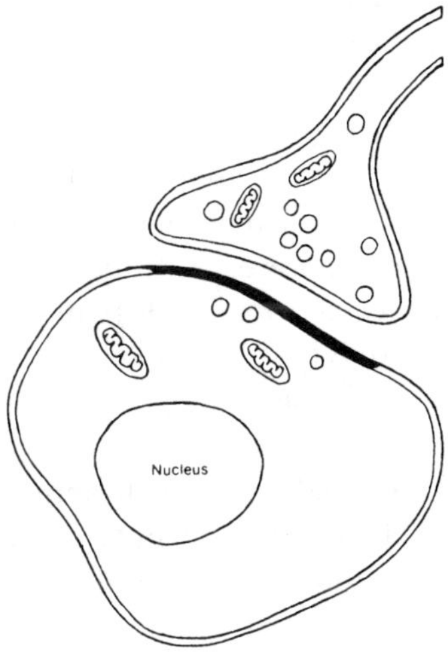

Multiple choice questions

For each of the following, choose the one best answer:

1. Which of the following drugs cannot safely be injected subcutaneously?
   a. epinephrine
   b. norepinephrine
   c. terbutaline
   d. bethanechol
2. Which of the following drugs is effective when administered orally?
   a. epinephrine
   b. norepinephrine
   c. dopamine
   d. ephedrine
3. Adrenergic drugs are substances that produce a physiologic response resembling that of
   a. parasympathetic stimulation
   b. parasympathetic inhibition
   c. sympathetic stimulation
   d. sympathetic inhibition
4. A cathecholamine is defined as a drug that
   a. mimics parasympathetic nervous system activity
   b. mimics sympathetic nervous system activity
   c. contains a steroid nucleus in its structure
   d. contains dihydroxybenzene in its structure

5. Toxic effects of adrenergic drugs include
   a. drowsiness
   b. insomnia
   c. pinpoint pupils
   d. cholinergic crisis
6. The drug most likely to cause a stroke is
   a. atropine
   b. ambenonium
   c. phentolamine
   d. norepinephrine
7. Epinephrine is usually administered
   a. orally
   b. by inhalation
   c. by injection
   d. transdermally
8. Dopamine is usually administered
   a. PO
   b. SC
   c. IV
9. Why is epinephrine mixed with local anesthetics?
   a. to prolong the numbing effect
   b. to increase circulation at the site
   c. to dilate local blood vessels
   d. to prevent infection
10. A side effect likely to occur with ergot alkaloids is
   a. an "aura"
   b. nausea
   c. cold painful extremities
   d. swelling of hands and feet
11. A food that can cause peripheral vascular insufficiency or abortion is
   a. hard cheese containing tyramine
   b. moldy flour containing ergot
   c. moldy food containing aflatoxins
   d. "sunburned" potatoes containing solanine
12. A hallucinogen chemically related to ergot is
   a. lysergic acid diethylamide (LSD)
   b. dichlorodiphenyltrichloroethane (DDT)
   c. tetrahydrocannabinol
   d. phencyclidine hydrochloride (PCP)
13. The body tends to store phenoxybenzamine in
   a. fat
   b. bone
   c. the thyroid gland
   d. the cerebrospinal fluid
14. A side effect of β-adrenergic blockers is a(n)
   a. increased heart rate
   b. impairment of response to stress
   c. decrease in respiratory secretions
   d. increased concentration of glucose in the blood
15. Clients receiving drug treatment for myasthenia gravis sometimes develop impaired respirations similar to those of the untreated disease. When this problem is caused by the medication it is called
   a. anaphylaxis
   b. tachyphylaxis
   c. myasthenia crisis
   d. addisonian crisis
   e. cholinergic crisis
16. The above condition is usually treated by mechanically assisted respirations and
   a. administration of atropine
   b. increasing the dose of cholinergics
   c. discontinuation of the cholinergics
17. Side effects of cholinergic drugs include
   a. bronchodilation
   b. relaxation of smooth muscle
   c. urinary retention
   d. increased peristalsis
18. A drug that is contraindicated in glaucoma is
   a. atropine
   b. pilocarpine
   c. morphine
   d. reserpine
19. The usual adult dose of atropine is
   a. 300–400 μg
   b. 300–400 mg
   c. 3–4 g
   d. 10–12 g
20. Nurses who handle atropine carelessly are likely to develop
   a. impairment of sexual function
   b. urinary retention
   c. contact dermatitis
   d. blurred vision
21. The first drug used in the treatment of anaphylaxis is usually
   a. atropine
   b. neostigmine
   c. propranolol
   d. epinephrine

Selection of options

For each of the following, select *all* appropriate responses. Circle the correct answers.

1. Adrenergic drugs tend to cause the following side effects:
   a. vasodilation
   b. central nervous system stimulation
   c. muscle tremor
2. In the autonomic nervous system the neurotransmitter acetylcholine is responsible for the transmission of impulses
   a. across most preganglionic synapses of the parasympathetic system
   b. across most postganglionic synapses of the parasympathetic system
   c. across most preganglionic synapses of the sympathetic system
   d. across most postganglionic synapses of the sympathetic system
   e. in most ganglionic synapses
3. Following transmission of an impulse, neurotransmitters in the synaptic gap are dissipated by
   a. rapid transport away from the area by lymphatic and venous drainage
   b. rapid breakdown by tissue enzymes
   c. active reuptake by the axon terminal
   d. absorption by the postsynaptic receptor area
4. Physiologic effects of epinephrine include
   a. stimulation of α-adrenergic receptors
   b. stimulation of β-adrenergic receptors
   c. miosis
   d. tachycardia
   e. bronchodilation
   f. release of histamine in allergic reactions
5. Routes used for administration of epinephrine include
   a. PO
   b. SC
   c. inhalation
6. Catecholamine drugs include
   a. ephedrine
   b. epinephrine
   c. norepinephrine
   d. amphetamines
7. Contraindications for the use of epinephrine include
   a. hypotension
   b. angina pectoris
   c. allergic reaction
   d. hyperthyroidism
   e. pheochromocytoma
8. Appropriate routes for administering norepinephrine include
   a. PA
   b. SC
   c. IM
   d. IV
9. Isoproterenol acts by stimulating
   a. α-adrenergic receptors
   b. β_1-adrenergic receptors
   c. β_2-adrenergic receptors
10. Sympathetic drugs that are effective when administered orally include
    a. amphetamine
    b. ephedrine
    c. epinephrine
    d. terbutaline
11. Adrenergic blocking agents are likely to produce the following cardiovascular effects:
    a. decreased blood pressure
    b. postural hypotension
    c. bradycardia
12. Side effects of sympathomimetic drugs include
    a. anorexia
    b. fatigability
    c. drowsiness
    d. dry skin
13. Ergot alkaloids should not be given to people suffering from
    a. arthritis
    b. hypotension
    c. phlebitis
    d. severe arteriosclerosis
14. Clients who are treated for migraine with ergot alkaloids should be monitored for
    a. warm sweaty extremities
    b. cold painful extremities
    c. peripheral numbness and tingling
15. Adverse reactions to cholinergics include
    a. bronchospasm
    b. urinary retention
    c. increased gastric acidity
    d. blurred vision secondary to midriasis
16. Side effects of anticholinesterases include
    a. dry skin
    b. salivation
    c. bradycardia
    d. bronchodilation

17. Those likely to experience adverse reactions to atropine include people with a history of
    a. bladder outlet obstruction
    b. glaucoma
    c. hypermotility of the bowel
    d. hyperthyroidism
    e. gastric hypersecretion

18. Autonomic drugs that act as miotics include
    a. cholinergic drugs
    b. anticholinesterases
    c. anticholinergics
    d. adrenergics

Short answer questions

1. Name the two main divisions of the central nervous system.

2. Identify the two main divisions of the brain.

3. Name at lease two physiologic "centers" in the brain stem that control visceral functions.

4. Name four subdivisions of the sympathetic nervous system.

5. Identify two subdivisions of the parasympathetic nervous system.

6. Give the four main classifications of autonomic drugs.

7. Identify four uses for cholinergic drugs.

8. What is the anatomic relationship between the cranial nerves and the autonomic nervous system?

9. Name three factors to consider when scheduling doses of cholinergic drugs prescribed to treat myasthenia gravis.

10. Define *tachyphylaxis.*

Enrichment experience

Interview an asthmatic client to determine the subjective effects of adrenergic medication used to control acute episodes of dyspnea. What does the client do to alleviate the adverse effects of these drugs?

17 ▪ *Central nervous system stimulants*

A mechanism known as the blood–brain barrier controls the distribution of drugs within the central nervous system. Response to drugs depends largely on the status of the person: underlying personality, physiologic function, and mental "set." Response is also influenced by the client's history and environment.

Matching

Match the description in the left-hand column with the appropriate drug in the right-hand column. Place your answer in the space provided.

_______	1. Ingredient of smelling salts	a. Strychnine
_______	2. Analeptic sometimes used to diagnose epilepsy	b. Picrotoxin
		c. Pentylenetetrazole (Metrazol)
_______	3. Ingredients of rat poison	d. Spirits of ammonia

Short answer questions

1. A xanthine used to treat apnea in premature infants is ________________________.
2. List at least three nursing measures helpful to clients receiving therapeutic doses of theophylline.

3. Name at least four signs and symptoms of xanthine toxicity.

4. What is the proper procedure for administering smelling salts?

5. List at least four beneficial effects of CNS stimulants.

6. Name at least four adverse reactions or toxic symptoms caused by CNS stimulants.

7. Give at least four therapeutic uses for amphetamines.

Correct the false statement

Indicate whether the following statements are true or false; if false, correct the underlined words.

_______ 1. Amphetamine exerts its pharmacologic action primarily by directly stimulating norepinephrine receptors in the nervous system.

_______ 2. Amphetamines are most likely to produce tolerance when high doses are used over long periods of time.

_______ 3. Among the physiologic effects of xanthine compounds are an increased basal metabolic rate and diuresis.

_______ 4. Xanthines can enhance the performance of motor skills that have been incompletely mastered.

_______ 5. The metabolism of levodopa by body tissues converts it to an inactive substance that is highly water-soluble.

_______ 6. Dopamine is not useful in treating Parkinson's syndrome because it is metabolized rapidly by the peripheral tissues.

_______ 7. Clients receiving phenytoin for control of seizures who develop Parkinson's syndrome may require a relatively low dose of levodopa to prevent adverse reactions.

_______ 8. Optimal response to levodopa therapy usually occurs 1 week to 10 days after treatment is initiated.

_______ 9. Smelling salts are used to prevent fainting.

_______ 10. The abuse of CNS depressants is more likely to be associated with homicidal and suicidal tendencies than is the use of CNS stimulants.

Multiple choice questions

For each of the following, choose the one best answer:

1. What is the blood–brain barrier?
   a. a lipid membrane that allows passage by diffusion of lipid-soluble chemicals only
   b. a semipermeable membrane that allows passage of ionized radicals only
   c. an active physiologic mechanism with functions similar to those of an active transport system
   d. all of the above
2. Stimulants should be used in small doses, if at all, for clients with
   a. asthma
   b. Addison's disease
   c. hypothyroidism
   d. hyperthyroidism
3. Amphetamines act as stimulants to
   a. the CNS
   b. α-adrenergic receptors
   c. β-adrenergic receptors
   d. all of the above
4. A client who took a large dose of amphetamines should be monitored for
   a. hypotensive shock
   b. bradycardia
   c. hyperthermia
   d. all of the above
5. Elimination of amphetamines is enhanced by
   a. stimulation of bile secretion
   b. lowering the pH of the urine
   c. raising the pH of the urine
   d. changes in the glomerular filtration rate
6. How do the amphetamines affect sleep?
   a. They delay or inhibit onset of sleep by increasing mental alertness.
   b. They suppress REM sleep.
   c. neither of the above
   d. both a and b above
7. In chronic or heavy users, withdrawal from amphetamines is followed by physical and emotional symptoms. Are amphetamines considered to cause dependence?
   a. Yes, they are believed to cause psychologic dependence but not physical dependence.
   b. Yes, they are believed to cause physical dependence but not psychologic dependence.
   c. Yes, they are known to cause both psychologic and physical dependence.
   d. The extent to which the withdrawal syndrome is caused by psychologic or physical dependence is unknown.
8. Are amphetamines acceptable for use in treating obesity?
   a. No, their use is forbidden by FDA regulation.
   b. Yes, provided the client is under close medical supervision.
   c. Sometimes, for the first 2 weeks of a weight reduction regimen.
   d. Yes, provided the client has been screened for factors that increase the risk of toxic effects.
9. What type of chemicals are the xanthines?
   a. inorganic salts
   b. catecholamines
   c. aldehydes
   d. alkaloids
10. At what blood concentration does theophylline usually produce toxic symptoms?
    a. 2 μg/ml or more
    b. 5 μg/ml or more
    c. 10 μg/ml or more
    d. 20 μg/ml or more

11. The primary medical use of the administration of the xanthine theophylline is to promote
    a. diuresis
    b. bronchodilation
    c. stimulation of the respiratory center
    d. stimulation of intestinal secretion
12. A drug used to treat convulsions caused by theophylline is
    a. diazepam (Valium)
    b. flurazepam (Dalmane)
    c. phenytoin (Dilantin)
    d. phenobarbital (Luminal)
13. A xanthine administered intravenously in the treatment of obstructive airway disease is
    a. caffeine sodium benzoate
    b. ethylenediamine (aminophylline)
    c. theobromine (Theo-Dur)
    d. xanthaline
14. To reduce the severity of side effects from levodopa, the drug is usually administered in conjunction with
    a. carbidopa
    b. phenobarbital
    c. diazepam (Valium)
    d. monoamine oxidase inhibitors
15. Caffeine withdrawal is likely to be accompanied by
    a. lethargy
    b. headache
    c. convulsions
    d. hallucinations
16. When levodopa treatment is begun, the first doses are usually
    a. larger than subsequent maintenance doses to saturate storage depots
    b. smaller than maintenance doses to avoid toxic reactions
    c. carefully calculated to establish the required maintenance dose
    d. given parenterally until a therapeutic response has been achieved
17. Individuals receiving levodopa for the treatment of Parkinson's syndrome should be advised to
    a. maintain a stable level of vitamin K in the diet
    b. maintain a stable level of pyridoxine in the diet
    c. avoid foods containing xanthenes
    d. eat plenty of green leafy vegetables
18. If tremors increase after initiation of levodopa therapy, the nurse should
    a. contact the physician
    b. withhold the drug and notify the physician
    c. suggest that the physician order a muscle relaxant
    d. inform the client that this sometimes occurs when medication is begun, but that it usually is temporary
19. Risus sardonicus is a sign of toxicity from
    a. amphetamines
    b. strychnine
    c. diazepam
    d. heroin
20. Clients receiving analeptics such as pentylenetetrazol (Metrazol) should
    a. receive concomitant tranquilizer medications
    b. be placed on seizure precautions
    c. be monitored for hypertension
    d. be monitored for signs and symptoms of psychosis

Selection of options

For each of the following, select *all* appropriate responses. Circle the correct answers.

1. Clients recovering from amphetamine overdose are likely to experience
   a. prolongation of REM sleep
   b. fatigue and lethargy
   c. episodic hyperactivity
   d. emotional depression
2. Which of the following foods contain xanthine stimulants?
   a. coffee
   b. ginger ale
   c. chocolate candy
   d. licorice candy
   e. tea
   f. cola beverages
   g. wine
3. Adverse reactions to levodopa include
   a. epigastric distress
   b. change in bowel function
   c. excess salivation
   d. restlessness
   e. inappropriate sexuality

4. Levodopa should not be given to people who
   a. are receiving allopurinol
   b. have a narrow-angle glaucoma
   c. have had malignant melanoma
   d. have heart disease

5. When levodopa therapy is initiated, the client should be monitored carefully for
   a. abnormal cardiac rhythms
   b. change in respiratory function
   c. signs of renal and liver impairment
   d. gastrointestinal upset

Learning experiences

1. Interview a school nurse to determine the extent of therapeutic use of amphetamines in the local school population. What is the nurse's attitude toward such drug therapy? If possible, interview a parent of one of the children treated with amphetamines. Does the parent feel the child has benefited from the medication? How does the child's response to treatment compare with his or her behavior before the drug was administered?

2. Prepare a lesson plan for teaching an elementary school class (ages 8–9) about use and abuse of stimulant drugs. Develop audiovisual aids such as posters that would be appropriate for the class. How would you measure the students' learning? Carry out your teaching plan and evaluate the results.

3. In a farm or garden supply store, investigate the pesticides offered for sale to determine if any contain strychnine. If none are displayed, ask if any are available on request. Are any special precautions taken when these poisons are sold?

4. Interview a local law enforcement officer to determine whether cocaine abuse is a problem in the local community. If so, what is being done to control it?

5. Observe a diagnostic or surgical procedure requiring the use of topical anesthesia with cocaine. Assist with the client's care following the procedure.

18 ▪ *Central nervous system depressants*

Among the central nervous system depressants discussed in Chapter 18 are many agents used to control pain and promote rest and sleep, as well as drugs of abuse. The following exercises deal with this material.

Short answer questions

1. Identify at least three characteristics common to toxic reactions to most central nervous system depressants.

2. List at least six types of drugs likely to be used when general anesthesia is required for surgery (include preoperative and anesthetic agents).

3. Under what schedule of the Controlled Substance Act of 1970 does pentazocine (Talwin) fall?

4. Does propoxyphene (Darvon) cause physical dependence?

5. Name at least four nursing measures to:
   a. Promote sleep:

   b. Decrease pain:

6. In terminal illness characterized by pain, the client may be given considerable control over analgesic drug therapy. Name at least four advantages and one disadvantage of this approach.

7. List the types of drugs usually used in conscious sedation.

8. Identify at least one disadvantage of continuous parenteral infusion of analgesic drugs.

9. What is the oral dose of meperidine (Demerol) that is equipotent to 75 mg administered parenterally?

10. List at least four assessment parameters useful to the nurse who is considering the administration of a PRN analgesic.

Sequences

Number the following goals in sequence of the relative priorities that should be assigned in situations of terminal illness characterized by pain, according to the philosophy expressed in the text.

_______ Prevention of drug dependence

_______ Minimization of tolerance to drugs

_______ Relief of pain and promotion of comfort

_______ Avoidance of excessive sedation

Situational exercises

Write your answers to the following questions in the spaces provided.

Your client's pain has not been well controlled on a regimen of 60 mg of morphine PO q4h. Continuous intravenous infusion of morphine has been ordered.

1. What is the IM morphine dose equipotent to 60 mg PO?
2. What is the dosage of morphine administered by continuous IV infusion that is equipotent to 60 mg PO q4h?
3. Would you anticipate that the continuous IV dosage of morphine ordered for your client would be the same as your answer to 2 above, less than that dosage, or greater than that dosage?

Personal exercises

1. What are your personal biases concerning the use of dependence-producing analgesics for the relief of pain? What life experiences led to their development? What effect are these biases likely to have on your nursing judgment in situations involving medication for clients in pain? What do you do to minimize their influence? Write your answer on a separate sheet of paper.
2. Consider your own attitude toward the use of analgesic drugs and the nature of past experiences contributing to it. Identify your biases. How do you think these biases will influence your nursing care of clients subject to pain? What can you do to prevent inappropriate nursing judgments from arising in clinical practice?

Find the hidden word

Hidden within the following grid are words and phrases from Chapter 18. They may be vertical, horizontal, or diagonal. Circle the letters as you find the words.

List of words and phrases

alcohol
analgesic
anesthetic
apnea
barbiturate
coma
dissociative
ether
halothane
heroin
hypnotic
meperidine
miosis
morphine
naloxone
neurolept
nitrous oxide
opioid
propoxyphene
REM sleep
reticular activating system
sedative
twilight sleep

m	o	r	p	r	o	p	o	x	e	h	e	r	o	e	t	h	e	r	e	r	h	t	e	i	r	b
m	e	p	e	n	e	h	p	q	a	n	a	n	i	t	v	s	l	e	e	a	n	a	l	i	g	a
a	n	e	s	t	h	e	t	i	c	m	o	r	t	i	n	i	l	c	l	x	j	u	p	s	e	r
p	i	n	t	w	i	l	m	o	r	p	h	x	a	n	o	p	t	o	p	i	u	s	e	d	a	b
e	d	i	i	i	x	w	r	a	n	g	e	r	o	u	t	i	t	a	s	h	e	r	o	d	s	i
r	i	t	r	l	o	c	n	o	c	t	r	a	i	l	e	h	e	r	i	e	a	n	a	v	a	s
i	r	i	p	i	d	a	i	l	i	w	t	h	e	m	a	r	c	o	v	c	r	e	h	p	r	o
d	e	m	a	h	l	s	e	d	a	p	y	t	o	n	o	n	s	i	c	r	o	s	p	o	r	p
e	p	s	r	g	a	j	e	n	e	p	a	r	e	r	p	a	t	i	i	a	h	s	e	d	a	e
p	e	r	e	t	i	c	u	l	a	r	a	c	t	i	v	a	t	i	n	g	s	y	s	t	e	m
r	m	s	i	s	i	c	o	m	u	l	e	n	a	i	d	o	n	e	a	l	c	i	p	i	n	e
e	i	v	r	l	n	r	i	t	c	i	n	m	o	e	n	i	t	r	o	u	s	o	x	i	d	e
c	c	g	u	e	u	a	i	o	r	a	i	l	s	p	o	m	a	s	p	o	t	o	n	p	y	h
o	i	l	e	e	a	b	h	n	p	y	h	a	y	l	p	n	t	a	i	p	e	l	o	r	a	l
d	t	a	n	p	r	o	p	o	x	y	p	h	e	n	e	h	i	m	o	e	h	t	e	l	o	h
e	e	n	m	a	l	e	p	t	w	i	r	e	h	t	h	e	r	o	i	n	u	h	o	c	l	a
i	r	a	b	a	r	b	i	t	w	i	o	p	i	a	n	a	p	c	d	i	t	t	r	o	m	l
t	e	r	e	t	i	c	u	a	c	t	m	e	p	e	r	i	d	i	n	e	h	s	e	d	a	f

Correct the false statement

Indicate whether the following statements are true or false; if false, correct the underlined words or phrases.

_______ 1. Codeine exerts its effect on the central nervous system <u>only after it has been transformed by the tissues to morphine</u>.

_______ 2. <u>Most</u> of a given dose of morphine crosses the blood–brain barrier.

_______ 3. Heroin <u>cannot</u> legally be prescribed for medicinal use in the United States.

_______ 4. People with <u>hypothyroidism</u> are relatively insensitive to opioids.

_______ 5. Opioids are generally contraindicated in <u>severe head injury and obstructive airway disease</u>.

_______ 6. In most states, narcotic control regulations require that opioid analgesics be stored in <u>locked cabinets</u>.

_______ 7. The hypnotic drugs currently preferred for reasons of safety are the <u>barbiturates</u>.

_______ 8. Prolonged residual effects of hypnotics ("hangover") are probably caused by persistence of <u>the unchanged drug</u> in body fluids.

_______ 9. Engaging in <u>vigorous exercise</u> before bedtime will promote rest and sleep.

_______ 10. Clients who use hypnotic drugs in the home should be advised to store the medicines <u>in a bedside table</u>.

_______ 11. The class of drugs most often prescribed worldwide for medicinal use is <u>central nervous system stimulants</u>.

_______ 12. The class of drugs most often abused worldwide for psychotropic effect is central nervous system stimulants.

_______ 13. According to the text, drugs affecting the central nervous system should be considered to be dependence-producing until proven otherwise.

_______ 14. Clients are unlikely to develop psychologic dependence on drugs that do not produce physical dependence.

_______ 15. The dosages of analgesics administered parenterally are usually smaller than equipotent oral dosages.

_______ 16. Overt evidence of discomfort is a reliable index to level of pain perception.

_______ 17. The pain threshold is defined as the strength of stimulus required for beginning pain perception.

_______ 18. Inflammation is likely to raise the pain threshold.

_______ 19. In similar circumstances, individual perception of pain tends to be similar from person to person.

_______ 20. Pain is usually less severe during the hours closest to the usual hour of sleep than during the hours immediately after awakening.

_______ 21. PRN analgesics should not be given to clients who are pain-free.

Multiple choice questions

For each of the following, choose the one best answer:

1. To protect the operating room and recovery room staff from adverse reactions to drugs, it is most important to equip these suites with
   a. ventilating systems that remove volatile drugs from the air
   b. cleansing systems that will wash drug residues from the walls and floors
   c. laminar air flow that will prevent contamination by antibiotic-resistant microorganisms
   d. incinerators to destroy drug residues in vials and ampules
2. A nursing intervention that helps to reduce the risk of cardiac arrest when a general anesthetic is given is
   a. preoperative teaching and emotional support to reduce the client's apprehension
   b. ensuring that the preoperative anticholinergic medication is given on time
   c. checking the ECG tracing for evidence of cardiac irritability
3. When general anesthesia is administered, which sense remains functional the longest?
   a. touch
   b. taste
   c. smell
   d. hearing
   e. vision
4. General anesthetics are most likely to be administered by
   a. topical application
   b. inhalation
   c. injection
   d. retention enema
5. Dosages of potent analgesics used postoperatively must be reduced if anesthesia involved the use of
   a. succinylcholine
   b. Innovar
   c. diazepam (Valium)
   d. nitrous oxide
6. Because they can block synaptic and neuromuscular transmission, some local anesthetics are employed medicinally as
   a. sedatives
   b. tranquilizers
   c. antihypertensives
   d. antiarrhythmics
7. A serious adverse reaction to some local anesthetics is
   a. coma
   b. hyperventilation
   c. anaphylaxis
   d. gastrointestinal atony
8. A drug often combined with local anesthetics for injection into soft tissues is
   a. cocaine
   b. epinephrine (Adrenalin)
   c. phentolamine (Regitine)
   d. diazepam (Valium)
9. Local anesthetics are eliminated primarily through
   a. the lungs
   b. the kidneys
   c. the liver
   d. tissue metabolism to water and carbon dioxide

10. The order in which sensory function in a peripheral nerve is interrupted by local anesthetics is

1. warmth	a. 5, 3, 1, 2, 4
2. cold	b. 1, 2, 5, 3, 4
3. pain	c. 3, 4, 1, 2, 5
4. deep pressure	d. 3, 2, 1, 5, 4
5. touch	

11. An overdose of a central nervous system depressant is characterized by
    a. paradoxic excitation and overactivity
    b. coma, apnea, and cardiovascular collapse
    c. hypnosis with little or no REM sleep
    d. respiratory paralysis without loss of consciousness
12. Withdrawal of opioids from dependent persons is often accompanied by hallucinations that are
    a. visual
    b. auditory
    c. olfactory
    d. tactile
13. Withdrawal of barbiturates from a dependent client poses a significant risk of
    a. convulsions
    b. coma
    c. severe fluid and electrolyte imbalance
    d. respiratory arrest
14. Nightmares and hallucinations sometimes occur on emergence from anesthesia induced by
    a. ether
    b. diazepam
    c. innovar
    d. ketamine
15. When administering nursing care during the night shift, care should be exercised to avoid awakening clients during
    a. the early hours of sleep
    b. the late hours of sleep
    c. the basic rest-activity cycles
    d. REM sleep
16. Which of the following beverages is most likely to promote sleep?
    a. hot coffee
    b. a carbonated cola drink
    c. warm cocoa
    d. warm milk
17. An absolute contraindication for the use of barbiturates and chloral hydrate is
    a. a history of allergy to hypnotics
    b. a history of cocaine use
    c. xanthine toxicity
    d. acute intermittent porphyria
18. Elimination of barbiturates from the body may be enhanced by
    a. increasing the pH of the urine
    b. decreasing the pH of the urine
    c. administering bile salts
    d. administering caffeine
19. "Daymares" (waking, daytime "nightmares") have occurred following administration of
    a. barbiturates
    b. benzodiazepines
    c. chloral hydrate
    d. paraldehyde
20. Dreaming is most likely to occur during
    a. basic rest-activity cycles (BRAC)
    b. REM sleep
    c. deep sleep
    d. the first hour or two of sleep
21. Diazepam is stored in the body
    a. in fatty tissue
    b. in the central nervous system
    c. by plasma protein binding
    d. none of the above; it is not stored in the body to a significant degree
22. What is the most likely effect when naloxone is administered to a person who is feeling "high" after an active exercise session?
    a. Few, if any, effects will be discernible.
    b. The "high" is likely to be decreased or abolished.
    c. The "high"is likely to be enhanced.
    d. Signs and symptoms of opioid withdrawal will develop.
23. A frequent side effect of opioid analgesics is
    a. hyperphagia
    b. rhinorrhea
    c. constipation
    d. photophobia
24. Naloxone is usually administered
    a. orally
    b. by inhalation
    c. by injection
25. According to the text, the risk of dependence on narcotic analgesics is least likely when
    a. escalation of dose is delayed as long as possible
    b. the client is taught to adapt to the pain with minimal medication
    c. adequate medication is administered to control pain

26. Gradual weaning from narcotic analgesics ameliorates but does not abolish signs and symptoms of withdrawal. The amount of time required for elimination of physical dependence is usually a few
 a. hours
 b. days
 c. weeks
 d. months
27. Signs and symptoms of allergy to opioids are usually manifested by
 a. bronchospasm
 b. rhinorrhea
 c. headache
 d. skin rash
28. Treatment of opioid overdose is most likely to require
 a. administration of norepinephrine to maintain blood pressure
 b. hemodialysis to lower blood concentrations of the drug
 c. mechanical ventilation to maintain respiration
 d. cardiopulmonary resuscitation to maintain tissue perfusion
29. Before administering an opioid analgesic, the nurse should assess
 a. the pulse rate
 b. the blood pressure
 c. respirations
 d. the client's level of dependence
30. Presence of residual opioids in a person with acquired tolerance to these drugs can be assessed most reliably by monitoring
 a. respirations
 b. blood pressure
 c. level of consciousness
 d. pupillary constriction
31. The drug(s) of choice for treating opioid overdose is (are)
 a. amphetamine
 b. xanthines
 c. pentylenetetrazol (Metrazol)
 d. naloxone (Narcan)
32. Opioid analgesics act by
 a. entering the nuclei of nerve cells and changing the action of messenger RNA
 b. occupying receptors on the membrane of nerve cells and influencing cytoplasmic enzymes
 c. altering the structure of nerve cell membranes and inhibiting impulse transmission
 d. blocking transmission of neurotransmitters across synapses
33. To be equipotent to parenteral doses, oral doses of opioid analgesics must usually be
 a. larger than parenteral doses
 b. smaller than parenteral doses
 c. equal to parenteral doses
 d. individually titrated
34. Abrupt withdrawal of drugs from dependent persons is likely to precipitate acute physiologic problems. The risk of death is greatest when the drug involved is
 a. an opioid
 b. alcohol
 c. a barbiturate
 d. cocaine
35. Legally, narcotics are defined as
 a. derivatives of opium
 b. strong analgesics likely to cause dependence
 c. drugs designated as narcotics by federal legislation
 d. class I drugs as defined by the Controlled Substance Act of 1970
36. Clients who use hypnotics over a long time should be monitored for
 a. hypotension
 b. respiratory acidosis
 c. lethargy
 d. personality change
37. The drugs most often ordered for treatment of severe acute pain are
 a. anti-inflammatories
 b. opioid analgesics
 c. tranquilizer sedatives
 d. hypnotics
38. According to the text, the primary goal of nursing care for clients experiencing pain should be to
 a. alleviate severe pain
 b. ensure that physical dependence on drugs does not develop
 c. prevent or relieve disabling pain and discomfort
 d. administer a minimum of pain-relieving drugs
39. To be most effective, a tentative plan for administering PRN pain medication should be projected over a period of at least
 a. the interval required between doses (e.g., 3–4 hours)
 b. an 8-hour shift
 c. a 24-hour day
 d. none of the above; the time for PRN medication cannot be anticipated

40. When is pain perception likely to be greatest?
   a. in the early morning hours after awakening
   b. in the late afternoon and evening
   c. when the client is subject to various stimuli, whether pleasant or unpleasant
   d. none of the above; pain perception tends to be constant
41. Following common surgical procedures such as appendectomy, the use of opioid analgesics is usually limited to a period of about
   a. 24 hours
   b. 3–5 days
   c. 1 week to 10 days
   d. 2 weeks
42. Clients receiving continuous intravenous infusion of opioid analgesics should be monitored closely for
   a. hypotension
   b. tachycardia
   c. bradypnea
   d. pupillary constriction
43. When severe respiratory depression occurs in clients receiving long-term opioid analgesic treatment for persistent severe pain, what is the most likely treatment approach?
   a. use of mechanical ventilation to maintain vital functions until excretion of the opioids has decreased blood concentrations below the toxic level
   b. administration of small doses of naloxone until respirations rise to 12 or more per minute
   c. administration of small amounts of naloxone until respirations reach 12 or more per minute and the client has regained consciousness
   d. administration of sufficient naloxone to counteract the opioid effects

19 ▪ *Drugs that control seizures*

Seizures are uncontrollable physiologic responses to abnormal electrical discharges in the central nervous system. Responses are usually sporadic and self-limiting. Drug treatment is directed at preventing normal nerve activity.

Correct the false statement

Indicate whether the following statements are true or false; if false, correct the underlined words or phrases.

_______ 1. If the aura preceding a seizure involves a visual hallucination, the focus at which the central nervous system impulses originate is likely to located in the temporal lobe of the brain.

_______ 2. Full development of a seizure may be prevented if the affected person exerts voluntary control.

_______ 3. A diagnosis of seizure disorder can be made only when symptomatic episodes involve loss of consciousness.

_______ 4. The temporal lobe is usually the area of origin of impulse waves in psychomotor seizures.

_______ 5. Most drugs used as anticonvulsants act as synaptic transmitters.

_______ 6. In some people, the use of phenytoin will increase the severity of diabetes mellitus.

_______ 7. Phenytoin is believed to be carcinogenic.

_______ 8. Phenobarbital and ethosuximide are frequently used in combination for the control of major motor seizures.

_______ 9. Phenobarbital is the drug of choice for initial treatment of petit mal seizures.

_______ 10. The initial treatment of status epilepticus usually involves the injection of diazepam.

_______ 11. The use of alcohol in moderation tends to improve the control of seizure disorders.

_______ 12. Phenobarbital can interact with other weak bases by competing with them for binding to plasma albumin.

_______ 13. The onset of action of phenobarbital is relatively rapid, with peak concentrations in the brain occurring 1–2 hours after oral doses.

_______ 14. Abrupt withdrawal of anticonvulsant drugs is likely to be followed by active seizures.

_______ 15. Valproic acid does not significantly bind to plasma proteins.

_______ 16. Carbamazepine is relatively less toxic than are other anticonvulsants.

_______ 17. When administered with meals, anticonvulsant drugs are less likely to cause gastrointestinal upset.

_______ 18. A diagnosis of seizure disorder does not carry a stigma similar to that of the old term "epilepsy."

_______ 19. Gabapentin promotes the release of GAPA.

_______ 20. The half-life of lamotrigine is increased when used with phenobarbital or phenytoin.

Short answer questions

1. Define *epilepsy.*

2. Define *seizure threshold.*

3. Name three factors affecting the occurrence of seizures.

4. List at least seven hygienic measures that can decrease the risk of seizures.

5. Identify at least two techniques used to minimize undesirable changes in appearance caused by hirsutism.

Matching

Match the drug in the left-hand column with all of its adverse reactions in the right-hand column. Place your answers in the space provided.

_______ 1. Phenytoin
_______ 2. Phenobarbital
_______ 3. Trimethadione
_______ 4. Ethosuximide
_______ 5. Valproic acid
_______ 6. Clonazepam
_______ 7. Gabapentin
_______ 8. Lamotrigine

a. Anemia
b. Nystagmus
c. Gastrointestinal upset
d. Hiccups
e. Lethargy and drowsiness
f. Cardiac arrhythmias
g. Liver abnormalities
h. Ataxia
i. Increased risk of fetal damage
j. Personality change
k. Muscle or joint pain
l. Psychologic depression
m. REM sleep deprivation
n. Visual disturbances
o. Gingival hypertrophy
p. Hirsutism
q. Alopecia
r. Blood dyscrasia
s. Irritability

Multiple choice questions

For each of the following, choose the one best answer:

1. A type of epilepsy for which phenytoin is *not* recommended is
   a. grand mal seizures
   b. jacksonian seizures
   c. psychomotor seizures
   d. petit mal seizures
2. Therapeutic blood concentrations of phenytoin range from
   a. 1 to 2 µg/ml
   b. 5 to 10 µg/ml
   c. 10 to 20 µg/ml
   d. 30 to 50 µg/ml
3. A drug frequently used in conjunction with phenytoin in the treatment of seizures is
   a. ethosuximide
   b. phenobarbital
   c. trimethadione
   d. valproic acid
4. When used to treat seizures, phenytoin is usually administered
   a. 4 or 5 times a day
   b. one to three times a day
   c. every 1 to 2 days

5. Intravenous solutions of phenytoin should be administered no faster than
   a. 5 g/min
   b. 500 mg/min
   c. 50 mg/min
   d. 5 mg/min
6. With which of the following solutions is phenytoin compatible?
   a. normal saline solution
   b. dextrose in water
   c. acidic solutions
   d. none of the above
7. The usual dosage of phenytoin for the maintenance of control of seizures in adults is
   a. 100 μg twice a day
   b. 100 mg two or three times a day
   c. 1 g daily, divided into two or three doses
   d. 600 mg, administered in one dose daily
8. Early signs of phenytoin toxicity include
   a. sluggishness or stupor
   b. circulatory shock
   c. nausea and vomiting
   d. nystagmus and diplopia
9. Toxic doses of phenytoin may cause
   a. lethargy and stupor
   b. spontaneous abortion in pregnant women
   c. osteomalacia
   d. central nervous system excitation
10. Toxic effects of phenytoin appear in most people when the blood concentration reaches
    a. 25 μg/ml
    b. 50 μg/ml
    c. 100 μg/ml
    d. 200 μg/ml
11. To prevent and minimize gingival hyperplasia secondary to anticonvulsant medication, the nurse should
    a. advise that the drug be taken with meals to prolong absorption time
    b. teach meticulous oral hygiene and gum massage
    c. refer the client to the physician for adjustment of the drug dosage
    d. refer the client to a dentist for special treatments
12. Therapeutic plasma concentrations of phenobarbital range from
    a. 1 to 2 μg/ml
    b. 5 to 10 μg/ml
    c. 10 to 25 μg/ml
    d. 40 to 50 μg/ml
13. Phenobarbital is contraindicated for clients with
    a. porphyria
    b. phenylketonuria
    c. glaucoma
    d. benign prostatic hypertrophy
14. Clients receiving phenobarbital for control of seizures should be advised to discontinue the drug and contact the physician immediately if
    a. lethargy develops
    b. insomnia occurs
    c. dreaming increases markedly
    d. skin rash appears
15. Therapeutic serum concentrations of dimethadione range from
    a. 1 to 2 μg/ml
    b. 10 to 25 μg/ml
    c. 50 to 100 μg/ml
    d. 700 to 800 μg/ml
16. Initial doses of dimethadione are usually
    a. carefully calculated for long-term maintenance effect
    b. relatively low, with succeeding doses increasing gradually
    c. relatively high, with succeeding doses decreasing in accordance with evidence of toxicity
17. Trimethadione (Tridione) is usually employed to treat
    a. absence seizures
    b. grand mal seizures
    c. psychomotor seizures
    d. jacksonian seizures
18. Toxic reactions commonly occur when the serum concentration of carbamazepine reaches or exceeds
    a. 2 μg/ml
    b. 5 μg/ml
    c. 10 μg/ml
    d. 50 μg/ml
19. When magnesium sulfate is administered as an anticonvulsant, it is usually given
    a. orally
    b. rectally, as an enema
    c. intravenously
    d. intrathecally
20. Magnesium sulfate is used most often as an anticonvulsant in the treatment of
    a. major motor seizures of grand mal epilepsy
    b. major motor seizures associated with toxemia of pregnancy
    c. absence seizures (petit mal)
    d. none of the above

21. Should women receiving anticonvulsants attempt to breastfeed their children?
   a. Yes, anticonvulsant drugs are not distributed in milk.
   b. Sometimes, although a few anticonvulsant drugs are distributed in milk in high concentrations.
   c. Usually not, because many anticonvulsant drugs are distributed in milk in high concentrations.
   d. No, the drugs will be distributed in milk in high concentrations.
22. During the treatment of status epilepticus, anticonvulsant drugs are most likely to be administered
   a. by mouth
   b. intramuscularly
   c. intravenously
   d. by inhalation
23. The agent of choice for petit mal seizures is
   a. phenytoin
   b. phenobarbital
   c. ethosuximide
   d. diazepam
24. Which of the following anticonvulsants is employed for the treatment of status epilepticus rather than for maintenance therapy?
   a. trimethadione
   b. valproic acid
   c. clonazepam
   d. diazepam
25. A class of anticonvulsants that are used to treat petit mal but not grand mal seizures is
   a. the barbiturates
   b. the hydantoins
   c. valproic acid
   d. the oxazolidinediones
26. Of the following anticonvulsant drugs, which is the most selective?
   a. phenobarbital
   b. phenytoin
   c. valproic acid
   d. trimethadione
27. An anticonvulsant that acts osmotically to decrease edema in the brain is
   a. phenytoin
   b. phenobarbital
   c. magnesium sulfate
   d. ethosuximide
28. The anticonvulsant drug that is used medicinally as a cardiac antiarrhythmic is
   a. phenobarbital
   b. phenytoin
   c. ethosuximide
   d. diazepam
29. The drug most likely to be prescribed to prevent recurrent seizures in children who have experienced febrile seizures is
   a. phenobarbital
   b. phenytoin
   c. ethosuximide
   d. diazepam
30. When counseling a young woman with a seizure disorder, who desires to start a family, you would inform her that
   a. once pregnancy has begun, the anticonvulsant drug will be withdrawn to avoid adverse effects on the fetus
   b. the dosage of drugs should be reduced to a minimum by the physician before conception is attempted
   c. seizures during pregnancy do not appreciably increase the risk of damage to or death of the fetus.
   d. it is inadvisable to attempt to conceive until anticonvulsant drugs have been withdrawn completely
31. In the United States, many states have adopted laws that restrict certain activities for persons prone to seizure disorders. At present, the restriction imposed most often affects
   a. the right of the person to marry
   b. the right of the person to have children
   c. entry into certain occupations
   d. the privilege of driving a motor vehicle
32. A person with obvious gingival hypertrophy is likely to be receiving as a medication
   a. phenytoin
   b. phenobarbital
   c. ethosuximide
   d. valproic acid
33. Is lifelong anticonvulsant therapy required for all clients with seizure disorders?
   a. yes; the seizure disorder recurs if medication is withdrawn
   b. by most clients, but not always by clients with childhood or posttraumatic epilepsy
   c. by most clients, but not always by clients with jacksonian seizures
   d. no, weaning from the drugs may be attempted for most clients after a seizure-free period of 2–4 years
34. Which of the following anticonvulsants is considered to be safe to administer during pregnancy?
   a. phenobarbital
   b. phenytoin
   c. trimethadione
   d. ethosuximide
   e. none of the above; all are reported to be teratogenic

Selection of options

For each of the following, select *all* appropriate responses. Circle the correct answers.

1. Among the physiologic effects of phenytoin are
   a. decreased movement of calcium ions across cell membranes
   b. decreased movement of sodium ions across cell membranes
   c. decreased movement of potassium ions across cell membranes
   d. increased movement of magnesium ions across cell membranes
   e. increased stability of cell membranes
2. What routes of administration are recommended for phenytoin?
   a. PO
   b. SC
   c. IM
   d. IV
3. Advantages of using phenobarbital in controlling seizures include
   a. economy
   b. minimal sedative effect, as compared with other anticonvulsants
   c. relatively few adverse reactions, as compared with other anticonvulsants
   d. relatively high effectiveness in many types of seizure disorders
4. Contraindications for phenobarbital include
   a. allergy to barbiturates
   b. bronchopneumonia
   c. central nervous system excitation
   d. porphyria
   e. acute depression
5. Generally, trimethadione is contraindicated for
   a. people with disease of the retina or of the optic nerve
   b. people with porphyria
   c. pregnant women
6. Clients receiving valproic acid for the treatment of seizures should be cautioned
   a. to avoid chewing the capsules before swallowing
   b. to buy the same name brand consistently
   c. to avoid alcohol intoxication
   d. not to discontinue the drug abruptly
7. Anticonvulsant drugs that do not bind significantly to plasma proteins include
   a. phenobarbital
   b. phenytoin
   c. trimethadione
   d. ethosuximide
8. Certain anticonvulsants are sometimes used in the treatment of
   a. cardiac arrhythmias
   b. neuralgia
   c. myasthenia gravis
   d. psychosis
   e. minimal brain dysfunction
9. Abrupt discontinuation of an anticonvulsant drug is likely to increase the risk of
   a. lethargy and stupor
   b. status epilepticus
   c. toxicity from the drug prescribed as a replacement

Enrichment experiences

1. Prepare a plan for teaching a client newly diagnosed as having a seizure disorder about self-care practices designed to minimize seizure activity. What recommendations will be included relative to the medication regimen?

2. Interview an adult client on prolonged anticonvulsant therapy. Ascertain the type of seizures experienced by the client, the medication regimen prescribed, and the client's response to medication. How does the client regard the disease and its treatment? Are there any adverse reactions to the medication? What does the client do about these responses?

20 ▪ Drugs that affect emotional and psychological functions

The development of psychoactive drugs and advances in psychopharmacology have radically changed treatment options for individuals with psychiatric and emotional disturbances. For individuals unresponsive to less invasive treatment interventions, psychoactive drugs may provide an alternative strategy to provide relief from debilitating symptoms including depression, psychosis, anxiety, and mood swings.

Multiple choice questions

For each of the following, choose the one best answer:

1. The goal of psychopharmacology is to
   a. provide symptomatic relief, ideally contributing to increased functional status and quality of life
   b. provide a cure to underlying causes of psychopathology
   c. reduce sensory stimulation
   d. replace psychosocial interventions
2. In general, psychoactive drugs exert their effect by influencing one or several of the following chemicals except for
   a. dopamine
   b. norepinephrine
   c. serotonin
   d. Urecholine
   e. GABA
3. The antipsychotic agents are primarily used to
   a. provide symptomatic relief of anxiety
   b. alleviate extrapyramidal symptoms (EPS)
   c. provide symptomatic relief of aggressive behavior
   d. provide symptomatic relief of paranoid thinking, disorganized speech, delusions, and hallucinations
4. The phenothiazines include the following compounds:
   a. aliphatic, piperazine, piperidine
   b. thioxanthenes, butyrophenones, diphenylbutylpiperidines
   c. tricyclics, tetracyclics, monoamine oxidase inhibitors (MAOI)
   d. clozapine, risperiodone, molindone
5. Chlorpromazine and fluphenazine are drugs in which class?
   a. thioxanthenes
   b. phenothiazine
   c. benzodiazepines
   d. butyrophenones
6. EPS are more likely to occur with drugs that have an increased capability to block
   a. D_2 receptors
   b. M_1 receptors
   c. α_1 receptors
   d. D_4 receptors
   e. α_2 receptors
7. Atypical antipsychotic agents differ from traditional antipsychotic agents in all of the following aspects, except for
   a. atypical agents decreased negative symptoms only
   b. atypical agents exhibit decreased EPS
   c. atypical agents result in improvement that is markedly different from that observed following traditional antipsychotic therapy
   d. atypical agents have a decreased risk for tardive dyskinesia (TD)
8. Anticholinergic effects include all of the following except
   a. constipation
   b. blurred vision
   c. nausea
   d. urinary retention
   e. dry mucous membranes

9. Pigmentary retinopathy, which can lead to blindness, is a possible adverse effect of
   a. thioridazine
   b. benztropine
   c. alprazolam
   d. sertraline
10. Clozapine therapy requires weekly monitoring of
   a. body weight
   b. white blood cell (WBC) count
   c. serum drug level
   d. body temperature
11. The most widely used prescribed drugs for anxiety are the
   a. phenothiazines
   b. benzodiazepines
   c. MAOIs
   d. tricyclics
12. Precautions for benzodiazepine use include all of the following except
   a. they have potential tolerance effects
   b. they have potential dependency effects
   c. they require gradual withdrawal
   d. the elderly are likely to be less sensitive to side effects
13. Selective serotonin re-uptake inhibitors (SSRIs) are, in many instances, the first choice for pharmacologic treatment of depression because of their
   a. ability to block serotonin re-uptake
   b. more desirable side effect profile
   c. lack of GABA activity
   d. ability to be well absorbed following oral administration
14. Because of the risk for serotonin syndrome, how many weeks should elapse following discontinuation of fluoxetine and starting an MAOI?
   a. two
   b. five
   c. eight
   d. none
15. Therapeutic blood levels of tricyclic agents are identified for all of the following except
   a. desipramine
   b. imipramine
   c. nortriptyline
   d. protriptyline
16. Which of the following statements is incorrect with regard to buproprion?
   a. Buproprion is associated with risk of seizures.
   b. Buproprion has little adverse effects on sexual functioning.
   c. Buproprion is contraindicated in bulimia nervosa.
   d. Buproprion is used to primarily treat psychosis.
17. Foods that interact with the MAOIs to induce a hypertensive crisis contain
   a. sodium
   b. potassium
   c. lithium salt
   d. tyramine
18. MAOIs include which of the following?
   a. phenelzine, tranylcypromine
   b. doxepin, desipramine
   c. ludiomil, remeron
   d. fluvoxamine paroxetine
19. The drug of choice for manic-depressive illness is
   a. lithium carbonate
   b. imipramine
   c. fluphenazine
   d. fluvoxamine
20. The serum lithium concentration range considered to be therapeutic is
   a. 0.5–1.0 mmol/liter
   b. 1.0–3.0 mmol/liter
   c. 1.0–1.2 mmol/liter
   d. 0.8–2.0 mmol/liter
21. Early symptoms of lithium toxicity include
   a. weight loss, arrhythmias
   b. blurred vision, slurred speech, tinnitus
   c. incoordination, muscle weakness, confusion, nausea
   d. polyuria, increased thirst
22. Lithium has an inverse relationship with
   a. sodium
   b. potassium
   c. H_2O
   d. tyramine
23. EPS are most commonly caused by
   a. antipsychotic agents
   b. anxiolytic agents
   c. antidepressant agents
   d. mood stabilizers

Matching

A. Match the terms in the left-hand column with the definitions in the right-hand column. Place your answer in the space provided.

_______ 1. Parkinsonism
_______ 2. Akathisia
_______ 3. Acute dystonic reaction
_______ 4. Tardive dyskinesia
_______ 5. Serotonin syndrome
_______ 6. Hypertensive crisis

a. Uncontrolled restlessness
b. Facial grimacing, stereotyped lipsmacking, protrusion of tongue, choreiform motions
c. Involuntary muscle contractions, oculogyric crisis
d. Muscle rigidity, cog-wheeling
e. Rigidity, agitation, hypertension, hyperthermia, fever, myoclonus
f. Stiff neck, diaphoresis, nausea, vomiting, headache, hypertension

B. Match the generic names of the following antipsychotic agents in the left-hand column with the trade names in the right-hand column.

_______ 1. Chlorpromazine
_______ 2. Fluphenazine
_______ 3. Perphenazine
_______ 4. Haloperidol
_______ 5. Clozapine

a. Prolixin
b. Clozaril
c. Thorazine
d. Trilafon
e. Haldol

C. Match the generic names of the following anxiolytic agents in the left-hand column with the trade names in the right-hand column.

_______ 1. Lorazepam
_______ 2. Alprazolam
_______ 3. Diazepam
_______ 4. Clonazepam
_______ 5. Buspirone

a. Buspar
b. Ativan
c. Xanax
d. Valium
e. Klonopin

D. Match the generic names of the following antidepressant agents in the left-hand column with the trade names in the right-hand column.

_______ 1. Fluoxetine
_______ 2. Amitriptyline
_______ 3. Nefazodone
_______ 4. Nortriptyline
_______ 5. Imipramine

a. Pamelor
b. Serzone
c. Prozac
d. Tofranil
e. Elavil

E. Match the side effect in the left-hand column most commonly associated with the blockade of the receptor in the right-hand column.

_______ 1. Postural hypotension
_______ 2. Constipation
_______ 3. Dry mouth
_______ 4. Weight gain
_______ 5. Sexual disturbance
_______ 6. Urinary retention
_______ 7. Blurred vision
_______ 8. Sedation

a. Histaminergic
b. Dopaminergic
c. Cholinergic
d. Adrenergic
e. Both a and d
f. Both b and d

Correct the false statement

Indicate whether the following statements are true or false; if false, correct the underlined words or phrases and place your answer in the space provided.

_______ 1. High potency antipsychotics are associated with <u>EPS</u>.

_______ 2. Traditional antipsychotic agents are <u>dopamine antagonists</u>.

_______ 3. Antipsychotic agents <u>accumulate</u> in body tissues when administered over time.

_______ 4. Diuretics <u>should not be taken</u> concurrently with lithium.

_______ 5. Foods, antacids, cigarette smoking, and possibly coffee can <u>decrease</u> the absorption of oral antipsychotic agents.

_______ 6. Antipsychotic agents are <u>not</u> bound to protein.

_______ 7. Males and younger age individuals are <u>at greater risk</u> for developing an acute dystonic reaction.

_______ 8. Gynecomastia can result during antipsychotic therapy because of drug action that decreases dopamine's ability <u>to inhibit prolactin release from the pituitary</u>.

_______ 9. Thioridazine dosage should not exceed <u>300 mg</u> per day.

_______ 10. Clients with depression <u>are at risk</u> for using their medications in an overdose-suicide attempt.

_______ 11. Psychoactive drugs <u>decrease</u> the seizure threshold.

_______ 12. Medications break down into metabolites that may be <u>even more</u> pharmacologically active than the parent drug.

_______ 13. Concomitant use of MAOIs and other seratonergic agents is generally <u>contraindicated</u>.

_______ 14. Ebstein's anomaly is associated with lithium use during the <u>first</u> trimester of pregnancy.

_______ 15. Nonsteroidal anti-inflammatory agents, including ibuprofen, interfere with lithium clearance thereby <u>increasing</u> the risk of lithium toxicity.

Short answer questions

1. Name at least six foods and beverages that contain tyramine and that interact with MAOIs.

2. Describe the necessary dietary considerations and reason of importance for clients on:
   a. Lithium

   b. MAOIs

3. Explain the concept of drug displacement and how this impacts on the use of psychoactive drugs.

4. In general, what problems are posed by the concomitant use of alcohol and psychoactive drugs?

5. Describe three situations in which consideration of the drug half-life is important.

UNIT SEVEN

Drugs affecting the cardiovascular and renal systems

21 ▪ *Drugs that manage heart failure*

Cessation of circulation for even a few minutes causes immediate and widespread cell death. Therefore, as the moving force behind circulation, the heart is absolutely vital to life. Many chemical substances affect cardiac function.

Correct the false statement

Indicate whether the following statements are true or false; if false, correct the underlined words or phrases and place your answer in the space provided.

_______ 1. Maintenance doses of digoxin are likely to be <u>considerably smaller</u> than are maintenance doses of other cardiac glycosides.

_______ 2. Digitalizing dosages of cardiac glycosides are likely to be <u>considerably larger</u> than are maintenance dosages.

_______ 3. Digitalis preparations produce diuresis by <u>stimulating tubular secretions of electrolytes in the kidneys.</u>

_______ 4. The digitalis drug <u>digoxin</u> is extensively metabolized by the liver.

_______ 5. Hemodialysis <u>will</u> remove cardiac glycosides from the blood.

_______ 6. Cardiac glycosides are the drugs of choice for the treatment of <u>myocardial infarction.</u>

_______ 7. The actions of cardiac glycosides are <u>curative</u> in nature.

_______ 8. Serum concentration of digoxin is <u>an absolute</u> indicator of toxicity.

_______ 9. When a client exhibits signs and symptoms of digitalis toxicity, the nurse <u>may withhold one or more doses of digitalis.</u>

Crossword puzzle

Across

1. A cardiac condition treated with digitalis
4. A marine source of digitalis
6. A frequently prescribed digitalis drug
7. See 3 down
8. A drink rich in potassium
9. Effect of digitalis on cardiac contractility
12. An electrolyte that accentuates effects of digitalis
13. A cardiotonic drug eliminated by the liver
14. Chemical nature of digitalis
15. A food rich in potassium
17. Effect of digitalis on urinary output
19. Effect of digitalis on cardiac conductivity
21. The process of building up serum levels of digitalis
22. A cardiac arrhythmia treated with digitalis

Down

2. A record of cardiac function
3. A symptom of digitalis toxicity
5. Effect of digitalis on cardiac rate
6. Drugs that can increase toxic effect of digitalis
9. A nutrient antagonistic to digitalis
10. Plant source of digitalis
11. A psychosomatic reaction that contributes to digitalis toxicity
16. An index to digitalis toxicity
18. See 16 down
20. See 15 across

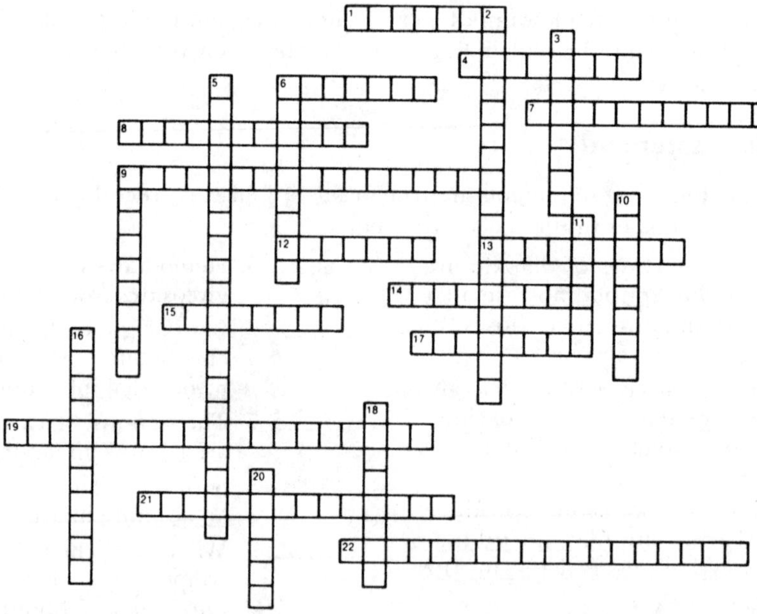

Matching

A. Match each chemical effect on the heart in the left-hand column with the property of the heart that is affected in the right-hand column. Place your answer in the space provided.

________ 1. Inotropic
________ 2. Dromotropic
________ 3. Chronotropic

a. Conductivity
b. Automaticity
c. Strength of contraction
d. Rate of contraction

B. Match the portion of the ECG tracing affected in the left-hand column with the effect of digitalis in the right-hand column.

_______ 1. T wave
_______ 2. Heart rate
_______ 3. P - R interval
_______ 4. Q - T interval
_______ 5. QRS complex

a. Depression or inversion
b. Acceleration
c. Deceleration
d. Shortening
e. Prolongation
f. Narrowing

Selection of options

For each of the following, select *all* appropriate responses. Circle the correct answers.

1. The function of the heart is influenced by
   a. the cortex of the brain
   b. the autonomic nervous system
   c. endocrine hormones
   d. the vagus nerve
   e. electrolytes in body fluids
2. The effects of digitalis drugs on the heart include a
   a. positive inotropic effect
   b. positive chronotropic effect
   c. negative chronotropic effect
3. Why is drug treatment sometimes initiated by administration of high ("loading") doses?
   a. to achieve a prompt therapeutic effect
   b. to saturate body tissue depots
   c. to raise serum concentrations quickly
   d. to stimulate metabolism and excretion of the dug
4. Factors influencing severity of toxicity from digitalis include
   a. serum concentration of the drug
   b. serum concentration of sodium ions
   c. age of the recipient
   d. pathologic status of the heart
   e. ratio between serum concentration of calcium and potassium ions
   f. level of stress response in the client
5. A drug considered to be "cumulative" is likely to exhibit the following characteristics:
   a. extensive storage in the tissues
   b. long serum half-life
   c. narrow safety margin
6. Therapeutic uses for cardiac glycosides include treatment of
   A. heart failure
   b. atrial fibrillation
   c. acute myocardial infarction
   d. paroxysmal tachycardia
7. Before administering digitalis, the nurse should always
   A. count the pulse
   b. assess the client's appetite
   c. measure the blood pressure
8. Signs and symptoms of *nontoxic* digitalis side effects include
   a. local tissue irritation
   b. post-medication nausea
   c. heart block
   d. skin rash
   e. decrease in neutrophils
   f. increase in eosinophils
   g. breast enlargement in males
9. Contraindications for cardiac glycosides include
   a. heart block
   b. heart failure
   c. hypertrophic subaortic stenosis
   d. myocardial infarction with severe myocarditis
10. Among the factors that tend to increase the risk of digoxin toxicity are
    a. immobility
    b. nausea and vomiting
    c. stress
    d. diarrhea
    e. renal impairment
11. Dietary changes most likely to be recommended to clients receiving digitalis drugs include
    a. ample use of foods rich in fiber
    b. limitation of foods rich in potassium
    c. limitation of foods rich in sodium
    d. ample use of foods rich in calcium
    e. control of calories

12. In an adult client receiving digitalis, a pulse rate greater than 100/min may signify
    a. incomplete therapeutic response to the drug
    b. beginning drug toxicity
    c. severe drug toxicity

13. Among the signs and symptoms of digitalis toxicity are
    a. anorexia
    b. nausea
    c. vomiting
    d. constipation
    e. bradycardia
    f. tachycardia
    g. changes in color vision

22 ▪ *Drugs that regulate cardiac rhythm*

Correct the false statement

Indicate whether the following statements are true or false; if false, correct the underlined words or phrases and place your answer in the space provided.

_______ 1. Bretylium can cause transient hypertension when therapy is initiated.

_______ 2. The antiarrhythmic drug likely to cause a syndrome resembling systemic lupus erythematosus is propafenone.

_______ 3. Drugs that are used to treat cardiac arrhythmias may increase the risk of other cardiac arrhythmias.

_______ 4. A complication that may follow cardioversion is venous embolism.

_______ 5. Treatment of cardiac arrhythmias by depressant drugs tends to increase the risk of congestive heart failure.

_______ 6. Bretylium and amiodarone exert their antiarrhythmic action through calcium channel blockade.

_______ 7. Quinidine is a drug used for dysrhythmias, angina pectoris, and hypertension.

_______ 8. The AV node is the normal pacemaker of the heart.

_______ 9. The refractory period is the time during the cardiac cycle when the heart is unable to respond to a new stimulus.

_______ 10. Atrial fibrillation is a serious type of arrhythmia that can be caused by several antiarrhythmic drugs.

Crossword puzzle

Across

5. Successful treatment of atrial fibrillation
7. A cardiac antiarrhythmic drug often administered intravenously
11. A compensatory process that predisposes the heart to fibrillation
12. An abnormally rapid cardiac rate
14. Extreme rapid, inefficient contractions of the heart
15. A property of the heart that increases the risk of arrhythmias
16. Areas outside the conduction system that initiate stimuli
18. A mechanical means of stimulating the heart
19. An antiarrhythmic drug that exhibits Class II and Class III effects
20. A cardiovascular drug that may cause dysrhythmias
21. An activity that increases vagal nerve stimulation

Down

1. An antiarrhythmic drug whose use is confined to critical care settings
2. A characteristic of the pulse of atrial fibrillation
3. A stress hormone that increases heart rate
4. The drugs used to correct arrhythmias often are also this type of drug
6. The most lethal of cardiac arrhythmias
8. The property of cardiac tissue that underlies spontaneous generation of impulses
9. An arrhythmia that predisposes to arterial embolism
10. A state in which sinoatrial impulses do not reach the ventricles
13. An antiarrhythmic drug that can cause cinchonism
17. An antiarrhythmic drug metabolized by 4 pathways in the liver
23. An adverse reaction common to several antiarrhythmic drugs

Across

22. An antiarrhythmic drug also used as an anticonvulsant
24. A necrotic area of heart muscle
25. An antiarrhythmic drug that can cause a reaction resembling that of systemic lupus erythematosus
26. An antiarrhythmic drug that can cause urinary retention

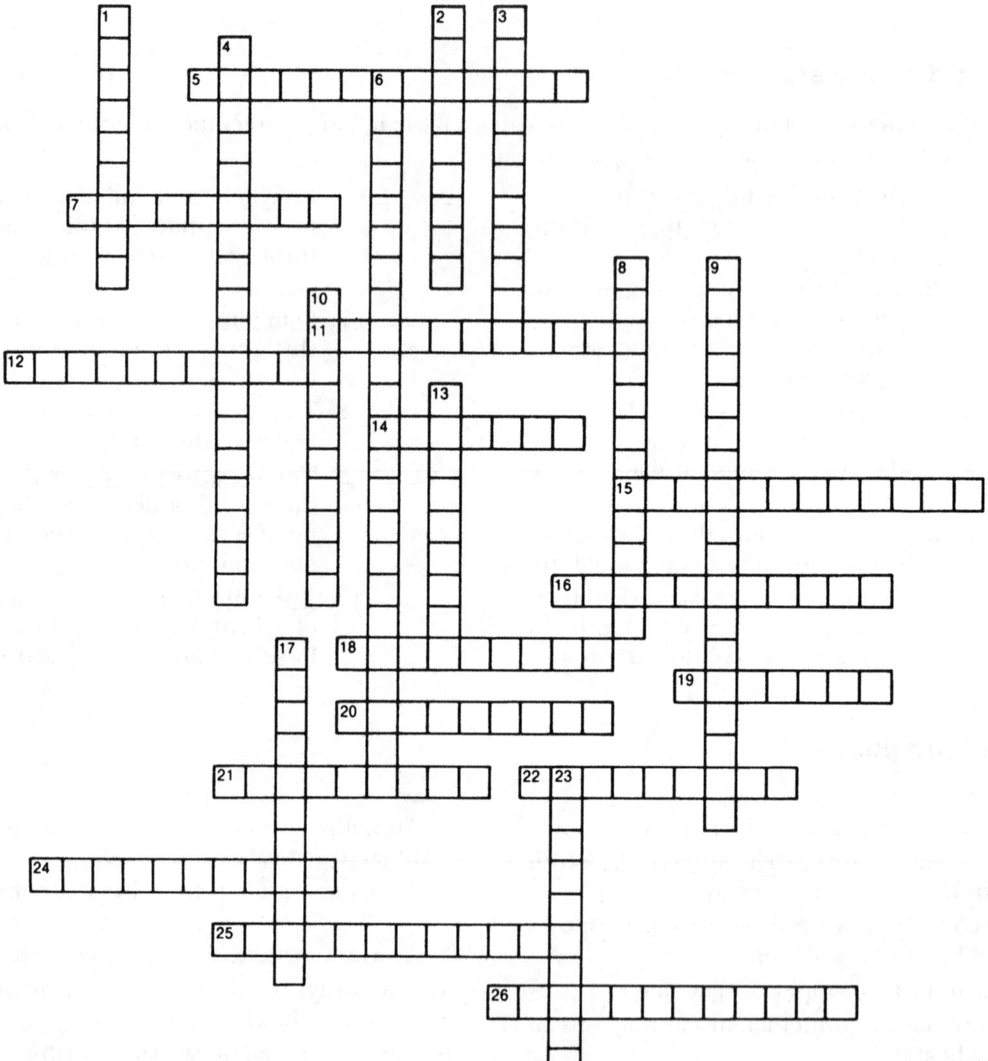

Selection of options

For each of the following, select *all* appropriate responses. Circle the correct answers.

1. Factors that increase the irritability of the myocardium include
   a. ischemia
   b. insomnia
   c. anxiety
   d. smoking
   e. sedative drugs

2. Adverse reactions to antiarrhythmic drugs include
   a. cardiac arrhythmias
   b. hypotension
   c. transient hypertension
   d. cardiac arrest
   e. mental changes

f. gastrointestinal upset
g. allergic manifestations

3. Drugs whose use is limited to acute care settings include
   a. bretylium
   b. propranolol
   c. phenytoin
   d. lidocaine
4. The families of clients receiving long-term antiarrhythmic therapy should be advised to
   a. be prepared to call emergency medical services
   b. become trained in emergency cardiopulmonary resuscitation
   c. learn to assess the blood pressure
   d. learn to assess pulses
5. Antiarrhythmic drugs that are used only in critical care settings with continuous ECG monitoring include
   a. procainamide
   b. lidocaine
   c. phenytoin
   d. bretylium
6. Antiarrhythmic drugs belonging to Class I include
   a. quinidine
   b. disopyramide
   c. propranolol
   d. bretylium

Learning experience

Read Part I of the critical thinking challenge in Chapter 22 in the textbook; then consider the following questions.

1. What would the usual bolus dose of lidocaine be for Mr. Smith? How soon after the initial bolus could you repeat the dose if needed? What would be the maximum dose you would expect to give in one hour? If a lidocaine blood level were to be measured, what would a therapeutic level be?
2. If you were to use a maintenance infusion, describe the steps you would take to prepare it and determine the rate of infusion.
3. Review lidocaine's mechanism of actions and explain how these mechanisms work to stop PVCs.
4. Why is lidocaine not administered orally?
5. Review the drugs that interact with lidocaine. If Mr. Smith's health history indicates that he was treated for an ulcer within the past year, what interactant drug would you specifically ask him about?

Refer to Part II of the critical thinking challenge in the textbook before considering the following:

6. How would you explain quinidine's mechanism of action to Mr. Smith?
7. Because he is to receive a sustained release form of the drug what should you tell Mr. Smith?
8. Because Mr. Smith is moving to Florida soon and there are three different forms of quinidine available, what advice would you give him?
9. What are the possible adverse drug effects of Mr. Smith's medication? If he should develop diarrhea, what strategies would you suggest to him? What laboratory data might his physician need to obtain if the diarrhea were severe and prolonged? What other adverse reactions should he report to his physician?
10. What drug-drug interactions are of concern with this medication? What should Mr. Smith do about the medication he has at home that he used for his ulcer early last year? What should he do if he thinks he is experiencing ulcer symptoms again?
11. What should any client on an antiarrhythmic be able to do on a frequent basis?

***Note:* You may wish to consult other medical-surgical and pharmacology sources in preparing your answers.**

23 ▪ Drugs that regulate lipid levels

Drugs may be used in addition to diet and exercise to combat atherosclerosis.

Correct the false statement

Indicate whether the following statements are true or false; if false, correct the underlined words or phrases and place your answer in the space provided.

_______ 1. HMG CoA reductase inhibitors commonly increase serum levels of glucose.

_______ 2. The most inexpensive HMG CoA reductase inhibitor is simvastatin.

_______ 3. Lovastatin is contraindicated during pregnancy because skeletal malformations have occurred in animals following its administration.

_______ 4. Anion exchange resins are absorbed from the gastrointestinal tract and act systematically.

_______ 5. Cholestyramine is used to treat pruritus associated with certain types of biliary disease.

_______ 6. Clients receiving bile acid-sequestering resins should be taught how to prevent constipation.

_______ 7. To prevent esophageal irritation and obstruction, bile acid-sequestering resins should be taken in the dry form.

_______ 8. Fat-soluble vitamins may be needed with long-term therapy with nicotinic acid.

_______ 9. Lovastatin is an example of a fibric acid derivative.

_______ 10. Nicotinic acid should be administered with meals.

_______ 11. An immediate reaction to large doses of nicotinic acid is epigastric pain.

_______ 12. Neomycin is sometimes used as an antilipemic agent.

_______ 13. The evidence that omega-3 fish oils can lower serum cholesterol and triglycerides includes well-controlled clinical trials.

_______ 14. Adverse reactions to gemfibrozil tend to be most severe when treatment is initiated and to subside with continued treatment.

Selection of options

For each of the following, select *all* appropriate responses. Circle the correct answers.

1. Among the hormones that tend to lower serum cholesterol and triglyceride concentrations are
   a. glucocorticoids
   b. estrogens
   c. testosterone
   d. thyroxine
   e. catecholamines
2. The effects of drugs used to regulate lipid levels include reduction of
   a. plasma triglyceride concentrations
   b. serum VLDL concentrations
   c. serum cholesterol concentrations
   d. serum LDL concentrations
3. Therapy with HMG CoA reductase inhibitors requires the following precautions to detect or prevent adverse reactions:
   a. regular complete blood counts
   b. regular liver function tests
   c. regular kidney function tests
   d. monitoring for neoplastic disease
   e. avoidance of pregnancy (for women)

4. Bile acid-sequestering resins include:
   a. cholestyramine
   b. colestipol
   c. lactulose
   d. kaolin
5. Adverse reactions to bile acid-sequestering resins include
   a. gastrointestinal upset
   b. hyperchloremic acidosis
   c. vitamin A toxicity
   d. vasodilation
   e. central nervous system disturbance
6. Which of the following drugs will be bound by anion exchange resins, with subsequent reduction in gastrointestinal absorption?
   a. digoxin
   b. anticoagulants
   c. vitamin C
   d. penicillin
   e. thiazide diuretics
7. Therapeutic actions for nicotinic acid (niacin) include a decrease in serum
   a. cholesterol concentration
   b. HDL concentration
   c. triglyceride concentration
8. Miscellaneous substances under investigation as antilipemic drugs include
   a. progestogens
   b. beta-sitosterol
   c. dextrothyroxine
   d. papaverine
   e. omega-3 fish oils
9. Vegetable fats that are highly saturated include
   a. coconut oil
   b. palm oil
   c. canola oil
   d. olive oil
   e. cocoa butter
10. Food substances that are more unsaturated include
   a. corn oil
   b. soybean oil
   c. peanut oil
   d. safflower oil

Short answer questions

1. How freely are drugs prescribed in the treatment of atherosclerosis?

2. Name at least three precautions necessary when bile acid-sequestering resins are administered.

24 ▪ *Drugs that affect circulation*

Drugs are an important component of therapy for ischemic heart disease and may be used for peripheral vascular disease of the arteries or veins.

Anagram

Unscramble the letters for the words below and enter them in the proper places in the scrabble grid, from top to bottom.

1. OSTNIYOHEPN
   MIBRHOT
   PONGLOI
   ROSSBIFI
   ERLTOSSIOREARCIS
   AFTICILANOCIC
   UPSRESER
   TROSEASHERLCOIS
   SCUTBORNITO
   AUPELQ
   MAVSAPOSS
   CERADSADE NETYCPA
   SOLS FO CLASTITYEI
   SOCHK
   RETONSIPHYEN

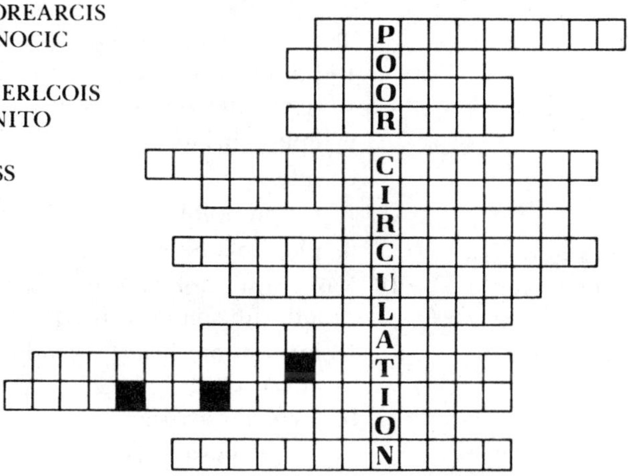

2. SESRTS
   VACNIYTIIT
   SEXECS SDLL
   GIMOSKN
   GIHH AFT TIDE
   BAITEDES
   HGHI DOBOL SOLTOHCEREL
   OSHYMPYROTDIHI
   OWL SHLD
   RENPIYHOSETN
   STYBEOI

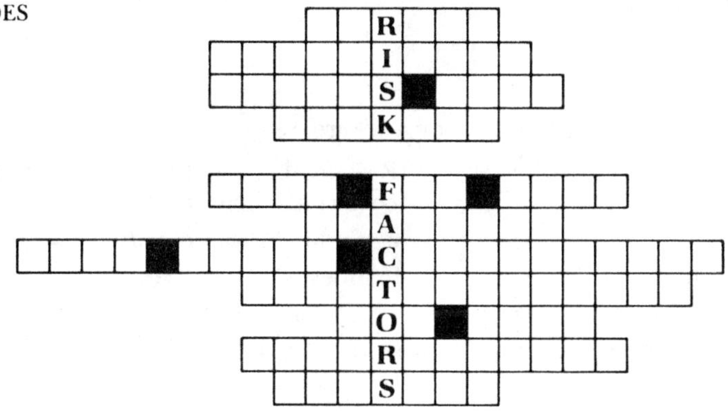

Multiple choice questions

For each of the following, choose the one best answer:

1. The main advantage of transdermal systems for administering nitroglycerin over nitroglycerin tablets given sublingually is
   a. avoidance of irritation to the oral and gastric mucosa
   b. prompt therapeutic response
   c. longer duration of action
   d. fewer adverse reactions
2. When nitroglycerin is used regularly, headaches tend to
   a. become more severe
   b. persist at the level experienced initially
   c. subside
   d. become irregular and intermittent
3. Following regular exposure to nitrates, withdrawal tends to cause
   a. flushing and throbbing headache
   b. myocardial ischemia and pain
   c. postural hypotension
   d. hypertension
4. An adverse reaction to nitrates seen only rarely is
   a. dizziness
   b. rash
   c. paradoxical hypotension
   d. methemoglobinemia
5. Clients beginning the use of nitroglycerin for the control of angina pectoris should be advised to
   a. consult the physician for a change in medication if headaches occur
   b. discontinue the drug and notify the physician if dizziness and weakness develop
   c. take the medication only when pain is experienced
   d. treat headache and postural hypotension symptomatically while continuing the medication for a trial period
6. Adverse reactions to nitroglycerin experienced when treatment is begun can be minimized if the client avoids
   a. the use of alcohol
   b. the use of analgesics such as acetaminophen
   c. overhydration
   d. inactivity
7. Pentoxifylline is classified as a
   a. sympatholytic vasodilator
   b. peripheral vasodilator
   c. vasopressor
   d. hemorrheologic
8. When sclerotherapy is undertaken, healthcare personnel must be prepared to treat sudden
   a. anaphylaxis
   b. embolism
   c. hemorrhage
   d. thrombosis
9. The emergency drug most likely to be required for treatment of adverse reaction to sclerosing agents is
   a. epinephrine
   b. nifedipine
   c. propranolol
   d. phentolamine
10. Vasoconstrictor solutions are often combined with solutions used for
    a. intravenous drugs used during anesthesia
    b. local anesthesia
    c. spinal anesthesia
    d. general anesthesia

Selection of options

For each of the following, select *all* appropriate responses. Circle the correct answers.

1. Vasoconstrictor drugs are useful in the treatment of
   a. hypertension
   b. hypotension related to anemia
   c. hypotension related to spinal anesthesia
   d. hypotension caused by neurogenic shock
2. Risk factors for the development of varicose veins include
   a. family history of varicose veins
   b. obesity
   c. pregnancy
   d. a vocation that involves prolonged standing

e. a vocation that involves a lot of walking
f. abdominal tumors
g. smoking
h. regular use of elastic garters to support hose

3. Complications of varicose veins include
   a. generalized rash
   b. leg ulcers
   c. gangrene

Short answer questions

1. Identify six drug categories, other than nitrites and nitrates, that are commonly involved in the management of ischemic heart disease.

2. Identify at least three measures that tend to delay or prevent the development of varicose veins.

25 ▪ *Drugs that regulate blood pressure*

Multiple choice questions

1. The percentage of adults in the United States with blood pressure above the "normal" range is probably
   a. 5 percent
   b. 20 percent
   c. 40 percent
   d. 50 percent
2. Which antihypertensive agent might be used with pheochromocytoma?
   a. carteolol
   b. pindolol
   c. clonidine
   d. phentolamine
3. Which is an example of a selective alpha-1 adrenergic blocking agent?
   a. tolazoline
   b. nadolol
   c. prazosin
   d. penbutolol
4. Reflex tachycardia is often experienced with
   a. diuretics
   b. angiotensin receptor antagonists
   c. direct-acting vasodilators
   d. beta-adrenergic blocking agents
5. Which is an example of a combined alpha and beta-adrenergic blocking agent?
   a. methyldopa
   b. dopamine
   c. labetalol
   d. carteolol
6. A common side effect of antihypertensive agents is
   a. irritability
   b. dehydration
   c. weight gain
   d. orthostatic hypotension
7. Which medication is available as a transdermal system?
   a. clonidine (Catapres TTS)
   b. methyldopa (Aldomet)
   c. prazosin (Minipress)
   d. reserpine (Serpasil)
8. Clients receiving minoxidil (Loniten) should be told
   a. to take the drug with food
   b. the drug increases thirst
   c. fine body hair may grow and thicken
   d. they should not take a diuretic concurrently
9. Hydralazine is an example of what type of antihypertensive agent?
   a. beta-adrenergic blocking agent
   b. direct-acting vasodilator
   c. ganglionic blocking agent
   d. monoamine oxidase inhibitor
10. The mechanism of action for captopril's antihypertensive effect is
    a. direct vasodilation
    b. inhibition of angiotensin converting enzyme
    c. blocking of calcium channels
    d. relaxation of smooth muscle
11. An example of an angiotensin receptor antagonist is
    a. diltiazem
    b. labetalol
    c. verapamil
    d. losartan
12. IV nitroprusside (Nitroprusside) is administered to a client with severe hypertension. How long will it take for this drug to act?
    a. almost immediately
    b. 60–120 sec
    c. 30 min
    d. 60 min

Selection of options

For each of the following, select *all* appropriate responses. Circle the correct answers.

1. Clients with hypertension can enhance control of the condition by
   a. reducing salt intake
   b. reducing water intake
   c. increasing physical activity as tolerated
   d. achieving and maintaining a lean body weight
   e. learning to manage stress well
2. Appropriate advice for those on antihypertensive drugs who experience undesirable changes in sexual function includes telling the client that
   a. sexual activity is risky in hypertension and decreased function is therapeutic
   b. impairment of sexual function is sometimes unavoidable but will become less pronounced with continued therapy
   c. the physician should be consulted for changes in drug prescriptions that may eliminate the problem
   d. the sexual problem may be ameliorated by counseling regarding alternative sexual expression
3. Therapeutic uses for trimethaphan include
   a. maintenance therapy for chronic hypertension
   b. treatment of hypertensive crisis
   c. producing controlled hypotension during surgery
   d. control of angina pectoris complicated by hypertension
4. Calcium channel blocking agents act by
   a. reducing serum levels of calcium ions
   b. raising body *p*H and decreasing ionization of calcium
   c. inhibiting flow of calcium ions into myocardial muscle cells
   d. inhibiting flow of calcium ions into vascular smooth muscle cells

Short answer questions

1. Discuss specific interventions a nurse could try to improve a client's compliance with the therapeutic drug regimen that is being used to manage hypertension.

2. Discuss specific instructions a nurse should give clients about orthostatic hypotension associated with taking their antihypertensive medication.

26 ▪ *Drugs that regulate hemostasis*

Hemostasis is a complex process. It involves vasospasm, formation of a platelet plug, and blood coagulation.

PART 1: HEMOSTATICS

Correct the false statement

Indicate whether the following statements are true or false; if false, correct the underlined words or phrases.

_______ 1. The development of a factor VIII inhibitor is usually associated with an increased response to antihemophilic factor.

_______ 2. Cryoprecipitate is the only form of concentrated fibrinogen available.

_______ 3. The agents used for treatment of hemophilia B include protamine sulfate.

_______ 4. Bacterial flora provide about half of the body's requirement for vitamin K.

_______ 5. For rapid reversal of anticoagulant-induced prothrombin deficiency, menadiol sodium diphosphate (Synkayvite) is used.

_______ 6. Vitamin K preparations are not helpful with bleeding associated with the use of heparin.

_______ 7. Aminocaproic acid is likely to be useful as an antidote for heparin.

_______ 8. Aminocaproic acid is representative of a group of compounds that facilitate fibrinolysis.

_______ 9. Tranexamic acid is much less potent than aminocaproic acid.

_______ 10. Rapid administration of protamine sulfate may cause acute hypertension.

Multiple choice questions

For each of the following, choose the one best answer:

1. The agent most likely to restore all coagulation factors to a normal level is
   a. fresh whole blood
   b. citrated blood
   c. plasma
   d. packed red blood cells
2. The active ingredient in antihemophilic factor is
   a. prothrombin
   b. factor VIII
   c. factor IX
   d. factor X
3. Antihemophilic factor is used to treat bleeding episodes caused by
   a. hemophilia A
   b. Christmas disease
   c. hemophilia B
   d. pseudohemophilia (von Willebrand disease)
4. When antihemophilic factor is infused intravenously, flow rates should be adjusted in accordance with changes in the
   a. blood pressure
   b. pulse rate
   c. prothrombin time
   d. visible bleeding

5. Proplex T or Proplex SX-T (prothrombin complex preparations) are used to treat
   a. hemophilia A
   b. hemophilia B
   c. hemophilia C
   d. pseudohemophilia (von Willebrand disease)
6. Vitamin K (phytonadione/AquaMEPHYTON) is effective in the reversal of impaired coagulation caused by
   a. pseudohemophilia (von Willebrand disease)
   b. platelet deficiency
   c. overdose of heparin
   d. oral anticoagulant-induced prothrombin deficiency
7. Aminocaproic acid acts by
   a. promoting prothrombin production by liver
   b. neutralizing warfarin sodium
   c. inhibiting plasmin (fibrinolysin) activity
   d. neutralizing heparin
8. Aminocaproic acid is eliminated through the
   a. urine
   b. bile into feces
   c. both of the above
   d. neither of the above
9. Aprotinin might be used in conjunction with coronary artery bypass graft surgery and is obtained from
   a. fish
   b. spider webs
   c. bovine lung
   d. porcine liver
10. When a bleeding episode occurs, clients with coagulation deficiency are most likely to experience
    a. anxiety related to potential death
    b. high risk for infection related to possible exposure to viruses in blood replacement product
    c. high risk for allergic hypersensitivity to drugs produced by recombinant DNA techniques
    d. pain: headache related to central nervous system irritation by hemostatic agent

Short answer questions

1. List, in order, the major steps in hemostasis.

2. List 10 foods that contain vitamin K. Determine portion sizes for each that would contain comparable levels of this nutrient.

PART 2: ANTICOAGULANTS

Correct the false statement

Indicate whether the following statements are true or false; if false, correct the underlined words or phrases.

_______ 1. anticoagulants prevent the formation and extension of clots <u>and dissolve clots already formed in the blood vessels</u>.

_______ 2. The desired therapeutic result of coumarin derivative anticoagulation is prothrombin time that is <u>about ten times</u> that of the normal control.

_______ 3. The International Normalized Ratio (INR) was introduced to resolve problems with <u>activated thromboplastin time</u> monitoring.

_______ 4. The anticoagulant used to prevent clotting in hemodialysis equipment is <u>sodium citrate</u>.

_______ 5. Enoxaparin was introduced as a <u>low-molecular-weight heparin</u> derivative.

_______ 6. An anticoagulant drug that can cause osteoporosis is <u>aspirin</u>.

_______ 7. Hirudin is the anticoagulant substance from the <u>medicinal leech</u>.

_______ 8. The client on warfarin sodium should <u>increase</u> intake of foods such as broccoli, cabbage, and spinach.

_______ 9. The "purple toe syndrome" is a potential adverse reaction to <u>enoxaparin</u>.

_______ 10. Hirudin and hirugen are inhibitors of <u>conversion of prothrombin to thrombin</u>.

Multiple choice questions

For each of the following, choose the one best answer

1. A client, hospitalized for treatment of deep vein thrombophlebitis of the right leg, is receiving both heparin and warfarin sodium. He tells you he is afraid of bleeding to death "because the medications may thin my blood too much." Your *best* reply would be:
   a. There is no danger of sudden death.
   b. The two drugs antagonize each other, reducing the risk of severe hemorrhage.
   c. The drugs do not really "thin" the blood.
   d. The two drugs slow clotting, but do not abolish the process.
2. The anticoagulant action of warfarin sodium is often influenced by drugs that:
   a. stimulate liver production of bile
   b. alter function of liver enzymes
   c. increase urinary output
   d. suppress normal intestinal flora
3. Clients on long-term oral anticoagulants should be cautioned against using
   a. acetaminophen
   b. aspirin
   c. antacids
   d. one-a-day vitamin preparations
4. The most common adverse reaction of heparin anticoagulation is
   a. allergic rash
   b. melena
   c. ecchymoses over venipuncture sites
   d. suppression of normal intestinal flora
5. Of the following drugs, which is most likely to cause adverse interaction with other drugs?
   a. thrombin
   b. heparin
   c. warfarin sodium
   d. urokinase
6. Allergic reaction to protamine sulfate is most likely in persons with known sensitivity to
   a. grains
   b. fish
   c. chocolate
   d. nuts
7. Following administration of protamine sulfate, clients should be watched for signs and symptoms of
   a. thrombophlebitis
   b. hemolysis and anemia
   c. pulmonary embolism
   d. rebound anticoagulation

Short answer questions

1. Is heparin effective when administered orally? Why/why not?

2. Why is heparin not administered intramuscularly?

3. What changes are necessary in subcutaneous injection technique when heparin is administered?

4. Are oral anticoagulants used during pregnancy? Why/why not?

5. Is it necessary to restrict/encourage vitamin K in the diets of clients receiving oral anticoagulants? Why/why not?

6. Explain the mechanism of action of protamine sulfate.

Completion exercise

Read the following carefully and place your answers in the space provided.

	Coumadin	Heparin
Mechanism of action	______	______
Route(s) of administration	______	______
Unit of measurement of doses	______	______
Frequency of dosage	______	______
Onset of action	______	______
Antidote(s)	______	______
Laboratory test(s) for monitoring	______	______
Adverse reactions	______	______

PART 3: DRUGS THAT AFFECT PLATELET AGGREGATION

Correct the false statement

Indicate whether the following statements are true or false; if false, correct the underlined words or phrases.

______ 1. Thromboxane A_2 inhibits platelet aggregation.

______ 2. In small doses, aspirin acts as an anticoagulant agent.

______ 3. Dipyridamole might be used for clients with mechanical prosthetic heart valves.

______ 4. The newest antiplatelet drug is ticlopidine (Ticlid).

PART 4: FIBRINOLYTIC AGENTS

Correct the false statement

Indicate whether the following statements are true or false; if false, correct the underlined words or phrases.

______ 1. Fibrinolytics are vitamin K analogs.

______ 2. To effectively dissolve intravascular clots, fibrinolytic therapy must begin within 6 hours of formation of the clot.

______ 3. When used to treat myocardial infarction, fibrinolytic drugs are likely to be administered orally.

______ 4. The most expensive fibrinolytic agent is urokinase.

______ 5. A fibrinolytic agent that is highly antigenic is tissue plasminogen activator/t-PA (alteplase/Activase).

______ 6. Commonly warfarin sodium is administered concomitantly with the fibrinolytic drugs.

Multiple choice questions

For each of the following, choose the one best answer:

1. During the natural process of clot dissolution, fibrin is degraded by
   a. plasminogen activator
   b. plasmin
   c. alpha 2-antiplasmin
   d. urokinase
2. Which of the following fibrinolytic drugs is the most "clot selective"?
   a. streptokinase
   b. urokinase
   c. tissue plasminogen activator
   d. abciximab

Short answer question

1. List at least four nursing behaviors that promote trust by clients in life-threatening situations.

PART 5: CHAPTERWIDE EXERCISES

Selection of options

For each of the following, select *all* appropriate responses. Circle the correct answers.

1. Indications for anticoagulant therapy include
   a. atrial fibrillation
   b. recent myocardial infarction
   c. pregnancy
   d. thrombophlebitis
2. Contraindications for anticoagulant therapy include
   a. active hemorrhage
   b. threatened abortion
   c. thrombophlebitis
   d. peptic ulcer
   e. intracranial hemorrhage
3. Drugs that inhibit platelet aggregation include
   a. aspirin
   b. phytonadione
   c. ticlopidine
   d. dipyridamole
   e. abciximab
4. Signs and symptoms of anticoagulant toxicity include
   a. hematuria
   b. tarry stools
   c. ecchymoses
   d. cold, pale extremities
   e. telangiectasia
   f. epistaxis
5. Clients on long-term oral anticoagulant therapy should be advised to
   a. avoid trauma
   b. avoid marked fluctuation in dietary iron intake
   c. avoid marked fluctuation in vitamin K intake
   d. wear a medical identification device
6. Adverse reactions to fibrinolytics include
   a. hemorrhage
   b. allergic reactions
   c. decreased fertility
   d. hypertensive crisis
7. Contraindications to fibrinolytic use include
   a. known bleeding diathesis
   b. recent intracranial surgery
   c. intracranial atrioventricular malformations
   d. renal disease
   e. GI bleeding ten years ago
   f. cholecystitis

27 ▪ *Drugs that affect the kidneys*

The kidneys eliminate fluids, electrolytes, nitrogenous wastes, and toxins. The kidneys keep the body's blood chemistry properly balanced by the selective excretion of unnecessary chemicals.

Correct the false statement

Indicate whether the following statements are true or false; if false, correct the underlined words or phrases.

_______ 1. The force responsible for maintaining glomerular filtration is <u>an osmotic diffusion gradient</u>.

_______ 2. The glomerular filtrate is <u>more concentrated than plasma</u>.

_______ 3. Normal glomerular filtrate contains <u>little or no protein</u>.

_______ 4. The presence of red blood cells in urine is <u>abnormal</u>.

_______ 5. Diuretics are usually <u>contraindicated</u> during pregnancy.

_______ 6. Hypokalemia tends to cause <u>cramping and diarrhea</u>.

_______ 7. In digitalized persons, the effect of hypokalemia on intestinal function <u>may be opposite</u> to that in a nonmedicated person.

_______ 8.Toxic reactions to diuretics are most likely to occur in <u>cold dry</u> environments.

_______ 9. <u>Potassium-sparing</u> diuretics are the strongest diuretics available.

_______ 10. To a degree, diuresis is <u>a positive feedback process (i.e., when diuresis begins it causes further diuresis)</u>.

_______ 11. The most frequent adverse reaction to diuretic therapy is <u>dehydration</u>.

_______ 12. Diuretics are often used because they <u>decrease</u> plasma volume.

_______ 13. Thiazide diuretics are the ones most often used for treatment of <u>acute conditions associated with edema</u>.

_______ 14. Aldosterone promotes <u>sodium excretion and potassium reabsorption</u>.

Matching

A. Match each of the physiologic segments of the renal tubule in the left-hand column with all appropriate responses in the right-hand column. Place your answer(s) in the space provided.

_______ 1. Proximal tubule

_______ 2. Descending portion of the thin segment of the loop of Henle

_______ 3. Ascending portion of the thin segment of the loop of Henle

_______ 4. Late distal tubule

_______ 5. Collecting tubule

a. Reabsorption of water
b. Active secretion of hydrogen ions
c. Reabsorption of vitamins
d. Reabsorption of chloride ions
e. Reabsorption of amino acids
f. Reabsorption of urea
g. Reabsorption of sodium
h. Reabsorption of potassium
i. Responds to antidiuretic hormone
j. Responds to aldosterone
k. Secretes potassium
l. Relatively little influence

B. Match each diuretic listed in the left-hand column with its major site of action in the kidney listed in the right-hand column.

_______ 1. Acetazolamide
_______ 2. Amiloride
_______ 3. Bumetamide
_______ 4. Chlorothiazide
_______ 5. Ethacrynic acid
_______ 6. Furosemide
_______ 7. Hydrochlorothiazide
_______ 8. Spironolactone
_______ 9. Triamterene
_______ 10. Methazolamide

a. Proximal tubule
b. Loop of Henle
c. Distal tubule

Find the hidden words

Hidden within the following letter grid are words and phrases from Chapter 27. They may be vertical, horizontal, or diagonal. Circle the letters as you find the hidden words.

List of words and phrases

absorption
acetazolamide
aldactone
amiloride
carbonic anhydrase
diabetes
Diamox
diffusion
diuretic
Diuril
Edecrin
edema
electrolyte
ethacrynic acid
fluid
furosemide
glomerulus
glycerol
gout
hydrochlorothiazide
hyperkalemia
hypokalemia
indoline
intake
Lasix
mannitol
nephrons
osmosis
output
reabsorption
secretion
sodium retention
spironolactone
triamterene
tubule
urea
weight
xanthine

c e e e r u i d o s a l i m a c e t a z o l a m i d e r i
a a l d a s i l u e c a r b l a s i n t u b u l i i d e p
a r e i u r e a b s o a a i d i a w b u t r i c n a e n o
b s c l e d i r o l i m a l a n d e n o t c a d l a s o s
d o t a a i n t a m e i b o c t r i n t a c i m a i r t o
s r r s m n t i e d r l s r h a m g i d i a m o x n e c m
m p o u o t e l e c t r o l y t e h p n o a e s a t a a s
o t l d i a a m i u r e r d d a y t y h n u r e a m b l d
s h y p o k a l e m i a p e r k a r h n k a t n i a s o b
e y t s r e a b s o r p t i o n c l i s a l a p m s o n r
c p e e a l d a o s e d i h c a g t u r l d n r u a c o a
r i p i b a i r d m a a o y h r o t m e e a o e p t a r c
e y r t s s e c i f b r n t l l d i u r i l p a i g d i e
h t e c i t e r u i d b e d o a m n e p h r y b l e l p d
y n a t r g d r m a n o c a r b o n i c a n h y d r a s e
s i s o m s o a r p e n r e o s m a n a o e c r e o s m o
e e e d e s i u e d r e a b t u b m t i r e o v r s n e p
c a r s e c r e t i o n e p h r o n s o r p p i e b a m i
a d i m d r r d e e d e d e i r i u u o n h y d i a m a n
r e i n t t e e n i e a e n a t f a l a s y h e n o t c a
b d s a n e a l t n l d m a z f t a m i l p r e a c e t a
e n b n b a b s i n t i i n i l u i d t d e l v c t r i a
t a a l a e s h o e u u a d d r b a i r e d e c r i n e p
h m l a i r t o n p g l o m e r u l u s k r e p i e e d o
a e d s a n e e y h y f c n e p l e r e a b e o m i d e n
c d d i a l d a s i n d o l i n e d e c a r b n a t n i a
r e a x a c e t o o s m o s e c r e d e c a r b e d e m o

Multiple choice questions

For each of the following, choose the one best answer:

1. Of the following elements, which exerts the most influence on fluid balance?
   a. calcium
   b. magnesium
   c. potassium
   d. sodium
2. How do osmotic diuretics affect blood volume?
   a. They increase blood volume.
   b. They decrease blood volume.
   c. Initially, they decrease blood volume and, subsequently, they increase it.
   d. Initially, they increase blood volume and, subsequently, they decrease it.
3. Mannitol is usually administered
   a. orally
   b. subcutaneously
   c. intramuscularly
   d. intravenously
4. Which diuretic has a significant adverse reaction of hyperkalemia?
   a. furosemide
   b. indapamide
   c. mannitol
   d. spironolactone
5. The diuretic used most frequently to prevent acute renal failure is
   a. furosemide
   b. glycerol
   c. hydrochlorothiazide
   d. mannitol
6. A common adverse reaction to osmotic diuretics is
   a. fluid overload
   b. delayed healing
   c. speech difficulties
   d. allergic reactions
7. The mechanism of action of acetazolamide is
   a. increased hydrostatic pressure in the glomerulus
   b. inhibition of carbonic anhydrase
   c. inhibition of active reabsorption of sodium in the tubule
   d. stimulation of active secretion of sodium in the tubule
8. A frequent side effect of acetazolamide is
   a. hyponatremia
   b. hyperkalemia
   c. metabolic alkalosis
   d. metabolic acidosis
9. In addition to increasing the volume of urine, a carbonic anhydrase inhibitor
   a. increases pH of urine
   b. decreases pH of urine
   c. increases response to hypoglycemics
   d. decreases excretion of acidic preparations
10. Clients at greatest risk for adverse reactions to carbonic anhydrase inhibitors are those predisposed to
    a. respiratory acidosis
    b. respiratory alkalosis
    c. hyperkalemia
    d. glaucoma
11. The site of action of "high-ceiling" diuretics is the
    a. proximal tubule
    b. loop of Henle
    c. diluting segment
    d. distal tubule
12. A major adverse reaction to thiazide diuretics is
    a. hypoglycemia
    b. metabolic acidosis
    c. hypermagnesemia
    d. hypokalemia
13. The mechanism of action of spironolactone is inhibition of
    a. aldosterone
    b. antidiuretic hormone
    c. carbonic anhydrase
    d. absorption of chloride
14. Clients most vulnerable to spironolactone are those with
    a. cardiac impairment
    b. hepatic impairment
    c. renal impairment
    d. adrenal hyperfunction
15. The most sensitive indicator of diuresis is
    a. body weight
    b. blood pressure
    c. fluid intake and output
    d. tissue turgor
16. Foods rich in potassium include
    a. apples and raisins
    b. bananas and oranges
    c. cranberries and boiled vegetables
    d. whole grain cereals

17. Hyperkalemia's effects on the gastrointestinal tract include
    a. vasodilatation and vascular congestion
    b. atony and intestinal obstruction
    c. increased motility and cramping pain
    d. prolongation of intestinal transit time

18. (A) dietary component(s) that can reduce the therapeutic effect of diuretics is (are)
    a. calories in the nutrients
    b. water and other fluids
    c. potassium
    d. sodium

Selection of options

For each of the following, select *all* appropriate responses. Circle the correct answers.

1. Compared to glomerular filtrate, urine usually contains a
   a. lower concentration of red blood cells
   b. lower concentration of water
   c. lower concentration of sodium
   d. higher concentration of nitrogenous wastes
   e. higher concentration of toxins
2. Mechanisms by which the kidney tubule controls the composition of urine include
   a. filtration
   b. passive diffusion
   c. carrier-mediated transport
   d. active transport mechanisms
3. Hormones that influence the function of the renal tubule include
   a. thyroxine
   b. aldosterone
   c. corticosteroids
   d. estrogen
   e. vasopressin
4. When a person on restricted sodium intake is overhydrated, physiological effects include
   a. increased production of urine
   b. increased loss of electrolytes in urine
   c. a tendency toward positive water balance
   d. decreased concentration of sodium in body fluids
   e. negative potassium balance
5. Therapeutic uses for osmotic diuretics include
   a. treatment of congestive heart failure
   b. prevention of acute renal failure following trauma
   c. treatment of pulmonary edema
   d. alleviating increased cerebrospinal fluid pressure
6. Assessment data that should be gathered regularly for clients receiving diuretics include
   a. fluid intake and output
   b. body weight
   c. vital signs
   d. tissue turgor
7. Diuretics that tend to cause hyperuricemia include
   a. acetazolamide
   b. benzothiazides
   c. loop diuretics
   d. spironolactone
8. Toxicity to various diuretics is sometimes characterized by
   a. sodium depletion
   b. sodium retention
   c. potassium depletion
   d. potassium retention
   e. low blood volume

Short answer questions

1. Name three disease conditions in which diuretics are used to control edema.

2. List two therapeutic uses for carbonic anhydrase inhibitors.

3. Name three qualities required of a drug for osmotic diuresis.

4. Identify two disease conditions that tend to increase in severity when diuretics are used.

5. How much will body weight decrease with a net loss of 1 liter of fluid?

UNIT EIGHT
Drugs affecting the gastrointestinal system

28 ▪ *Drugs that affect the upper gastrointestinal tract*

Large quantities of nonprescription drugs for self-treatment of problems of the upper gastrointestinal tract are purchased over the counter. This fact makes consumer education very important. Nurses must be familiar with nonprescription drugs so that they can help clients use them safely. In addition, they must understand prescription drugs to assist with medical treatment.

Matching

A. Match the agent in the left-hand column with the actions or properties it exhibits in the right-hand column.

_______ 1. Sodium perborate	a. Causes toxicity when ingested
_______ 2. Hydrogen peroxide	b. Acts as an oxidizing agent
_______ 3. Potassium permanganate	c. Discolors the membranes
	d. Must be used while solutions are fresh
	e. Can cause "hairy tongue" when used for a prolonged period

B. Match the metallic ion contained in antacids in the left-hand column with all of its appropriate adverse effects in the right-hand column.

_______ 1. Sodium	a. Diarrhea
_______ 2. Calcium	b. Constipation
_______ 3. Magnesium	c. Water retention
_______ 4. Aluminum	d. Neurotoxicity
	e. Potentiation of digitalis
	f. Gastrointestinal or renal concretions
	g. Hypertension

Crossword puzzle

Across

5. A trade name for ranitidine
6. An erosion of gastrointestinal mucosa that is exposed to gastric secretions
7. Generic name of one of the histamine$_2$-receptor antagonists
10. Frequency of ranitidine dosage
12. The site of action of ranitidine and cimetidine
14. A condition treated by both antacids and histamine$_2$-receptor antagonists
15. A side effect of ranitidine
16. A trade name for cimetidine
18. A gastric enzyme that is most active in an acid medium
19. Drugs used to neutralize hydrochloric acid in the stomach
20. The first histamine$_2$-receptor antagonist approved for medical use

Down

1. An adverse reaction to cimetidine
2. The generic name for Zantac
3. A form of medication that may be prematurely released when taken with antacids
4. A medication that forms a nonabsorbable complex when taken with calcium antacids
8. Usual timing of cimetidine dosage for treatment of peptic ulcer
9. A drug that forms a mechanical barrier between peptic ulcer sites and gastric secretions
11. The effect of cimetidine on liver microsomal enzymes
17. An undesirable side effect caused by all three histamine$_2$-receptor antagonists

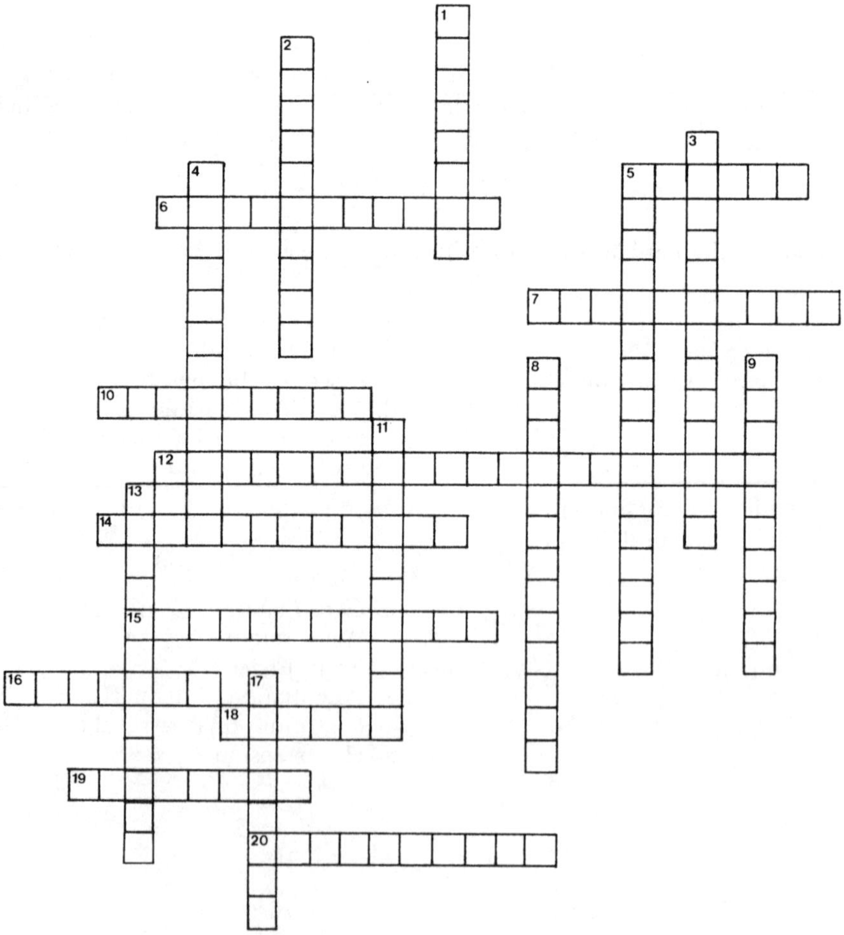

Correct the false statement

Indicate whether the following statements are true or false; if false correct the underlined words or phrases.

_______ 1. In people with normal dietary intake and good habits of hygiene, persistent offensive breath odors are most likely to be caused by systemic conditions.

_______ 2. Fluorides are incorporated into the crystalline structure of tooth enamel only when they are ingested for systemic effect.

_______ 3. Fluoride rinses are recommended for children age 3 years and older.

_______ 4. Foods most likely to promote tooth decay are those containing fatty acids.

_______ 5. A good mouthwash will mask breath odor for 3 hours.

_______ 6. Clients using oral lozenges should be advised to remove the lozenge from the mouth as soon as discomfort subsides.

_______ 7. Digestants are essential for the breakdown of food into insoluble particles.

_______ 8. Pepsin facilitates the breakdown of protein in the stomach.

_______ 9. Pancreatin contains the enzymes lipase, amylase, and trypsin.

_______ 10. Pancreatic enzymes are taken on an empty stomach.

_______ 11. 10% hydrochloric acid solution is diluted before its administration.

_______ 12. Bile aids in the digestion of fats.

_______ 13. Digestive enzymes can be easily destroyed by a basic environment.

_______ 14. Bile is secreted by the duodenum.

_______ 15. Emulsification reduces surface tension of foods.

_______ 16. Vitamin K is water-soluble.

_______ 17. The ingestion of food stimulates hydrochloric acid secretion.

_______ 18. An autogenous biochemical that directly stimulates gastric acid secretion is epinephrine.

_______ 19. Histamine$_2$-receptor antagonists act in the same way as antihistamines.

_______ 20. Histamine$_2$-receptor antagonists inhibit gastric acid secretion in response to food as much as they inhibit basal secretion of hydrochloric acid.

_______ 21. In persons with normal liver function, oral doses of both cimetidine and ranitidine undergo first-pass metabolism of half or more of the dose.

_______ 22. Histamine$_2$-receptor antagonists readily cross the blood–brain barrier.

_______ 23. Both cimetidine and ranitidine are distributed to milk.

_______ 24. Dosage of histamine$_2$-receptor antagonists should be reduced for clients with renal impairment.

_______ 25. In clients with renal failure, histamine$_2$-receptor antagonists should be administered after the hemodialysis treatments.

_______ 26. Ranitidine does not exert the same antiandrogenic effects that are seen with cimetidine.

_______ 27. A therapeutic response to histamine$_2$-receptor antagonists rules out gastric malignancy.

_______ 28. Histamine$_2$-receptor antagonists are considered safe for use during pregnancy.

_______ 29. Antacids sold over the counter are considered nontoxic and free from serious adverse side effects.

_______ 30. Liquid preparations of oral antacids are generally more effective than tablets.

_______ 31. In the treatment of peptic ulcers, a disadvantage of antacids not shared by histamine$_2$-receptor antagonists is a shorter duration of action.

_______ 32. The use of antacids in the treatment of hiatal hernia is primarily a comfort measure.

_______ 33. The action of sucralfate is systemic rather than local.

_______ 34. Before an emetic is administered, nothing should be given by mouth.

_______ 35. Adverse reactions to trimethobenzamide occur infrequently and seldom require discontinuation of the drug.

_______ 36. When antiemetics are ordered to be given PRN, the nurse may administer the drug prophylactically to prevent vomiting.

_______ 37. Prokinetics are used to stimulate the lower GI tract.

_______ 38. Misoprostol aids in protection at the gastric mucosa by inhibiting prostaglandin synthesis.

Multiple choice questions

For each of the following, choose the one best answer:

1. Halitosis ("bad breath") may arise from
   a. inability to eat and drink
   b. lack of rudimentary oral hygiene
   c. ingestion of strong-flavored foods or alcoholic drinks
   d. systemic disease
   e. all of the above
2. An ingredient of toothpaste that can reduce the incidence of tooth decay is
   a. calcium carbonate
   b. alcohol
   c. propylene glycol
   d. stannous fluoride
3. The authority that endorses fluoride toothpastes as effective deterrents to dental decay is the
   a. Food and Drug Administration
   b. Council on Drugs of the American Medical Association
   c. Council on Dental Therapeutics of the American Dental Association
   d. United States Public Health Department
4. Salt and soda bicarbonate tooth powder should not be recommended to clients
   a. prone to respiratory acidosis
   b. prone to metabolic alkalosis
   c. on restricted fluid intake
   d. on restricted sodium intake
5. All oxidizing agents used to clean the mouth act by
   a. sterilizing the mouth
   b. breaking down foreign material in the mouth
   c. effervescing and mechanically washing away debris
   d. all of the above
6. A sodium perborate solution suitable for use as a mouthwash would have the following concentration:
   a. 0.2%
   b. 1%
   c. 2%
   d. 5%
7. To prepare a hydrogen peroxide mouthwash from 3% hydrogen peroxide, you should
   a. mix one part of 3% peroxide with two parts of water
   b. mix one part of 3% peroxide with one part of water
   c. use the 3% peroxide undiluted
   d. obtain a stronger solution; hydrogen peroxide mouthwash should be a 5% solution
8. The mouth cleaners most likely to reduce the normal flora of the mouth significantly are
   a. solutions of sodium perborate
   b. lozenges containing antiseptics
   c. rinses containing potassium permanganate
   d. solutions of hydrogen peroxide
9. When administered as a digestant, hydrochloric acid is preferred from a
   a. 0.9% solution
   b. 1% solution
   c. 1.5% solution
   d. 5% solution
   e. 10% solution
10. When administered orally, hydrochloric acid should be given
    a. at least 1 hour before meals
    b. just before meals
    c. with meals
    d. after meals
11. When administered as a digestant, the usual adult dosage range for 10% hydrochloric acid is
    a. 1–2 ml
    b. 4–8 ml
    c. 15–30 ml
    d. 30–50 ml
12. When administered orally, hydrochloric acid solutions should be diluted to a strength of about
    a. 0.5%
    b. 1%
    c. 5%
    d. 10%

13. What is the source of pancreatin?
   a. chemical synthesis
   b. animal tissue
   c. plant extract
   d. bacterial culture
14. The usual dosage of pancreatic enzymes is defined in terms of
   a. trypsin
   b. amylase content
   c. lipase content
   d. all of the above
15. What is the chemical structure of most enzymes?
   a. acid
   b. base
   c. steroid
   d. protein
16. Digestive enzymes should be administered
   a. before meals with cold fluids
   b. before meals with hot fluids
   c. after meals with cold fluids
   d. after meals with hot fluids
17. Bile acids act as
   a. acids
   b. enzymes
   c. active transport carriers
   d. surfactants
18. Bile salts are most important to digestion of
   a. sugars
   b. starches
   c. proteins
   d. fats
19. The source of bile acids used medicinally is
   a. chemical synthesis
   b. animal tissue
   c. plant extract
   d. bacterial culture
20. What type of substance is dehydrocholic acid?
   a. an inorganic acid
   b. a bile acid
   c. a bile salt
   d. an enzyme
21. The conversion of pepsinogen to active pepsin is most rapid at a pH of
   a. 2
   b. 5
   c. 7
   d. 8
22. Gastric pH normally ranges between
   a. 0 and 2
   b. 2 and 5
   c. 5 and 7
   d. 7 and 8
23. The main protection for the gastric mucosa against acid secretions is
   a. the buffering action of food
   b. the buffering action of saliva
   c. thin mucus
   d. viscid mucus
24. A secondary effect of histamine$_2$ antagonists is
   a. stimulation of gastric mucosa secretion
   b. stimulation of gastric pepsin secretion
   c. inhibition of gastric mucus secretion
   d. inhibition of gastric pepsin secretion
25. If cimetidine is administered to clients receiving opioid analgesics, the nurse should observe the clients carefully for
   a. hypotensive shock
   b. respiratory depression
   c. jaundice
   d. restlessness and hyperactivity
26. When cimetidine therapy is reduced or withdrawn, the dose that is likely to be the last one discontinued is the
   a. morning dose
   b. noon dose
   c. late afternoon dose
   d. bedtime dose
27. Antacids administered orally tend to cause
   a. respiratory acidosis
   b. respiratory alkalosis
   c. metabolic acidosis
   d. metabolic alkalosis
   e. little change in acid-base balance, unless they are absorbed systemically
28. The antacid most likely to cause acute gastric distention is
   a. calcium carbonate
   b. aluminum hydroxide
   c. magnesium hydroxide
   d. sodium bicarbonate
29. At the present time, the incidence of adverse reactions to sucralfate is believed to be
   a. less than 5 percent
   b. about 10 to 15 percent
   c. about 20 to 25 percent
   d. about 30 to 50 percent
30. What percentage of sucralfate is absorbed systemically from the gastrointestinal tract?
   a. less than 1 percent
   b. 3 to 5 percent
   c. approximately 50 percent
   d. 70 to 90 percent

31. Two classes of drugs with useful antiemetic properties are
    a. opioids and barbiturates
    b. anticholinergics and antihistamines
    c. sympathomimetics and xanthines
32. The most common adverse reaction to benzquinamide is
    a. hyperphagia
    b. drowsiness
    c. myoclonus
    d. pallor
33. An antiemetic likely to be used in treatment of Menière's is
    a. benzquinamide
    b. diphenidol
    c. metoclopramide
    d. scopolamine
34. An antiemetic that sometimes causes visual and auditory hallucinations is
    a. benzquinamide
    b. diphenidol
    c. metoclopramide
    d. atropine
35. An antiemetic whose use is limited to acute care settings is
    a. diphenidol
    b. metoclopramide
    c. scopolamine
36. An prokinetic for the management of gastrointestinal motility disorders is
    a. benzquinamide
    b. diphenidol
    c. metoclopramide
    d. scopolamine
37. An antiemetic likely to be used for the control of chronic nausea and vomiting is
    a. benzquinamide
    b. diphenidol
    c. metoclopramide
    d. trimethobenzamide
38. To decrease the morning sickness of pregnancy, the nurse may recommend
    a. eating dry crackers before arising
    b. drinking effervescent beverages
    c. drinking large amounts of water
    d. the use of over-the-counter antiemetics
39. Dosages of over-the-counter antiemetics used to prevent carsickness should be taken
    a. immediately prior to starting the trip
    b. at least 15 minutes before the beginning the trip
    c. at least 30 minutes before beginning the trip
    d. at least 1 hour before beginning the trip

Short answer questions

1. How would you prepare an effective, low-cost tooth powder?

2. Using household measures, how would you prepare 100 ml of the following?
    a. 2% solution of sodium perborate:

    b. 1% solution of sodium bicarbonate:

    c. 0.9% solution of sodium chloride:

3. What concentration of sodium chloride in water would be isotonic?

4. Define the term *digestant.*

5. Name four major categories of digestants.

6. Briefly describe instructions that you would give to the patient receiving 10% hydrochloric acid solution.

7. List at least five factors predisposing to problems associated with hyperacidity.

8. Name at least six mechanisms by which the genetic predisposition to hyperacidity may be expressed.

9. What is acid rebound?

10. Why should clients receiving histamine$_2$-receptor antagonists be observed closely for changes in psychologic, intellectual, and affective status?

11. Identify at least four environmental factors that increase the risk of problems attributed to hyperacidity.

12. Should water be administered with liquid antacids? Why or why not?

13. How frequently are oral antacids usually administered?

14. Are over-the-counter antacids cheaper overall than the legend drug cimetidine for the treatment of peptic ulcer?

15. Is it advisable to leave antacid medications at the bedside for clients to administer to themselves?

16. May one over-the-counter antacid be substituted for another?

17. How is sucralfate eliminated from the body?

18. How should oral antacids in tablet form be administered?

19. Define *emetic*.

20. Define *antiemetic*.

21. The anticholinergic most often used as an antiemetic is:

22. Name three signs or symptoms that require immediate discontinuation of diphenidol.

23. How can vomiting be differentiated from regurgitation?

24. Is the use of antiemetics recommended for the treatment of nausea and vomiting of pregnancy?

Personal exercise: Self-medication

Common drug advertisements deal with signs and symptoms of indigestion. How do you decide which remedy is best for you?

Enrichment experiences

1. **Prepare 2 ounces of salt and sodium bicarbonate tooth powder. Use it for dental hygiene until the supply is exhausted. Compare the cost of using commercial toothpaste during this time period with the cost of preparing the tooth powder. Was the tooth powder an adequate cleanser? Was it anesthetically acceptable? Would you recommend such a preparation to your clients?**
2. **Contact the health department and ascertain whether the local water supply is fluoridated. If it is, determine the quantities of chemicals added to the water and the methods used to control the levels of concentration. If the water is not fluoridated, ascertain whether fluoridation was ever considered. What arguments have been offered for and against fluoridation?**
3. **With classmates, develop criteria for evaluating advertisements that promote hygienic aids as mouthwashes. Assign one commercial product to each class member, and ask each member to evaluate printed advertisements in magazines, newspapers, or on billboards and media advertisements on television or radio. Discuss the evaluations in class. What claims were made for the products?**

   What values were implied in the advertisements without being expressly stated? What are the techniques used to condition the public through advertisements? How can nurses assist their clients in evaluating such products objectively?
4. **Examine antacid preparations offered for over-the-counter sale in a drugstore. Choose three preparations containing different metallic salts and compare the metallic salts contained in each, the recommended dose of each, precautions listed on each label, and cost of each daily dosage. What recommendations would you offer a client seeking information and advice on the use of one of these preparations?**
5. **Many third-party payment plans will not pay the cost of over-the-counter preparations such as vitamins or antacids, even when prescribed by a physician. How might this influence a physician's choice of drugs and the client's compliance with the physician's recommendations?**
6. **Interview three people to ascertain how each would define vomiting, regurgitation, and reaching. What elements are common to all three? How do they differ?**
7. **With your classmates, develop a list of essential information for determining the true nature of symptoms related to nausea and vomiting (i.e., the dimensions of these symptoms).**

29 ▪ *Agents affecting the lower gastrointestinal tract*

The following exercises relate to the material in the textbook on antiflatulents, laxatives, and antidiarrheals.

Correct the false statement

Indicate whether the following statements are true or false; if false, correct the underlined words or phrases.

_______ 1. Flatulence and abdominal cramping caused by lactulose tend to subside with continued administration of the drug.

_______ 2. Hyperosmotic laxatives containing magnesium are preferred for treating constipation in clients with renal failure.

_______ 3. The laxatives whose actions mimic most closely the physiologic process of fecal elimination are the surfactant laxatives.

_______ 4. The use of psyllium hydrophilic mucilloid tends to reduce plasma cholesterol concentrations.

_______ 5. The use of laxatives tends to be habit-forming.

_______ 6. An initial defecation reflex tends to persist for 5–10 minutes.

_______ 7. Reducing stress levels may help to correct constipation in persons in whom stress increases parasympathetic nervous activity.

_______ 8. For the treatment of recurrent chronic constipation, the nurse may recommend regular long-term use of lubricant laxatives.

_______ 9. Phenolphthalein sometimes changes the color of urine or stools.

_______ 10. Aloin is an herbal remedy that is effective and safe for use as a laxative.

_______ 11. Mineral waters are effective laxatives.

_______ 12. Adsorbent antidiarrheals act by neutralizing irritants and toxins in the intestine.

Crossword puzzle

Across

3. A laxative food
4. A type of drug likely to be used to treat diarrhea during narcotic withdrawal
8. Term used for the strongest type of laxative
10. A chemical reaction in the intestine that generates gas
11. A food substance that promotes intestinal fermentation and flatus
13. Chemical nature of most antiflatulents
16. A nutrient likely to become deficient when mineral oil is used regularly.
18. A folk remedy that is effective in relieving flatulence
22. Type of bean used as a laxative
24. An organism in the normal gastrointestinal flora that protects against some kinds of diarrhea
26. A laxative food enjoyed by most children
27. Drugs that act as antiflatulents

Down

1. A folk remedy for diarrhea
2. A potentially lethal result of careless handling of dry bulk laxatives
5. A defoaming antiflatulent
6. Term used for a strong laxative
12. A food component that promotes fermentation in the gut
14. A nonnutritive lubricating laxative
15. A beverage that is useful for diarrhea
17. A nursing measure to relieve gas in the colon
19. A food that acts as a laxative
20. A black drug in the "black and white" laxative
21. A food useful in reducing diarrhea caused by broad-spectrum antibacterial anti-infectives
23. The chemical formed from castor oil that produces its laxative effect
25. Pain in newborns associated with flatulence

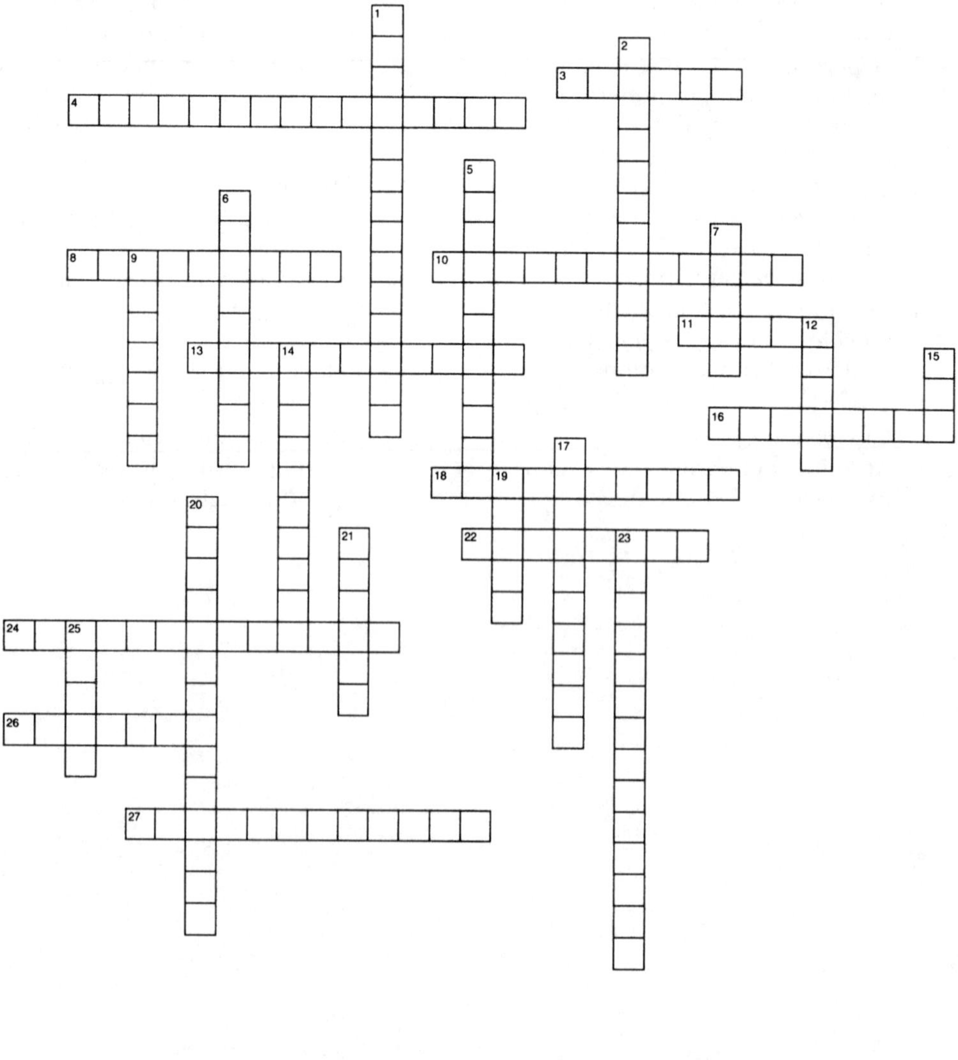

Multiple choice questions

For each of the following, choose the one best answer:

1. The chemical nature characteristic of most carminatives is
   a. aromatic oil
   b. inorganic salt
   c. protein
   d. steroid
2. A hormone remedy used as a carminative is
   a. oil of cloves
   b. lemon extract
   c. peppermint
   d. wintergreen
3. The mechanism of action of peppermint when used as a carminative is
   a. adsorption
   b. demulcent
   c. irritant
4. A common effect of carminative medications is
   a. anorexia or nausea
   b. eructation
   c. constipation
   d. alcoholic intoxication
5. An autogenous chemical that increases the tone and action of the intestines is
   a. acetylcholine
   b. epinephrine
   c. norepinephrine
   d. atropine
6. The laxative ingredient in rhubarb is
   a. acetylcholine
   b. oxalic acid
   c. senna
   d. tannin
7. Use of the diphenylmethane laxative phenolphthalein may increase the risk of developing
   a. appendicitis
   b. hepatitis
   c. serous skin eruptions
   d. ulcerative colitis
8. Stimulant laxatives such as phenolphthalein should not be used by children younger than
   a. 6 months
   b. 1 year
   c. 3 years
   d. 6 years
9. A laxative likely to be used to prevent constipation caused by the use of sodium polystyrene is
   a. cascara
   b. milk of magnesia
   c. psyllium hydrophillic mucilloid
   d. sorbitol
10. When administering bulk laxatives, the nurse should be sure to
    a. follow the drug with ample amounts of fluid
    b. mix the dry drug thoroughly with fluid before administration
    c. caution the client against excessive fluid intake
11. Dysphagia is a contraindication for
    a. irritant laxatives
    b. hyperosmotic laxatives
    c. bulk-forming laxatives
    d. lubricant laxatives
12. Most lubricant laxatives are
    a. irritants
    b. mucilloids
    c. oils
    d. surfactants
13. A laxative used as a retention enema, but not administered orally, is
    a. magnesium sulfate
    b. mineral oil
    c. sodium phosphate
    d. vegetable oils
14. The enema solution that is least irritating is
    a. tap water
    b. normal saline
    c. sodium phosphate
    d. soap suds
15. When is the best time to administer mineral oil?
    a. on arising
    b. with meals
    c. 2 hours before bedtime
    d. at bedtime
16. The laxatives that are least harmful when used in conjunction with weight reduction regimens are
    a. bulk-forming laxatives
    b. hyperosmotic laxatives
    c. irritant laxatives
    d. lubricants

17. In most diarrheas, the most important therapeutic measure in treatment is
    a. adsorption of the intestinal irritants
    b. inhibition of peristalsis
    c. reduction of the frequency of stools
    d. replacement of fluid and electrolyte loss
18. A contraindication for the use of kaolin is
    a. cramping abdominal pain
    b. fever
    c. watery stools
    d. a positive stool culture
19. Most antidiarrheal foods act as
    a. adsorbents
    b. anticholinergics
    c. astringents
    d. demulcents
20. Excessive loss of intestinal contents caused by diarrhea, laxatives, or enemas tend to cause serious depletion of body
    a. calcium
    b. carbohydrates
    c. sodium
    d. potassium
21. An adverse reaction likely to develop when astringent antidiarrheals are employed is
    a. constipation
    b. central nervous system depression
    c. central nervous system stimulation
    d. overhydration
22. The most urgent need of a client with acute severe diarrhea is
    a. correction of the underlying pathology
    b. correction of the fluid and electrolyte imbalance
    c. reduction in the frequency of stools
    d. relief of pain
23. Clients at greatest risk for rapid dehydration and electrolyte depletion from diarrhea are
    a. infants and small children
    b. pubescent youngsters
    c. young adults
    d. adults 40–60 years of age
    e. adults older than 60 years of age

Short answer questions

1. Identify at least three nursing measures to decrease flatulence.

2. Define the following terms:
    a. Diarrhea:

    b. Constipation:

    c. Laxative:

    d. Adsorbent:

3. How do the terms *purgative, laxative,* and *cathartic* differ?

4. List at least three characteristics of the ideal laxative.

5. What are four situations in which a laxative should not be used?

6. Name at least four laxative foods.

7. Because it is inactive until changed chemically by the body, castor oil may be considered to be a prodruct. How does the body "activate" castor oil, and what chemical is produced by this process?

8. Name at least four hyperosmotic laxatives.

9. Identify four hygienic measures that help to reduce constipation.

10. List at least five factors that increase the risk of constipation in institutionalized populations.

11. Name at least three foods and three types of drugs that can contribute to constipation.

12. Name at least three adsorbent antidiarrheals.

13. Identify one undesirable side effect of adsorbent antidiarrheals.

14. What is the effect of artificial sweeteners (saccharin and cyclamates) on the colon?

15. Name at least four foods that should be avoided by clients prone to chronic diarrhea.

Enrichment experiences

1. **Interview an elderly client to determine the influence of folk or traditional medicine on that client's health practices. Ask specifically about home remedies used for indigestion or excessive flatulence. Later, analyze the remedies described by the client to ascertain the active pharmacologic agents (if any) involved and the influence of associated factors, such as method of administration or concomitant applications of heat. Discuss with your classmates what nursing approaches should be used when caring for clients who use folk remedies frequently.**
2. **Investigate remedies for promoting fecal elimination offered for sale by a local drugstore. How many different products are displayed on the shelves? How many are stool softeners? How many are laxatives? Choose examples of irritant, hyperosmotic, bulk-forming, lubricant, and stool-softening laxatives; compare the cost per dose of each type of laxative. Are any preparations available that combine different types of laxatives? Compute the daily cost of using a stool softener for prevention of constipation. How does this compare with the cost of laxatives?**
3. **Observe advertisements for laxatives in magazines or on television. With your classmates, discuss aspects of these advertisements that may be confusing to laypeople.**
4. **List the indications for use of stool softeners and laxatives. Under what conditions is each type of laxative preferred? Develop guidelines for counseling clients who have problems with fecal elimination.**
5. **Prepare teaching posters on hygienic measures to correct constipation and foods that promote good bowel habits.**

UNIT NINE

Drugs affecting the endocrine system

30 ▪ *Drugs that regulate steroidal hormone levels*

Hormones are glandular secretions, produced by organs and tissues, that are transported through the bloodstream to other tissues, in which they alter the rate of cellular processes. Steroid hormones help maintain blood volume and blood pressure, influence metabolic processes, and determine sexuality and sexual function. The following exercises deal with corticosteroids and sex hormones.

Matching

Match each therapeutic use listed in the left-hand column with the appropriate glucocorticoid dosage schedule in the right-hand column.

_______ 1. Treatment of severe acute allergic reactions
_______ 2. Replacement therapy
_______ 3. Treatment of collagen diseases
_______ 4. Prevention of cerebral edema
_______ 5. Prevention of sympathetic ophthalmia

a. Dosage at fixed intervals around the clock
b. Administration of doses every other day
c. Administration of a dose daily on arising
d. Administration of a dose daily at the hour of sleep

Correct the false statement

Indicate whether the following statements are true or false; if false, correct the underlined words or phrases.

_______ 1. In most treatment situations, the drug action of the glucocorticoids is palliative rather than curative.

_______ 2. Allergic reactions to the glucocorticoids rarely, if ever, occur because these drugs suppress the immune system.

_______ 3. Persons receiving glucocorticoid replacement therapy should increase their drug dosage twofold or more when experiencing unusual stress.

_______ 4. When glucocorticoids are prescribed once daily, or once every other day, the drugs should be given after breakfast.

_______ 5. Glucocorticoid therapy may produce psychological dependence because of its stimulant and euphorigenic properties.

_______ 6. When long-term therapy with prednisone is prescribed, for anti-inflammatory effect, antirheumatic drugs such as phenylbutazone are contraindicated for all members of the family.

_______ 7. Clients receiving high doses of glucocorticoids are likely to experience daytime drowsiness.

_______ 8. The likelihood of systemic reaction to over-the-counter ointments and creams containing cortisone is minimized because cortisone is not absorbed transdermally.

_______ 9. When therapeutic glucocorticoids are prescribed for persons with a history of tuberculosis, antimycobacterial drugs are very likely to be prescribed also.

_______ 10. Mineralocorticoids probably alter kidney function by enhancing the effects of antidiuretic hormone.

_______ 11. Mineralocorticoids such as aldosterone affect renal function by promoting potassium reabsorption and sodium excretion.

_______ 12. Clients receiving parenteral mineralocorticoids should be monitored for irritation or inflammation at injection sites.

_______ 13. A diagnostic test that is unlikely to be ordered for clients receiving mineralocorticoids is fasting blood sugar.

_______ 14. When mineralocorticoid therapy is initiated for the treatment of Addison's disease, clients are apt to exhibit a high sensitivity to the drugs.

_______ 15. High doses are avoided when mineralocorticoid therapy is initiated because of a high risk of hypotensive shock.

_______ 16. Desoxycorticosterone should usually be given with a fine-gauge needle.

_______ 17. A mineralocorticoid preparation that also has glucocorticoid properties is desoxycorticosterone.

_______ 18. In general, clients receiving glucocorticoids for replacement therapy are less likely to recover endocrine function than are those receiving replacement mineralocorticoids.

_______ 19. Sex hormones are produced endogenously only by the gonads.

_______ 20. Normal genital development *in utero* is dependent in part on testosterone in both sexes.

_______ 21. Production of androgens in males is higher *in utero* than is production of the hormones during prepubescent childhood.

_______ 22. Sex hormones generally enhance catabolism.

_______ 23. In both sexes, high levels of sex hormones tend to stimulate epiphyseal closure and halt growth.

_______ 24. Androgens prescribed for anabolic effects are free of masculinizing properties.

_______ 25. The addition of androgens to drug regimens of clients receiving anticoagulants tends to cause decreased therapeutic response to the anticoagulant.

_______ 26. The hormones most often used in the treatment of cancer of the prostate are androgens.

_______ 27. Oral administration of natural androgens is more effective than is oral administration of synthetic androgens.

_______ 28. Adverse reactions to buccal or sublingual administration of androgens include tissue irritation at the site of administration.

_______ 29. The production of sex hormones in the body fluctuates more markedly in young men than it does in young women.

_______ 30. In a young adult woman with adequate estrogen concentrations, the skin is thicker than it is in estrogen-deficient women.

_______ 31. Estrogens can function as both estrogenic and antiestrogenic substances.

_______ 32. An estrogen that is stored in large amounts in fatty tissue is estriol.

_______ 33. Estrogens applied topically do not exert systemic effects.

_______ 34. Risks of adverse effects of hormone contraceptives are usually as high as those stemming from pregnancy.

_______ 35. Estrogen therapy is contraindicated during pregnancy and lactation.

_______ 36. During menopause, hot flashes tend to subside as time passes.

_______ 37. Following menopause, most women will need to use more soap for skin care than they did at younger ages.

_______ 38. Natural progesterone is metabolized more rapidly by the liver than are synthetic or semisynthetic progestogens.

_______ 39. Contraindications for progesterone are similar to those for <u>estrogens</u>.

_______ 40. The use of progestogen contraceptives tends to <u>decrease</u> the incidence and severity of acute asthma.

Short answer questions

1. List at least four signs or symptoms of primary corticosteroid deficiency.

2. When cortisone ointments or creams are administered topically, are the drugs absorbed systemically?

3. List at least ten adverse signs or symptoms of high doses of cortisone.

4. Identify at least eight baseline data parameters that should be assessed before glucocorticoid therapy is begun.

5. Why is stress management important for clients receiving glucocorticoids?

6. What effects do mineralocorticoids have on fluid and electrolyte balances?

7. Identify at least ten signs or symptoms of mineralocorticoid toxicity.

8. List at least six parameters that should be monitored in clients receiving mineralocorticoids.

9. What risks are imposed by the use of androgens in young males?

10. How useful are androgens in the treatment of delayed maturation in young males?

11. Are anabolic androgens safe for use by male athletes to enhance muscular development?

12. What type of diet should be given to clients receiving anabolic androgens?

13. Which hormones have stronger anabolic effects, estrogens or androgens?

14. Which sex hormones are considered to be diabetogenic?

15. Is impotence an unavoidable consequence of effective estrogen therapy for cancer of the prostate?

16. Are estrogens used to treat acne in pubescent women?

17. Name three factors usually considered to be indications for the use of estrogen replacement therapy in postmenopausal women.

18. List three conditions whose risks appear to be increased by ample estrogen levels in postmenopausal women.

19. Identify two recommendations appropriate for women who wish to correct postmenopausal hirsutism.

20. Name one antiestrogenic drug currently available for clinical use.

Multiple choice questions

For each of the following, choose the one best answer:

1. Most hormone drugs that are administered by mouth are
   a. salts
   b. proteins
   c. steroids
   d. iodinated amines
2. When glucocorticoids are administered as replacement therapy, what adjustments in dosage are required to compensate for environmental factors affecting hormone need?
   a. Dosage is increased in accord with increased dietary intake.
   b. Five to fifteen extra units are administered, depending on results of urine glucose tests.
   c. Dosage is decreased by a third to a half when environmental stress stimulates endogenous stress hormone secretion.
   d. Dosage is increased twofold to threefold according to the level of environmental stress.
3. The physiologic effects of prednisone include
   a. a tendency to develop hypoglycemia
   b. delayed coagulation
   c. inhibition of the growth of pathogenic microorganisms
   d. reduction in the inflammatory response
4. A chronic inadequacy of corticosteroid secretion may cause
   a. hypertension
   b. inhibition of adrenocorticotropin secretion
   c. signs and symptoms of pregnancy
   d. masculinization in females
5. Anabolic androgens are approved for medicinal use to
   a. stimulate tissue rebuilding in debilitating diseases
   b. increase muscle mass in professional athletes
   c. replace male sex hormones in deficient postpubertal men
   d. stimulate sexual maturation in cases of male hormone deficiency
6. Estrogen replacement hormone therapy of postmenopausal women is avoided by many physicians because maintenance of high estrogen levels for prolonged periods after menopause increases the risk of
   a. infertility
   b. osteoporosis
   c. cardiovascular disease
   d. uterine malignancies
7. Side effects of estrogen administration to men include
   a. genital atrophy
   b. priapism
   c. urinary retention
   d. hair loss
8. The preferred treatment of dyspareunia caused by vaginal atrophy in postmenopausal women is
   a. avoidance of intercourse
   b. topical lubricants applied vaginally prior to intercourse
   c. topical estrogen creams applied vaginally following intercourse
   d. systemic estrogens to supply complete hormone replacement

9. Fluctuation in therapeutic response to mineralocorticoids may be minimized by manipulation of the intake of
   a. carbohydrates
   b. fluids
   c. phosphate
   d. sodium
10. Abrupt withdrawal of high doses of glucocorticoids is likely to cause
   a. hypertensive crisis
   b. hypotension and a tendency toward shock
   c. formation of abnormal clots and emboli
   d. inhibition of pituitary secretion of corticotropin
11. The glucocorticoid preparation most likely to be used to prevent cerebral edema is
   a. cortisone
   b. dexamethasone
   c. hydrocortisone
   d. prednisone
12. The major role of the glucocorticoids in normal physiology is
   a. maintaining strong bones
   b. maintaining adequate immune response
   c. moderating coagulation to prevent abnormal clots
   d. assisting the body to adapt to stress
13. Glucocorticoids used as antineoplastics are most effective in the treatment of
   a. solid tumors
   b. genital malignancies
   c. skin cancer
   d. lymphomas
14. When used in the treatment of adrenogenital syndrome, glucocorticoids reduce the signs and symptoms of masculinization by
   a. inactivating androgens in the body
   b. enhancing estrogenic responses in the body
   c. inhibiting pituitary secretion of adrenocorticotropin
   d. inhibiting androgen production in the testes
15. Hormones useful in the treatment of postpartum afterpains are
   a. estrogens
   b. antiestrogens
   c. androgens
   d. progestogens
16. What effect do the glucocorticoids have on wound healing?
   a. They accelerate it by promoting cell division.
   b. They delay it by inhibiting cell division.
   c. They prevent delay in wound healing caused by inflammation.
   d. They prevent delay in wound healing caused by infection.
17. The physiologic effects of progesterone are dependent in part on adequate tissue concentrations of
   a. androgens
   b. estrogens
   c. cell membrane receptors
   d. somatotropin
18. What effect do androgens have on body lipids?
   a. They increase LDH and VLDL serum concentrations.
   b. They increase HDL serum concentrations.
   c. They increase subcutaneous fat deposits.
   d. They increase body stores of cholesterol.
19. Sex hormones are normally deactivated in the body by
   a. metabolism for energy through the Krebs cycle
   b. chemical transformation by the target cells
   c. liver enzyme metabolism
   d. urinary excretion
20. Mineralocorticoids are most likely to be prescribed for persons with
   a. Addison's disease
   b. Cushing's syndrome
   c. heat exhaustion
   d. diarrhea
21. A mineralocorticoid preparation that is effective when given orally is
   a. cortisone
   b. desoxycorticosterone
   c. fludrocortisone
   d. prednisone
22. Anabolic androgenic hormones are used therapeutically to treat
   a. postpubertal cryptorchidism
   b. aplastic anemia
   c. male impotence
   d. postpartum breast engorgement

23. A potentially fertile female baby may be born with external genitalia that appear to be male if, *in utero,*
    a. estrogen levels were deficient
    b. progesterone levels were deficient
    c. androgen levels were deficient
    d. androgen levels were excessive

Selection of options

For each of the following, select *all* the appropriate responses. Circle the correct answers.

1. The effects of glucocorticoids on the central nervous system include
    a. general stimulation
    b. blunting of sensory perception
    c. inhibition of antidiuretic hormone secretion
    d. inhibition of somatotropin secretion
2. Glucocorticoid therapy is often employed in the treatment of
    a. autoimmune diseases
    b. atherosclerosis
    c. hypertension
    d. acute allergic reactions
    e. malignant neoplasms
    f. transplant rejection
    g. infections
    h. intracranial trauma
3. Although the general action of glucocorticoids is to increase water retention and edema, their anti-inflammatory action effectively reduces harmful edema in persons with
    a. brain trauma
    b. intracranial metastases
    c. lymphatic metastases
    d. pyelonephritis
    e. glomerulonephritis
4. Drugs that should be avoided when glucocorticoids are administered for drug effect include
    a. antihistamines such as Chlor-Trimeton
    b. histamine$_2$-receptor antagonists such as cimetidine
    c. antirheumatics such as aspirin or phenylbutazone
    d. potassium-sparing diuretics such as spironolactone
    e. vaccines and toxoids
    f. anticoagulants
5. The use of drug dosages of glucocorticoids is likely to be associated with increased need for
    a. antacids such as aluminum hydroxide
    b. antimycobacterials such as isoniazid
    c. antibiotics such as penicillin
    d. hemostatic agents such as clotting factor VIII
    e. sodium in the diet
    f. calcium in the diet
    g. potassium in the diet
6. Caution must be exercised when glucocorticoids are prescribed for
    a. postmenopausal women and elderly men
    b. persons with seizure disorder
    c. persons with liver impairment
    d. persons with renal impairment
    e. persons with osteoporosis
7. Relative contraindications for glucocorticoid therapy include
    a. childhood
    b. pregnancy
    c. lactation
    d. advanced age
    e. positive tuberculin reaction
8. Persons receiving glucocorticoids should be monitored for signs and symptoms of
    a. hypertension
    b. hypotension
    c. infection
    d. delayed healing
    e. inflammation
    f. peptic ulcer
    g. thromboemboli
    h. diabetes mellitus
    i. sodium imbalance
    j. potassium imbalance
    k. abnormal moods
    l. drowsiness
    m. weight gain
    n. cardiac abnormalities

9. Clients receiving pharmacologic doses of glucocorticoids should be advised to take a diet that is
   a. low in sodium
   b. low in potassium
   c. high in calories
10. The addition of prednisone to drug regimens increases the risk of toxicity from
   a. antibiotics
   b. digitalis
   c. potassium-sparing diuretics
   d. potassium-wasting diuretics
11. What effect do estrogens have on body lipids?
   a. They decrease LDH and VLDH serum concentrations.
   b. They decrease HDL serum concentrations.
   c. They increase biliary excretion of cholesterol.
   d. They increase subcutaneous fat deposits.
   e. They increase body stores of cholesterol.
12. Functions of androgens in females include
   a. normal reproductive development *in utero*
   b. enhancement of anabolic processes such as muscle building
   c. enhancement of libido
   d. stimulation of gonadotropin secretion by the pituitary
13. What drugs are likely to be prescribed to alleviate postpartum breast engorgement in nonnursing mothers?
   a. estrogens
   b. progestogens
   c. androgens
   d. glucocorticoid antagonists
14. Androgen therapy in men can cause
   a. gynecomastia
   b. urinary retention
   c. priapism
   d. permanent elevation of the voice register
   e. impaired sexual response
15. Young men receiving androgen replacement therapy should immediately report the development of
   a. sudden spurts in growth
   b. high fever
   c. a deepening of the voice
   d. priapism
16. Side effects of progesterone include
   a. breakthrough vaginal bleeding
   b. suppression of part of the immune response
   c. enhancement of the effects of prolactin
   d. formation of a mucous plug in the cervix
   e. a rise in body temperature
17. Normal young adult women who take exogenous estrogens are at increased risk for
   a. hypercholesterolemia
   b. cholelithiasis
   c. thrombophlebitis and thromboembolism
   d. hemorrhage
18. Body storage depots for estrogens include
   a. serum proteins
   b. the gonads
   c. fatty tissue
   d. the enterohepatic circulation
19. Estrogens are eliminated from the body by
   a. metabolism for energy through the Krebs cycle
   b. fecal elimination through bile
   c. excretion in urine
   d. chemical destruction by the target cells
20. Currently, estrogens are often used therapeutically
   a. to alleviate acute symptoms of menopause
   b. as contraceptives
   c. to treat hormone-dependent breast cancers in postmenopausal women
   d. to treat cancer of the prostate in men
21. Risks of adverse reactions to estrogen therapy are increased in women who
   a. smoke cigarettes
   b. drink alcoholic beverages
   c. are more than 35 years of age
   d. are less than 20 years of age
   e. have never had children
22. Estrogen therapy may increase the severity of
   a. hypercholesterolemia
   b. thromboemboli
   c. migraine
   d. manic depressive psychosis
   e. seizure disorders
   f. peptic ulcer disease
   g. diabetes mellitus
   h. cholelithiasis

23. Women at high risk for estrogen deficiency after menopause tend to
  a. be more obese then their age peers
  b. have smaller bones than their age peers
  c. weigh less than their age peers
24. Young women at high risk for post-menopausal estrogen deficiencies may reduce the eventual need for high-dose estrogen therapy by
  a. increasing their consumption of protein
  b. increasing their consumption of calcium
  c. engaging in active weight-bearing exercise
  d. restricting vitamin D intake
25. Signs and symptoms that should be reported immediately when they occur in women receiving estrogen therapy include
  a. nausea
  b. tenderness in the calf
  c. bloating
  d. pain on dorsiflexion of the foot
  e. sudden neurologic deficit (paralysis, aphasia)

31 ▪ *Drugs that affect sexual behavior and reproduction*

Fertility and sexual responses are affected by many factors, including the health status of the person, hormonal levels, psychosocial influences, and growth and development.

Multiple choice questions

For each of the following, choose the one best answer:

1. Luteinizing hormone (LH) stimulates
   a. lactation
   b. ovulation
   c. placental growth
   d. uterine contractions
2. The decrease in serum levels of estrogens at menopause increases the risk of
   a. mental illness
   b. hypertension
   c. memory loss
   d. coronary thrombosis
3. To prevent osteoporosis, menopausal women should be encouraged to ingest adequate
   a. calcium
   b. iron
   c. protein
   d. vitamins
4. A common complication resulting from osteoporosis is
   a. atherosclerosis
   b. bone fractures
   c. dysmenorrhea
   d. hypercalcemia
5. Treatment commonly prescribed for premenstrual syndrome (PMS) includes
   a. estrogen
   b. progesterone
   c. high calcium snacks
   d. vitamin D
6. The reason estrogen is prescribed in a cyclic fashion with progestogen is to reduce the risk of
   a. endometrial carcinoma
   b. ischemic heart disease
   c. osteoporosis
   d. vaginal atrophy
7. Which guidelines should be followed for the use of a condom to prevent pregnancy?
   a. Additional contraceptive protection must be used to increase effectiveness greater than 90 percent.
   b. Coverage should extend over the entire penis with no space at the tip.
   c. Additional spermicide must be used if the condom is reused.
   d. The same condom can be reused only if intercourse takes place again within five minutes.
8. Drugs that have adverse effects causing impairment of sexual function include
   a. bethanechol
   b. lithium
   c. phenytoin
   d. ranitidine

Sequences

Arrange the following by numbering in order of occurrence during the ovarian cycle.

_______ Degenerating corpus luteum
_______ Mature corpus luteum
_______ Primary follicle
_______ Ovulation
_______ Growing follicle
_______ Mature follicle
_______ Early corpus luteum

Completion exercises

Read each question carefully and place your answer in the space provided.

1. A female hormone that affects height in growing girls is _____. An increase in this hormone at puberty limits height through two actions, which are ______________________________.
2. Two female sex hormones produced in the interior lobe of the pituitary gland during the menstrual cycle are ______________________________ and ______________________________.
3. In the following table, describe the action and time of the highest level of each of these hormones during the menstrual cycle.

Hormone	Action	Time of Highest Level
FHS	______________________	______________________
LH	______________________	______________________

Correct the false statement

Indicate whether the following statements are true or false; if false, correct the underlined words or phrases.

_______ 1. In high doses, alcohol <u>increases sexual desire</u>.
_______ 2. Thiazides may cause <u>impotence</u>.
_______ 3. β-blockers <u>have no effect on sexual response</u>.

Matching

Match the method of contraception in the left-hand column with the descriptive phrase in the right-hand column. Place your answer in the space provided.

_______	1. Nonpharmacologic methods	a. Predictive test for ovulation
_______	2. Barrier methods	b. Absolute compliance
_______	3. Monoclonal antibody test	c. May be irreversible
_______	4. Oral contraceptives	d. Fertility awareness
_______	5. Surgical methods	e. Used in conjunction with spermicide

Short answer questions

1. Systemic illness may cause sexual problems. Name one sexual problem that can be anticipated in each of the following disorders:
   a. Diabetes mellitus: ______________________________
   b. Cardiovascular disease: ______________________________
   c. Kidney disease: ______________________________
   d. Thyroid deficiency: ______________________________
2. List at least five factors that may affect sperm production in a 25-year-old man.

3. Name at least three medications that are helpful in treating dysmenorrhea and describe their actions.

4. Identify two nonpharmacologic methods for decreasing premenstrual symptoms.

5. Osteoporosis sometimes occurs secondary to menopause. List two possible preventive measures.

32 ▪ *Drugs that regulate blood glucose levels*

The following exercises deal with substances used pharmacologically to control blood glucose levels.

Correct the false statement

Indicate whether the following statements are true or false; if false, correct the underlined words or phases.

______ 1. Protein hormones tend to act more rapidly than do steroid hormones.

______ 2. Protein hormones are degraded at the receptor site by the target tissue.

______ 3. The effects of insulin are anabolic rather than catabolic.

______ 4. Insulin is frequently administered orally.

______ 5. Insulin preparations require constant refrigeration.

______ 6. Porcine insulin is generally less antigenic than is bovine insulin.

______ 7. Insulin has a relatively low therapeutic index.

______ 8. Hyperglycemic ketoacidosis usually develops more rapidly than does hypoglycemic insulin reaction.

______ 9. If solid deposits are visible in an insulin solution, the vial should be rotated gently to redissolve the precipitate.

______ 10. The action of glucagon is generally similar *to* that of insulin.

______ 11. The structure of glucagon of animal origin differs somewhat from that of human glucagon.

______ 12. Glucagon has a wide margin of safety.

Short answer questions

1. Name at least two hormones with simple protein structures.

2. How are protein hormones and their metabolites excreted?

3. Identify the physiologic change that stimulates insulin secretion.

4. Identify two risk factors for allergy to insulin.

5. Why is it desirable to warm refrigerated insulin prior to injection?

6. Is it advisable for a newly diagnosed diabetic to be refracted for corrective eyeglasses?

7. Name at least five effects of insulin.

8. List at least three conditions required for proper storage of the insulin bottle in current use.

9. Name two antidotes for insulin toxicity.

10. When preparing mixtures of regular and modified insulin, which type of insulin should be drawn into the syringe first?

11. How frequently can successive doses of glucagon be administered?

12. How long does it take for injected glucagon to exert peak action?

13. How long does the blood sugar level remain elevated following onset of action of glucagon?

Questions 1–5 are based on the following situation. Choose the one best answer for each question.

Situation: Mrs. D. has responded well to treatment for diabetic ketoacidosis during her 6-day hospital stay. She has recovered from the infection that precipitated the episode, and is to be discharged as soon as she has been stabilized on a new regimen of insulin and diet. For the past 2 days she has been on a 1,500-calorie ADA diet and has been receiving 20 units NPH (isophane) insulin before breakfast daily, with regular insulin coverage for AC or HS glycosuria.

1. When NPH insulin is administered once daily, before breakfast, hypoglycemic reactions are most likely to occur
   a. 2 hours after the drug is injected
   b. at midday (before lunch)
   c. before the third meal of the day (supper)
   d. during early morning sleep
2. Factors that reduce the body's need for insulin include
   a. exercise
   b. increase in stress levels
   c. interrupted therapy
   d. none of the above—the need for insulin is affected only by the level of pancreatic islet function and calorie intake
3. While you are making rounds at the beginning of the evening shift (4 P.M.), Mrs. D. complains of a headache and slight nausea. When taking her pulse, you note that her hand trembles slightly and feels cool and moist. It is most likely that Mrs. D. is experiencing
   a. a relapse into ketoacidosis
   b. an insulin reaction
   c. respiratory alkalosis from hyperventilation
   d. none of the above; there are insufficient data given to indicate the problem
4. In preparation for discharge, it would be appropriate to teach Mrs. D. that
   a. insulin action is not influenced by changes in stress levels
   b. exercise decreases the risk of insulin reaction
   c. the bedtime snack provided in her diet will help prevent insulin reactions in the early night hours
5. The day Mrs. D. is to be discharged, she is notified that her husband is in the emergency room after experiencing chest pain at work. Her reaction to this sudden stressor is likely to
   a. increase the risk of insulin reaction
   b. increase the risk of hyperglycemia
   c. both a and b
   d. neither a nor b

For each of the following, choose the one best answer:

6. Hormones derived from an amino acid include
   a. epinephrine
   b. luteinizing hormone
   c. norepinephrine
   d. thyrotropin
   e. thyroxine
7. By what gland is insulin secreted?
   a. the pituitary
   b. the thyroid
   c. the adrenal cortex
   d. the pancreas
8. A drug that masks the symptoms of insulin reaction is
   a. aspirin
   b. vitamin C
   c. IV saline solution
   d. propranolol
9. Clients who are to receive only one insulin injection daily usually take it
   a. before breakfast
   b. during lunch
   c. early evening
   d. at bedtime
10. Clients receiving daily doses of long-lasting insulin in the morning are most likely to experience hypoglycemia
    a. before breakfast
    b. before lunch
    c. before supper or at bedtime
    d. during sleep
11. To treat insulin reaction in a conscious client, the nurse should administer
    a. orange juice
    b. grape juice
    c. a protein
    d. Gatorade
12. The wife of an insulin-dependent diabetic asks you, "What should I do if my husband appears to be ill but I cannot tell whether he has high or low blood glucose?" Your best reply is:
    a. Delay treatment until the signs and symptoms clearly indicate the problem.
    b. Treat both possible problems by administering food and insulin.
    c. Administer insulin to prevent dangerous hyperglycemia.
    d. Administer food to prevent dangerous hypoglycemia.
13. To correct hypoglycemia, glucagon is usually administered
    a. orally
    b. subcutaneously
    c. intramuscularly
    d. intravenously
14. The most critical need of the client in hypoglycemic insulin reaction is correction of
    a. glucose deprivation in the brain
    b. fluid volume deficit
    c. acid-based imbalance
    d. central nervous system depression
15. Insulin preparations that can be added to glucose solutions for intravenous administration are distinguishable from other insulin preparations by
    a. their origin as products of recombinant DNA techniques
    b. their origin as biological products of animal slaughter or bacterial cultures
    c. their duration of action, which is prolonged by addition of a metallic ion
    d. their solubility as shown by the clarity of the solution
16. Most parenteral solutions of insulin contain drug concentrations of
    a. 1 mg/ml
    b. 100 U/ml
    c. 200 U/ml
    d. 500 U/ml
17. When insulin is to be given IV, what preparation is used?
    a. NPH
    b. Protamine zinc
    c. Lente
    d. Regular
18. Which of the following is most likely to contribute to the development of diabetes mellitus?
    a. Hyperlipemia
    b. Obesity
    c. Hypertension
    d. Vitamin D deficiency
19. The incomplete metabolism of which of the following leads to ketoacidosis?
    a. Carbohydrates
    b. Fats
    c. Proteins
    d. Minerals
    e. Vitamins

20. Which of the following is characteristic of IDDM rather than of NIDDM?
    a. It usually is the milder of the two types of diabetes
    b. The pancreas still produces insulin
    c. Mostly older adults are affected
    d. It usually develops in childhood
21. Hypoglycemia during night sleep is most likely to be manifested by
    a. convulsions
    b. diaphoresis
    c. coma
    d. hyperpnea (Kussmaul breathing)
22. When insulin syringes are used for more than one injection, their use should generally be limited to
    a. a period not exceeding 3 days
    b. a maximum of five injections
    c. injection of regular (crystalline zinc) insulin
    d. doses that do not exceed 0.5 ml in volume
23. Insulin used for "coverage" is usually
    a. isophane insulin
    b. lente insulin
    c. protamine zinc insulin
    d. regular insulin
24. Physiologic effects of insulin include:
    a. decrease in blood sugar levels
    b. decrease in glycogen stores
    c. decrease in fat deposition
    d. decrease in energy production
    e. decrease in protein and nucleic acid synthesis
    f. ketoacidosis
25. Among the signs and symptoms of IDDM is
    a. Weight gain
    b. Thirst
    c. Nervousness
    d. Edema
26. Sometimes sodium bicarbonate is given to a client in diabetic coma. The purpose of this treatment is to reduce
    a. fluid overload
    b. metabolic acidosis
    c. metabolism of carbohydrates
27. Which of the following is a fast-acting insulin?
    a. Lente
    b. NPH
    c. Protamine zinc
    d. Regular
28. Use of alcohol by clients receiving oral hypoglycemics may cause
    a. a disulfiramlike reaction
    b. severe gastric irritation
    c. excessive sedation
    d. an increased risk of hyperglycemia
29. To prevent lipohypertrophy from insulin injections, the client should
    a. encourage regular daily exercise
    b. rotate the injection sites
    c. administer insulin intramuscularly
    d. store insulin in the refrigerator
30. Among the signs and symptoms of a suddenly lowered blood sugar is
    a. trembling
    b. polyphagia
    c. thirst
    d. frequent urination
31. To treat a coma induced by insulin overdose, administer
    a. oral glucagon
    b. sodium bicarbonate
    c. sweetened orange juice
    d. IV glucose
32. Among the signs and symptoms of diabetic ketoacidosis are
    a. a sudden onset of symptoms
    b. warm, dry, flushed skin
    c. anxious, excited behavior
    d. excessive sweating
33. Which of the following is most likely to precede an insulin reaction?
    a. Weight gain
    b. Missed meal
    c. A febrile illness
    d. A stressful situation
34. Long-term treatment with sulfonylurea hypoglycemics increase the risk of
    a. Kidney failure
    b. Liver failure
    c. Heart disease
    d. Lung disease
35. After initial resolution of acute hypoglycemia in an insulin-dependent diabetic, recurrent insulin toxicity may be prevented by
    a. alleviating the client's stress
    b. feeding the client
    c. having the client exercise
    d. withholding food from the client

36. Glucagon is not administered orally because
   a. its onset of action by this route is too slow
   b. it is highly irritating to the gastric mucosa
   c. its structure is destroyed by digestive enzymes
   d. it is metabolized in high quantities by first pass through the liver
37. Glucagon injections to correct a hypoglycemic episode may be repeated
   a. once only
   b. up to 3 times
   c. up to 5 times
   d. not at all; only one dose is used
38. Doses of glucagon are measured in
   a. grams
   b. grains
   c. micrograms
   d. units
39. Following successful treatment with glucagon of hypoglycemia caused by exogenous insulin, clients should be given
   a. a sweet food
   b. starches and proteins
   c. fats such as cream or butter
   d. ample fluids
40. Following successful treatment of hypoglycemia with glucagon, most clients should be given
   a. sugar, candy, or jelly to eat
   b. a meat sandwich or crackers and cheese to eat
   c. a fatty food such as artificially sweetened ice cream
   d. low-calorie fluids such as dietetic Kool-Aid

Selection of options

For each of the following, select *all* of the appropriate responses. Circle correct answers.

1. Chemical structures of nonsteroidal endocrine hormones include:
   a. simple proteins
   b. glycoproteins
   c. lipoproteins
   d. amino acid derivatives
2. Hormones derived from a single amino acid include:
   a. epinephrine
   b. luteinizing hormone
   c. norepinephrine
   d. thyrotropin
   e. thyroxine
   f. triiodothyronine
3. Physiologic effects of insulin include:
   a. decrease in blood sugar levels
   b. decrease in glycogen stores
   c. decrease in fat deposition
   d. increased energy production
   e. increased protein and nucleic acid synthesis
   f. ketoacidosis
4. Therapeutic effects of insulin in persons with diabetes mellitus include:
   a. decrease in blood sugar levels
   b. increased energy production from carbohydrate metabolism
   c. increased energy production from protein metabolism
   d. decreased breakdown of fatty tissue for energy
   e. decreased ketoacidosis
   f. enhanced growth in children
   g. a slowing of cardiovascular degeneration
5. Factors that enhance the action of insulin include:
   a. active exercise
   b. reduction in adiposity
   c. limitation of vitamin C intake
   d. reduction in stress
6. Of the following insulins, which may be administered intravenously?
   a. crystalline zinc insulin
   b. isophane insulin
   c. lente insulin
   d. protamine zinc insulin
   e. regular insulin
7. Drugs that tend to reverse the acute effects of insulin reaction include:
   a. cortisone
   b. epinephrine
   c. glucagon
   d. sugar

8. Hypoglycemia can be differentiated from hyperventilation syndrome because hypoglycemia is characterized by
   a. central nervous system stimulation
   b. little change in respirations
   c. headache
   d. flushing of the skin
9. Serious physiologic imbalances characteristic of diabetic acidosis include:
   a. hyperosmolarity of body fluids
   b. dehydration
   c. metabolic acidosis
   d. glucose deprivation in the brain
   e. hyperkalemia with depletion of body stores of potassium
   f. general tissue malnutrition
10. During titration of insulin dosages, clients should
    a. avoid excessive stress
    b. avoid active exercise
    c. maintain a normal diet
11. When using insulin, clients should
    a. keep all bottles of insulin refrigerated
    b. rotate the bottle gently to ensure even distribution of the drug in the solution
    c. warm the insulin bottle in warm water before drawing up the dose
    d. avoid injecting bubbles of air into the insulin solution
12. Insulin doses can be measured precisely with
    a. insulin syringes with scales marking even-numbered units of dosage
    b. insulin syringes with scales marking single units of dosage
    c. tuberculin syringes
    d. subcutaneous syringes with scales marking dosages in tenths of a milliliter
13. When administering insulin, the angle of insertion of the needle varies with
    a. the needle gauge
    b. the needle length
    c. the thickness of the client's skin
    d. the client's adiposity
14. Insulin preparations are produced by
    a. extraction from animal tissues
    b. chemical alteration of animal hormones
    c. genetic recombination techniques
    d. chemical synthesis
15. Oral hypoglycemics in current use in the United States include:
    a. acid-resistant insulin
    b. biguanide compounds
    c. sulfonamides
    d. sulfonylureas
16. Clinical indications for the use of oral hypoglycemics include:
    a. insulin-dependent diabetes mellitus
    b. non-insulin-dependent diabetes mellitus
    c. inability to control diabetes mellitus by diet
    d. presence of cardiovascular pathology
    e. pregnancy
17. Drugs that interact with oral hypoglycemics to enhance their effects include:
    a. anti-inflammatory steroids
    b. oral anticoagulants
    c. sulfonamides
    d. salicylates
18. Adverse reactions to sulfonylurea drugs include:
    a. agranulocytosis
    b. cardiovascular disease
    c. stroke caused by severe hypoglycemia
    d. jaundice
19. Clients receiving sulfonylurea hypoglycemics should avoid the use of
    a. alcohol
    b. antibiotics
    c. glucocorticoids
    d. salicylates
20. The effects of glucagon on glucose balance include:
    a. increased blood concentration of glucose
    b. increased glycogenesis
    c. increased glycogenolysis
    d. increased gluconeogenesis
21. Because glucagon maintains a steady supply of glucose to tissues that are obligate users of this nutrient, it protects energy metabolism in the
    a. brain
    b. gonads
    c. skeletal muscles
    d. retina
22. An excess of glucagon would cause
    a. decreased severity of diabetes mellitus
    b. increased severity of diabetes mellitus
    c. impairment of brain metabolism
    d. decreased glycogenesis
23. Therapeutic uses of glucagon include:
    a. treatment of hypoglycemia
    b. treatment of hyperglycemia
    c. preparation for intestinal x-ray examination
    d. stimulation of intestinal motility

33 ▪ *Drugs that affect the thyroid, parathyroid, pituitary, and hypothalamic glands*

In addition to questions dealing with the content of Chapter 33, the following material includes exercises relating to all endocrine hormones (Chapters 30–32).

Matching

Match the hormone in the left-hand column with the function or factor that inhibits its production, thus completing a negative feedback mechanism, in the right-hand column.

_______ 1. Thyrotropin
_______ 2. ACTH
_______ 3. ADH
_______ 4. Gonadotropins
_______ 5. Mineralocorticoids
_______ 6. Calcitonin
_______ 7. Parathormone

a. Increased concentration of sex hormones
b. Increased serum concentration of glucocorticoids
c. Inceased osmolarity of body fluids
d. Increased serum concentration of thyroid hormone
e. Increased blood pressure
f. Decreased sodium concentration in body fluids
g. Increased calcium ion concentration in the serum
h. Decreased calcium ion concentration in the serum

Correct the false statement

Indicate whether the following statements are true or false; if false, correct the underlined words or phrases.

_______ 1. The effects of hormones used as drugs are highly specific, with a single hormone usually producing a single effect in the body.

_______ 2. Steroid hormones are destroyed by digestion and are usually administered parenterally.

_______ 3. Exogenous protein hormones rarely produce allergic reactions.

Short answer questions

1. The chemical structures of hormones are most often either _______________ or ____________.
2. What biochemical is the basic building block for steroid hormones?

3. Define Addison's disease.

4. Give at least two reasons why client assessment is particularly important when hormone therapy is in progress.

Multiple choice questions

For each of the following, choose the one best answer:

1. Steroid hormones are usually metabolized to inactive substances by the
   a. liver
   b. kidneys
   c. target cells on which they act
   d. digestive process
2. For the most part, steroid hormones and their metabolites are excreted
   a. in feces, by way of bile
   b. in urine
   c. by the lungs
   d. none of the above; these substances are metabolized for energy
3. A sex hormone with catabolic properties is
   a. estrone
   b. progesterone
   c. testosterone
   d. insulin

Crossword puzzle

Across

3. A glucocorticoid drug used to prevent cerebral edema
6. One name for ACTH
8. A drug that inhibits synthesis of thyroid hormones
11. A hormone that increases calcium concentration in body fluids
13. The metabolic process of body tissue breakdown
16. The hormones that exert the greatest effect on renal reabsorption of sodium and potassium
17. An antiestrogenic drug used as a fertility drug
18. The pituitary hormone that stimulates thyroid gland function
20. A radionuclide used to diagnose and treat thyroid pathology
23. A common adverse reaction to antithyroid drugs
25. Abbreviation for a trophic pituitary hormone
26. A drug preparation used to treat diabetes insipidus
29. A substance that causes thyrotropin secretion because of its inhibition of thyroid gland function
30. The hormones responsible for male secondary sex characteristics
31. An antiestrogenic drug used to treat cancer of the breast

Down

1. A disease characterized by deficiency of ADH
2. A hormone that increases basal metabolism
3. Abbreviation for a synthetic estrogen associated with increased risk of vaginal cancer in women exposed to it *in utero*
4. The metabolic process of building up body tissue
5. The pituitary hormone that stimulates glucocorticoid production by the adrenals
6. A unit for measuring radioactivity
7. A goitrogenic substance found in infant formulas
8. Abbreviation of the name of long-lasting insulin
9. A thyroid hormone used as a drug
10. A class of drug used to diagnose and treat thyroid pathology
12. A hormone that decreases calcium concentration in body fluids
14. The most frequently prescribed preparation of insulin
15. A pituitary hormone used medicinally to stimulate labor
19. The amino acid incorporated into thyroid hormone molecules
21. Growth hormone
22. A hormone whose actions reverse the effects of insulin
24. The hormone responsible for female secondary sex characteristics
27. A glucocorticoid drug used to treat chronic collagen disease
28. A nutrient that functions as an antidote for insulin toxicity

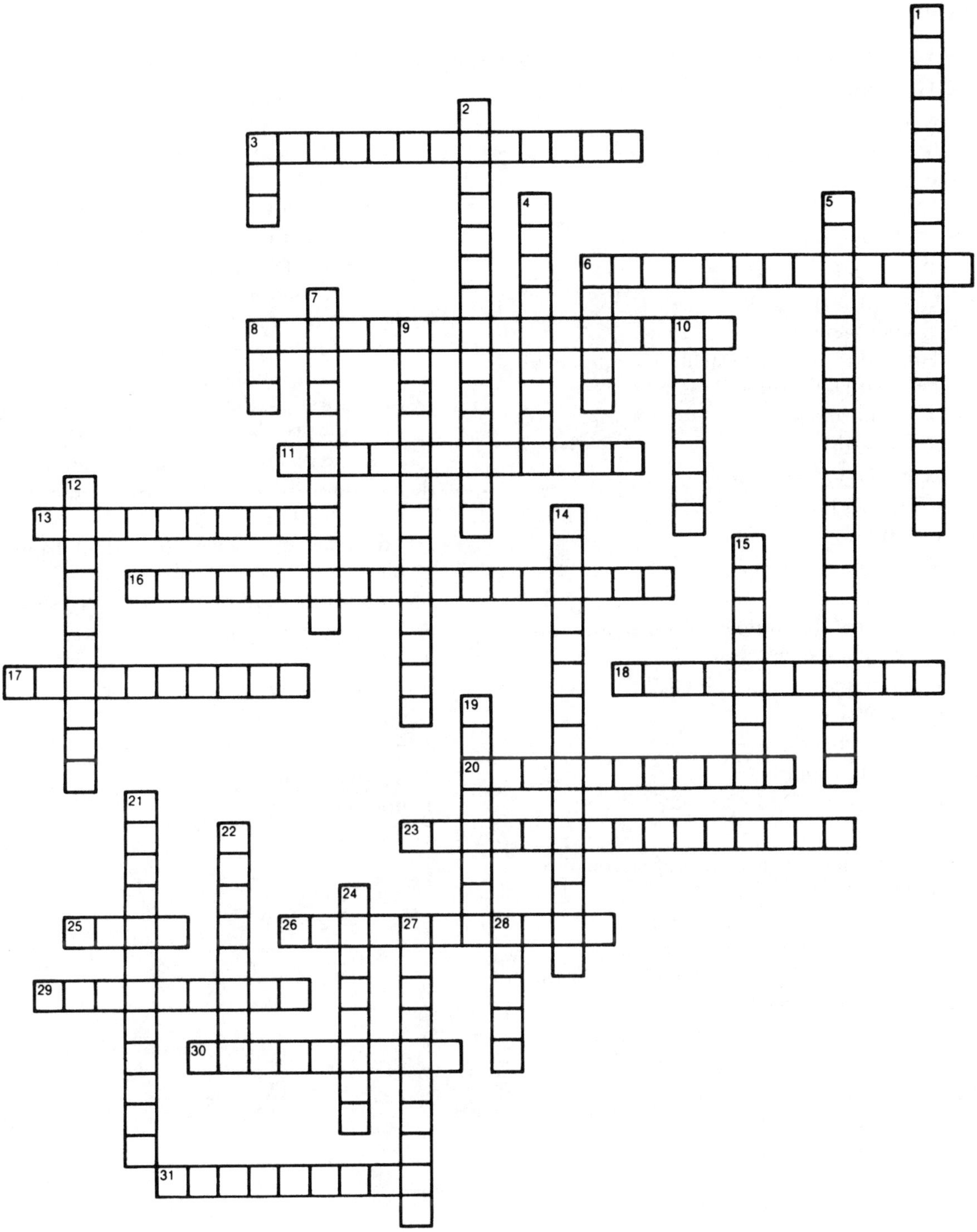
1
2
3
4
5
6
7
8
9
10
11
12
13
14
15
16
17
18
19
20
21
22
23
24
25
26
27
28
29
30
31

Selection of options

For each of the following, select *all* appropriate responses. Circle the correct answers.

1. Hormones with steroid structures include
   a. cortisone
   b. insulin
   c. thyroxine
   d. somatotropin
   e. aldosterone
   f. estrogen
   g. progesterone
   h. androgens
2. Hormones that are usually considered to be essential for survival include
   a. sex hormones
   b. glucocorticoids
   c. mineralocorticoids
   d. thyroid hormone
   e. insulin
   f. antidiuretic hormone
   g. somatotropin
3. Which of the following hormones are known teratogens?
   a. androgens
   b. estrogens
   c. progestogens
   d. somatotropin
   e. thyroxine
   f. ADH
4. The mechanism of action of steroid hormones usually involves
   a. interaction with a receptor site on the membrane of the target cell
   b. penetration of the cell membrane by the hormone molecule
   c. interaction with a cytoplasmic receptor protein
   d. alteration of the function of nuclear chromatin
   e. alteration of the nature of cell function
   f. alteration of the rate of cell function
5. Which of the following statements is (are) true of cholesterol?
   a. It is a toxic biochemical that performs no useful biologic function.
   b. When blood concentrations of cholesterol are high, there is an increased risk of cardiovascular degeneration.
   c. It is essential to life (in mammals).
   d. For humans, it is an essential dietary component.
   e. The body can make cholesterol from many other nutrient substances.
6. Hormones that are destroyed by digestive enzymes include
   a. androgens
   b. antidiuretic hormone
   c. epinephrine
   d. estrogens
   e. luteinizing hormone
   f. norepinephrine
   g. thyroxine

UNIT TEN
Drugs affecting the immune system

34 ▪ *Drugs that control allergies*

Allergic reactions may occur in persons sensitive to specific substances, including foods, fibers, environmental contaminants, and chemicals.

Completion exercises

Read each question carefully and place your answer in the space provided.

1. The most important factor in making an accurate diagnosis of an allergy is ________________ or, if a healthcare professional is present when the allergy develops, ____________ of symptoms.
2. Accurate reporting to the prescriber should include ________________ and ______________.
3. When possible, clinical verification should be avoided because ____.
4. Common food allergies are ________________________________.
5. Common medication allergens are ____.
6. Environmental factors causing allergies are ____.
7. Three body areas in which atopic eczema manifests itself in children are ________________, ________________, and ________________.
8. Treatment of allergic reactions, whenever possible, centers on ____________________, which requires accurate diagnosis.
9. Severe reactions may require medical intervention. One such intervention for anaphylactic shock is ________________________________.
10. Complete the following table of drugs that may cause a reaction.

Drug	Possible Side Effects or Secondary Effects	Possible Idiosyncrasy
Penicillin	________________	________________
Anticonvulsants	________________	________________
Chloramphenicol	________________	________________
Mercurial diuretics	________________	________________
Aspirin	________________	________________

Multiple choice questions

For each of the following, choose the one best answer:

1. Symptoms of urticaria include
   1. erythema
   2. skin elevation that blanches with pressure
   3. scaliness
   4. possible pruritis
   a. all of the above
   b. 1, 2, 4
   c. 2, 3, 4
   d. only 2
2. Drug reactions may be a result of which of the following?
   1. overdose because of synergism
   2. overdose because of client's condition
   3. lack of compliance
   4. personal idiosyncrasy
   5. side effects
   a. 1, 2, 4
   b. 3, 4, 5
   c. 1, 2, 5
   d. 2, 3, 4
   e. all of the above
3. Anaphylactic shock results most frequently from use of
   a. chloramphenicol
   b. thiazides
   c. penicillin
   d. aspirin
   e. all of the above
4. Thrombocytopenia may be associated with use of
   a. phenothiazines
   b. chloramphenicol
   c. phenacetin
   d. penicillin
   e. aspirin

Personal exercise: Allergies

Read each question carefully and write your answers on a separate sheet of paper.

1. Do you have any allergies? If so, in what form?
2. What medication do you take for this allergy?
3. Make up an allergy history for yourself, including such consideration as when allergies occur, possible causes, and how you treat them. (If you do not have an allergy, you may want to interview a friend or family member who has allergies.)

35 ▪ *Drugs that moderate the immune system*

The use of immunomodulating agents, such as immunizing agents, immunostimulants, and immunosuppressants, should take the individual status of the person into account, including such factors as age, medical conditions, allergies, and possible adverse reactions that might result with exposure to the agent.

Short answer questions

1. Immunization programs should be instituted during infancy, as recommended by the Committee of Infectious Diseases of the American Academy of Pediatrics, and continued through childhood. Give the appropriate age schedules for the following immunizations:
   a. DTP

   b. Td

   c. OPV

   d. MMR

2. Explain the rationale for the following statements:
   a. Smallpox vaccinations are no longer given routinely.

   b. Neonates at high risk for hepatitis B should be given HBV at birth.

   c. Mumps vaccine should be given to an unimmunized boy before adolescence.

   d. Anyone receiving immunization should be observed for 30 minutes following the procedure.

   e. Programs for HBV for healthcare workers have been instituted throughout the United States.

   f. Immunization programs should receive ongoing reevaluation.

Correct the false statement

Indicate whether the following statements are true or false; if false, correct the underlined words or phrases and place your answer in the space provided.

_______ 1. <u>All</u> infants are born with natural immunity.

_______ 2. Malnutrition is one factor <u>reducing the body's defenses</u> against disease.

_______ 3. Antibodies are supplied <u>only through the placenta, in colostrum, or by immunization with appropriate materials</u>.

Completion exercises

Read each question carefully and place your answer in the space provided.

1. Antibodies transmitted through the _______________ protect newborns against certain diseases to which their mothers have immunity.
2. Additional protection to the newborn is provided through _______________.
3. The antibody response occurs in reaction to a _______________.
4. The best protection against pertussis in newborns is adequate immunization of _______________.
5. Immunizations are contraindicated if the child has _______________.
6. Children should be instructed not to rub the site of an injection because _______________.
7. The client is receiving filgrastim (Neupogen) which is an example of a _______________.
8. Epoetin alfa might be used for the client with _______________.
9. A family of glycoproteins, the _______________, are produced by cells such as T-lymphocytes.

Multiple choice questions

For each of the following, choose the one best answer:

1. A child's defense system is usually activated between
   a. 9 and 12 months of age
   b. 6 and 15 months of age
   c. 16 and 30 months of age
   d. 3 and 15 months of age

2. What is the primary function of cytokines?
   a. production of immunoglobulins
   b. defense of body against bacteria
   c. phagocytosis
   d. immunopotentiation

36 ▪ *Drugs that treat inflammation*

The inflammatory process is composed of multiple physiologic responses to a stimulus and is primarily a protective mechanism essential for survival. Fever and pain are cardinal signs and symptoms of inflammation that may require intervention, including the use of certain medications. Some of the medications have an antipyretic action as one of their actions, meaning that they can reduce abnormally high body temperatures by suppressing inflammation or by resetting the hypothalamic thermostat toward normal levels. The drugs reviewed in this chapter include the salicylates, acetic acids, propionic acids, fenamates, pyrazoles, oxicams, para-aminophenol derivatives, gold compounds, certain drugs used in management of gout, and uricosurics.

Find the hidden words

Hidden within the following letter grid are words and phrases from Chapter 36. They may be vertical, horizontal, or diagonal. Circle the letters as you find the hidden words.

List of words and phrases

acetaminophen
aspirin
antipyretic
chill
crisis
dantrolene
fever
glucocorticoids
hypothalamic thermostat
hypothermia blanket
indomethacin
lysis
phenacetin
phenylbutazone
pyrogen
salicylates
thermometer
willow bark

```
l a n t k r a b w o l l i w c h d t o r a b d e l e
y s c l y s i n n a s a l i c y l a t e s a c l y n
s p h e n a c e t i n l l n p p c p n h p r o w s o
i i n d t l g l u i y g l u c o c o r t i c o i d s
r r i n d a e e m m p m p r d t h e r m r h n l a a
c i s e r d m r u y o y i n d h t l y s e o y l i c
a n l y e e c i i d h s r e f e v y s a o e l o h r
n d p h e r r n n d e l e e c r i s i s f d e e y i
t o y a i e d i e o y a v h t m c i n e a t u b n n
i m r s l t h e r h p e c r i i a s d e h e c a y e
f e v e r e t h e r p h h e c a c h i l l h r r e o
e t d e l m u u h y p o e a l b y y n y p z o k t m
t h e r m o b d d h p h e n y l b u t a z o n e h r
t a t s o m r e h t c i m a l a h t o p y h a t p e
a c e t o r l p y r r c c e s n h y p e r e s y w h
w i h h y e y h y p i h l a n k e t h y p y r o p t
a n t i y h n i p s p y r o g e n h y y n n s h y n
p h e n l t h e i n d o l l i t w o l l i s a l i c
```

 Study Guide to Accompany Clinical Pharmacology and Nursing Management, 5th edition

Matching

Match the following preparations listed by their generic name in the left-hand column with the trade names listed in the right-hand column. Place your answer in the space provided.

_______ 1. Phenylbutazone
_______ 2. Indomethacin
_______ 3. Ibuprofen
_______ 4. Naproxen
_______ 5. Nabumetone
_______ 6. Mefenamic acid

a. Tolectin
b. Butazolidin
c. Ponstel
d. Orudis
e. Relafen
f. Dolobid
g. Indocin
h. Nalfon
i. Clinoril
j. Naprosyn
k. Motrin

Multiple choice

For each of the following, choose the one best answer:

1. At the same time a chill begins, body temperature is most likely to be
   a. below normal
   b. normal, or slightly above normal
   c. markedly elevated
   d. rapidly fluctuating
2. Aspirin and acetaminophen reduce body temperature by
   a. directly stimulating perspiration
   b. inhibiting skeletal muscle contractility
   c. inhibiting contractility of smooth muscle in peripheral blood vessels
   d. resetting the hypothalamic thermostat to a lower setting
3. The use of antipyretics during a febrile illness may be delayed or restricted because fever
   a. mobilizes the body's defense systems
   b. often is harmful to pathogenic organisms causing such illnesses
   c. is a valuable diagnostic sign, and early reduction of body temperature may obscure diagnosis
   d. increases the inflammatory response significantly
4. Arrange the following series of events during a chill in chronologic order:
   1. a rise in body temperature
   2. vascular constriction and shivering
   3. an elevation of the "set" of the hypothalamic thermostat
   a. 1, 2, 3
   b. 1, 3, 2
   c. 2, 1, 3
   d. 3, 2, 1
5. A drug that is *not* used routinely, because of its adverse reactions, is
   a. acetylsalicylic acid
   b. phenylbutazone
   c. acetaminophen
   d. indomethacin
6. Colchicine is used in the management of
   a. gout
   b. ankylosing spondylitis
   c. rheumatic fever
   d. osteoarthritis
7. Ibuprofen is an example of a
   a. salicylate
   b. para-aminophenol derivative
   c. pyrazole
   d. propionic acid
8. Allopurinol (Zyloprim) achieves its therapeutic effects by
   a. increasing excretion of uric acid
   b. decreasing production of uric acid
   c. inhibiting prostaglandin synthetase activity
   d. interfering with platelet aggregation
9. Clients taking gold compounds should be assessed for
   a. stomatitis
   b. constipation
   c. nose bleeds
   d. tachycardia

Selection of options

For each of the following, select *all* appropriate responses. Circle the correct answers.

1. Drugs employed to control fever include
   a. thyroxin
   b. epinephrine
   c. ibuprofen
   d. morphine
   e. propoxyphene
   f. acetaminophen
   g. dantrolene
2. Headache can be a significant adverse reaction to
   a. indomethacin
   b. acetaminophen
   c. fenoprofen
   d. ibuprofen
3. Aspirin can cause adverse reactions of
   a. suppression of immune toxicity
   b. ototoxicity
   c. asthma as an allergic manifestation
   d. bleeding
   e. liver damage

Short answer questions

1. Identify at least four harmful effects of very high fevers.

2. Describe two effective methods for reducing body temperature in clients who do not respond to antipyretic drugs.

3. Explain the role of prostaglandins in the inflammatory process.

4. At what point in the process of prostaglandin synthesis do many drugs discussed in this chapter appear to interfere? How does this action help the client?

5. Identify three interventions to use when giving anti-inflammatory medications to lessen gastric irritation.

6. How do the therapeutic properties of the para-aminophenol derivatives differ from those of acetylsalicylic acid?

7. Review the process of acute poisoning with acetaminophen. How would it be managed?

8. What is the difference between primary and secondary gout?

9. Describe the mechanism of action of allopurinol.

10. Describe the use of probenecid as adjunct therapy with penicillin.

11. How can alkalinization of the urine be accomplished? Why might it be recommended?

UNIT ELEVEN
Drugs affecting other body systems

37 ▪ *Drugs that affect the respiratory tract*

A patent airway is the number one priority in nursing care. However, many general nursing measures also involve respiratory care of clients. Nurses are important in assisting clients to manage their respiratory disorders and to lead productive lives.

Short answer questions

1. Identify the following:
   a. P

   b. PO_2

   c. PCO_2

   d. PaO_2

   e. $PaCO_2$

2. Define the following:
   a. Oxygen tension:

   b. Oxygen saturation:

   c. Airway resistance:

   d. Bronchospasm:

e. Carbon dioxide narcosis:

f. Surfactant:

g. Hypoxia:

h. Hyperpnea:

i. Hypocapnia:

j. Diffusion capacity:

k. Cyanosis:

l. Anoxia:

m. Cor pulmonale:

3. Why is the nose important?

4. Describe why the nurse must be concerned if the nose is bypassed (i.e., in a mouth breather or a person with an endotracheal tube or tracheostomy tube).

5. Describe the action and importance of the mucociliary system and the mucous blanket.

6. List etiologic factors that inhibit mucociliary transport.

7. Explain the physiology of breathing.

8. Diagram in equation form an allergic person's response to an antigen leading to bronchospasm and bronchoconstriction.

9. Explain how the following produce bronchodilation:
   a. Sympathomimetics

   b. Anticholinergics

10. Discuss the relationship of hydration and sputum viscosity.

11. What is the effect of expectorants on the mucous blanket?

12. Describe the factors that inhibit or prevent learning in clients with respiratory dysfunctions.

13. List at least five goals for the client with a nursing diagnosis of respiratory impairment.

14. In which types of clients is the use of a spacer indicated?

15. Explain how surfactants produce therapeutic effects in premature infants with RDS.

Sequences

Arrange the following parts of the body in the order in which air from the atmosphere passes through in the breathing process by numbering each in sequence.

_______ Trachea
_______ Nose
_______ Pharynx
_______ Alveoli
_______ Bronchi
_______ Bronchial tree
_______ Larynx

Completion exercise

Read each question carefully and place your answer in the space provided.

1. Complete the following table on sympathomimetic drugs.

Drug	Receptor	Action	Adverse Reactions
Epinephrine	_______	_______	_______
Albuterol	_______	_______	_______
Metaproterenol	_______	_______	_______
Terbutaline	_______	_______	_______

Using the following word list, identify the parts of the upper and lower respiratory system shown in the two figures.

Nasal concha
Glottis
Bronchiole
Trachea

2. a. ____________________
   b. ____________________
   c. ____________________
   d. ____________________
   e. ____________________
   f. ____________________

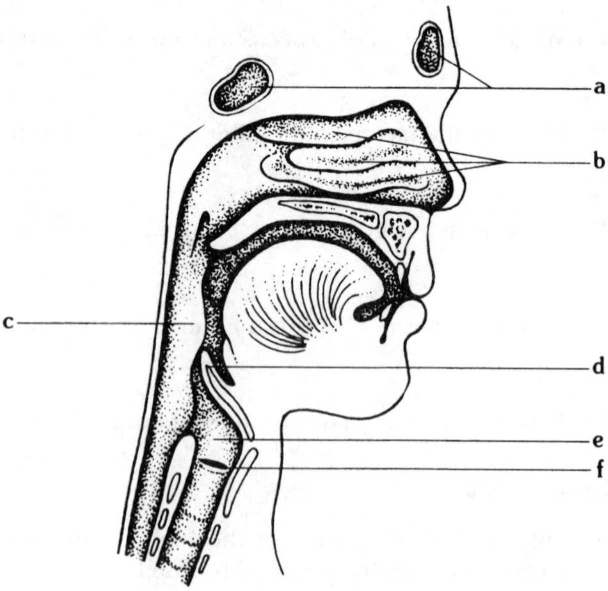

Bronchus
Larynx
Epiglottis
Alveolus
Pharynx

3. a. ____________________
   b. ____________________
   c. ____________________
   d. ____________________

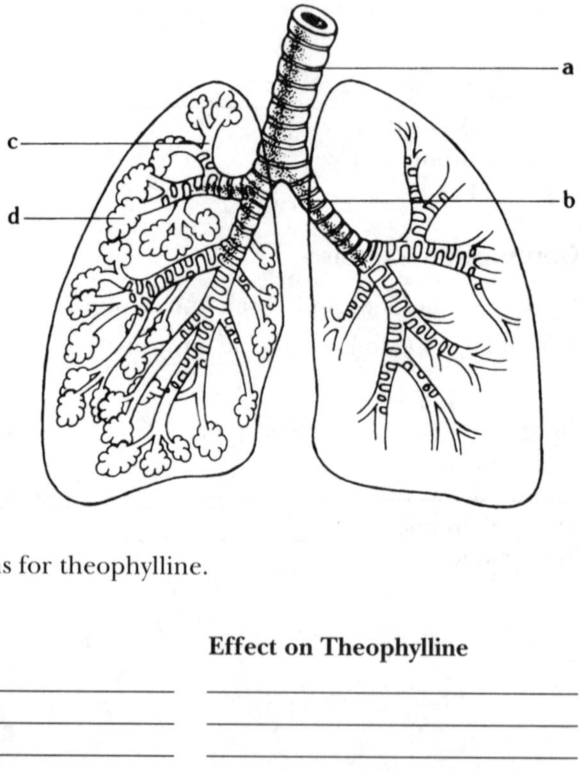

4. Complete the table of drug–drug interactions for theophylline.

	Drug	Effect on Theophylline
Cimetidine	____________________	____________________
Furosemide	____________________	____________________
Propranolol	____________________	____________________
Phenobarbital	____________________	____________________
Phenytoin	____________________	____________________
Smoking	____________________	____________________

Situational exercises

What would you do in the following situations? Write your answer in the space provided.

1. Mr. P.'s blood gases are as follows: pH, 7.31; PaO_2, 105; bicarbonate, 36.
   a. Postulate what stimulates this person's respiratory drive.

b. Compare with a normal person's respiratory drive.

c. List six symptoms that you would expect to find with Mr. P., based on his blood gases.

2. Mrs. G. is receiving theophylline. Her blood level is 25 μg/ml. What adverse reactions would you anticipate?

3. Mrs. S. has a diagnosis of asthma. She is being started on cromolyn sodium. What should she be taught with respect to its use prophylactically in contrast to use of other drugs for acute attacks?

4. Mr. T., who has long-standing emphysema, is cyanotic and dyspneic, and his blood gases reveal a PO_2 of 40 and PCO_2 of 110. Why would oxygen be used with extreme caution?

Personal exercises: Respiratory system

Read each question carefully and write your answers on a separate sheet of paper.

1. Try an intermittent positive breathing machine in a pulmonary laboratory. What does it feel like? Try a spirometer and determine the tidal volume. How does this compare with normal values?
2. Develop a teaching plan that you could use in showing a client the proper use and administration of some type of inhalant therapy.
3. Develop a care plan that would promote respiratory function for a client suffering from obstructive lung disease.

Learning experiences

1. **There are many terms and words with which you may become familiar. Define *trachea, oxygen tension, oxygen saturation, lung compliance, airway resistance, blood gases, bronchospasm, pulmonary function tests, carbon dioxide narcosis, surfactant, hypoxia, hypoxemia, hyperpnea, shunting, dead space, hypercapnia, hypocapnia, cor pulmonale, intermittent positive-pressure breathing machine, mucous blanket, alveolus, expectorant, antibody, antigen, perfusion-ventilation abnormalities, diffusion capacity, cyanosis, anoxia, and spirometer.***
2. **Review the anatomy and physiology of respiration in an anatomy and physiology text. Review Chapter 16, Drugs That Affect the Autonomic Nervous System. Review the autonomic nervous system. Review the immunological system of the body. Review pulmonary function tests.**
3. **Compare normal respiratory drive with the respiratory drive of a person with chronic lung disease with high PCO_2 levels. Postulate the typical arterial blood gases you would expect to see with such a person.**
4. • **Make a chart comparing the actions of the sympathetic and parasympathetic nervous systems.**
   • **Make a chart comparing the actions of norepinephrine, epinephrine, metaproterenol, albuterol, and isoproterenol with respect to $beta_1$ receptors, alpha receptors, and $beta_2$ receptors.**
5. **Look up your predicted expiratory flow rate (PEFR) in a table with values for height and gender. What value (percent of PEFR) would indicate a need for urgent action if you had asthma?**

38 ▪ *Drugs that affect the musculoskeletal system*

Different kinds of drugs are capable of relaxing skeletal muscles and treating spasticity. Skeletal muscle relaxants are used to decrease pain and increase mobility of affected muscles in acute musculoskeletal disorders. Antispastic agents are used for such disorders as cerebral palsy, multiple sclerosis, and spinal cord injury. There is no completely satisfactory form of therapy for alleviating skeletal muscle spasticity.

Matching

A. Match the generic names of the common skeletal muscle relaxants in the left-hand column with the trade names in the right-hand column. Place your answer in the space provided.

_______	1. Carisoprodol	a. Lioresal
_______	2. Chlorzoxazone	b. Dantrium
_______	3. Methocarbamol	c. Quinamm
_______	4. Orphenadrine	d. Rela, Soma
_______	5. Cyclobenzaprine	e. Flexeril
_______	6. Baclofen	f. Robaxin, Robaxisal
_______	7. Dantrolene	g. Paraflex, Parafon Forte
_______	8. Quinine	h. Norflex, Norgesic, Norgesic Forte

B. Match the drug in the left-hand column with its adult oral dose in the right-hand column.

_______	1. Rela, Soma	a. 10 mg t.i.d
_______	2. Robaxin	b. 1 g q.i.d
_______	3. Methocarbamol	c. 5 mg t.i.d. to 80 mg q.d.
_______	4. Orphenadrine	d. 25-400 mg q.d.
_______	5. Dantrium	e. 260 mg qhs
_______	6. Quinamm	f. 350 mg q.i.d.

Completion exercises

Identify the ingredient(s) in the following compounds and place your answer in the space provided.

1. Soma compound: ______________________________
2. Robaxin: ______________________________
3. Norgesic: ______________________________

Short answer questions

1. List at least six specific conditions that cause muscle spasms intense enough to warrant medication.

2. Common side effects with all the skeletal relaxants are drowsiness and dizziness. Describe what advice about the side effects a nurse should give to a client who is just starting one of these medications.

3. Identify significant or unusual adverse reactions associated with the following drugs:
   a. Maolate:

   b. Dantrium:

   c. Robaxin:

   d. Norflex:

   e. Flexeril:

4. List at least five nonpharmacological measures to use with skeletal muscle relaxants or, possibly, instead of skeletal muscle relaxants.

39 ▪ *Drugs that affect the eyes and ears*

The eyes and ears are sensory organs with direct connections to the central nervous system. In general, the medications used to treat disorders of the eyes and ears are topical. These medications used in the eyes must be sterile, as the eye is quite susceptible to local infections. Nurses must be familiar with the techniques for applying medications to the eyes and ears, as well as being aware of the side effects and adverse reactions of the medication used.

Personal exercise: Eye and ear medications

Have you ever personally used eye or ear medications? Do you remember how difficult applying the medication was? Self-administration of ear drops generally requires the use of a mirror. Application of both types of medications is often uncomfortable.

Using a short piece of drinking straw, and your finger to seal one end, try getting a drop of water into your ear canal without touching the tip of the straw to your ear or hair (i.e., without "contaminating" the tip). If the water won't come out after you have succeeded, a drop of rubbing alcohol such as you can squeeze from an alcohol wipe, will dissolve in the water, lowering the surface tension and allowing the water to run out of your ear.

If you have access to some sterile saline solution or a sterile ophthalmic lubricant, such as natural tears, try getting a single drop in each eye, again without contaminating the tip of the bottle.

Did you blink and miss your eye?

Short answer questions

1. Activation of which receptors causes mydriasis?

2. Blocking of which receptors also causes mydriasis?

3. What is cycloplegia and what is its result?

4. Where is aqueous humor generated and where does it go?

5. Name three of the classes of drugs used to treat glaucoma.
   a.
   b.
   c.
6. The two common uses for ear drops are:
   a.
   b.

40 ▪ *Drugs that affect the integumentary system*

More than 2,000 skin disorders are recognized. A wide variety of agents are applied to the skin and used to treat integumentary disorders and are not used for other medical problems. At the same time, drugs used for major medical problems may also have uses with disorders of the integumentary system (such as corticosteroids, cytotoxic and immunosuppressive drugs, antimalarials, antimicrobials, antihistamines, and minoxidil).

Matching

A. Match the preparations in the left-hand column with the integumentary system disorder for which they might be used in the right-hand column. Place your answer in the space provided.

______	1. Medicated bar soap	a. Deodorant use
______	2. Shake lotion	b. Dandruff
______	3. Topical antibiotic	c. Dry skin for hydration
______	4. Keratolytic	d. Pruritus
______	5. Topical steroid	e. Acute localized inflammatory eruption
______	6. Wet soaks	f. Drying of oozing eruption
______	7. Ointment	g. Acne vulgaris
		h. Head lice
		i. Wart removal

B. Match the disorder in the left-hand column with the preparation that would be useful in the right-hand column. Place your answer in the space provided.

______	1. Photoaging	a. Mupirocin (Bactroban)
______	2. Impetigo	b. Benzoyl peroxide
______	3. Psoriasis	c. Azathioprine (Imuran)
______	4. Wound healing	d. Formulation of tretinoin (Renova)
______	5. Wound cleansing	e. Duo-Derm Dressing
______	6. Pain following shingles	f. Dextranomer (Debrisan)
______	7. Alopecia	g. Minoxidil (Rogaine)
		h. Capsaicin (Zostrix)
		i. Calcipotriene (Dovonex)

C. Match the term in the left-hand column with the definition in the right-hand column. Place your answer in the space provided.

______	1. Astringent	a. Infestation of skin by lice
______	2. Pruritus	b. Infestation of skin with mites
______	3. Keratolytic	c. Suspension of powder in ointment
______	4. Lotion	d. Mixture of powder in ointment
______	5. Gel	e. Itching
______	6. Paste	f. Emulsion of oil-in-water
______	7. Cream	g. Water-in-oil emulsion
______	8. Pediculosis	h. Solution used for drying and cooling effect
		i. Agent that causes sloughing of epidermal cells
		j. Active ingredient in semisolid preparation

Short answer questions

1. List at least six functions of the skin.

2. The client has been prescribed tretinoin (Retin-A) for acne vulgaris. List at least five self-care measures the client should carry out while using this preparation.

3. List at least (a) four pruritic integumentary disorders and (b) four pruritic systemic disorders.

UNIT TWELVE
Drugs affecting inflammation and infection

41 ▪ *Antimicrobial drugs that affect bacterial cell wall synthesis*

Antimicrobial drugs are a major class of curative drugs frequently used in clinical medicine. Treatment protocols are fairly well developed for many agents but certain aspect of therapy such as client education have not always been fully addressed. The nurse's role is vital to the success of chemotherapy involving these drugs.

Personal exercise: Antimicrobials

Review the list of drugs developed for Exercise 1 in the workbook material for Chapter 1. Were any antimicrobials on the list? In relation to this or to some other antimicrobial treatment given to you, evaluate the prescribed regimen. Did the health care provider inform you fully about the effects of the medicine(s)? Was the drug regiment clearly explained? Did you experience any adverse reactions to the drug(s)? What type were they? How severe? Do you now wear a medical identification device warning of adverse reaction to antimicrobials? Should you?

Short answer questions

1. List the six properties of an ideal antimicrobial.
   a.

   b.

   c.

   d.

   e.

   f.

2. Identify five bacterial cell structures or processes that are damaged or disrupted by antimicrobial drugs.

3. Name four processes by which resistance to anti-infectives develops and spreads among microbial populations.

4. Define spectrum of activity.

5. The drug of choice for initiating treatment of anaphylaxis is ______________________.
6. List the characteristics that distinguish cephalosporins of the three generations.
First-generation cephalosporins: ______________________
Second-generation cephalosporins: ______________________
____
Third-generations cephalosporins: ______________________
____

Multiple choice questions

For each of the following, choose the one best answer.

1. Which of the following is true of bacteriostatic and bactericidal antimicrobial?
   a. bactericidal antimicrobial require that the client's immune system be functioning
   b. the use of bacteriostatic antimicrobial will decrease the effectiveness of a bactericidal antimicrobial
   c. whether a drug is bacteriostatic or bactericidal is not dependent on dosage or route
2. A common site for superinfection is:
   a. bowel
   b. skin
   c. stomach
   d. eyes
3. Superinfection is more likely to occur:
   a. when antimicrobial are used in serious infections caused by streptococci
   b. when clients are receiving bacteriocidal antimicrobials
   c. within the first 24 hours of antimicrobial therapy
   d. when broad spectrum antimicrobial are used
4. Bacterial resistance occurs:
   a. only in pathogens
   b. when the client's immune system is able to control the infection
   c. when bacteria mutate so that an antimicrobial no longer affects it
   d. when higher and higher doses of the antimicrobial are required in order to achieve the same therapeutic effect
5. Penicillin is most effective in combating
   a. gram-positive organisms
   b. gram-negative organisms
   c. acid-fast organisms
   d. fungi
6. Penicillin is
   a. bacteriostatic
   b. bactericidal
   c. both bacteriostatic and bactericidal
   d. neither bacteriostatic and bactericidal
7. Severe adverse reactions to penicillin usually take the form of
   a. acute hepatitis
   b. anaphylaxis
   c. aplastic anemia
   d. loss of hearing
8. Drugs that are most effective in the treatment of infections caused by gram-negative organisms are the
   a. penicillins
   b. aminoglycosides
   c. cephalosporins
   d. erythromycins
9. An antimicrobial drug that is contraindicated in pregnancy
   a. penicillin
   b. sodium sulfasuxidine
   c. streptomycin
   d. tetracycline

10. Immunosuppressed clients who experience infections require treatment with
    a. narrow-spectrum bactericides
    b. narrow-spectrum bacteriostatics
    c. broad-spectrum bactericides
    d. broad-spectrum bacteriostatics
11. Your neighbor's child has been receiving penicillin for a strep sore throat. Her mother tells you she has recovered now and asks what should be done with the rest of the prescription. You would advise her to
    a. save the medication and resume treatment if the symptoms return
    b. discard the medication and destroy by burning
    c. continue to administer the drug until the original prescription is used up
    d. contact the physician for specific instructions about the medicine.
12. When antimicrobials are prescribed for the treatment of infection
    a. the initial dose of antimicrobial must be given without delay
    b. cultures should be taken before the initial dose of antimicrobial administered
    c. cultures are never taken after antimicrobial treatment is in progress
    d. it is irrelevant when cultures are taken in relation to antimicrobial therapy
13. Is antibiotic therapy with a combination of a bactericidal drug and a bacteriostatic drug an example of synergism?
    a. Yes, the effect will be greater than the sum of the effects of each drug used alone.
    b. No, the effect is additive.
    c. No, the effect is less than the effect of either drug alone.
    d. No, the effect of one drug decreases the effectiveness of the other drug.

Selection of options

For each of the following, select *all* appropriate responses. Circle the correct answers.

1. Probenecid inhibits the excretion of
    a. penicillin
    b. streptomycin
    c. tetracycline
2. How does penicillin become an environmental contaminant?
    a. It is used in animal husbandry and is found in meat and milk.
    b. It is found in the urine if persons taking the drug.
    c. It is spilled into the environment during preparation of doses for administration.
3. Which of the following statements are valid recommendations for the use of antimicrobials?
    a. Antimicrobial therapy should be discontinued when symptoms disappear so as to decrease the development of resistant strains of organisms.
    b. Antimicrobial drugs should not be used prophylactically.
    c. The use of chloramphenicol should be avoided except for the treatment of serious infections caused by resistant organisms.
4. Assessment of clients receiving aminoglycosides for adverse drug reactions should include monitoring of
    a. CBCs
    b. Urinary output, BUN, creatinine levels, and urinalysis
    c. eighth cranial nerve function
    d. respiratory function

42 ▪ *Antimicrobial drugs that affect protein synthesis*

Multiple choice questions

For each of the following, choose the one best answer:

1. Which of the following is true of tetracyclines?
   a. can be taken without regard to meals
   b. should not be taken with milk or cheese
   c. client can take tetracycline with an antacid if gastric irritation occurs
2. Tetracyclines should not be used in
   a. children over 8 years of age
   b. pregnant woman
   c. clients with Chlamydia infection
   d. clients with constipation
3. Erythromycin
   a. should be taken with meals
   b. is primarily bactericidal
   c. often is used to treat persons allergic to penicillin
   d. can be used safely with clarithromycin
4. Which of the following is an adverse effect of chloramphenicol?
   a. gray syndrome in newborns
   b. damage to tooth development
   c. granulocytosis
   d. ototoxicity
5. A life-threatening adverse reaction likely to occur in clients receiving chloramphenicol is
   a. anaphylaxis
   b. bone marrow depression
   c. kidney impairment
   d. liver degeneration

Selection of options

For each of the following, select *all* appropriate responses. Circle the correct answers.

1. Drugs derived from sulfonamides include
   a. antimycobacterials
   b. antifungals
   c. diuretics
   d. hypoglycemics
   e. antithyroid compounds
   f. antihistamines
2. Probenecid inhibits the excretion of
   a. penicillin
   b. streptomycin
   c. tetracycline
3. Drugs that are toxic to the eighth cranial (acoustic) nerve include
   a. streptomycin
   b. tetracycline
   c. kanamycin
4. Assessment of clients receiving aminoglycosides for adverse drug reactions should include monitoring of
   a. CBCs
   b. urinary output, BUN, creatinine levels, and urinalysis
   c. eighth cranial nerve function
   d. respiratory function

This puzzle includes information and concepts from Chapters 41 and 42.

Crossword puzzle

Across

2. Drugs that exhibit cross-sensitivity with penicillins
3. Incorporation by a microbe of genes from the environment that were previously released by another microbe
4. Staining property characteristic of microbes affected by penicillin
6. An early antimicrobial currently used most often to treat and prevent urinary tract infections
7. A serious side effect of prolonged aminoglycoside therapy
9. An enzyme produced by penicillin-resistant organisms
10. The property that enables microbes to thrive in the presence of an antimicrobial drug
13. Laboratory test used as a guide to choice of anti-infective medication
17. A juice administered to produce an acid urine
18. A basic requirements for infection control in healthcare institutions
19. Exchange of genetic material by two microbes connected by a corridor from cytoplasm to cytoplasm
20. The number and types of organisms affected by an antimicrobial
21. Route of drug administration most likely to induce allergic sensitivity in the recipient
22. An antibiotic that should not be given to young children
23. Body organ most likely to be damaged by sulfonamide therapy
24. Transfer of genetic material from one organism to another by a virus

Down

1. A drug that may cause gray syndrome in babies
3. One method by which resistance is spread from one organism to another without direct contact
5. A macrolide anti-infective used to treat the eyes of newborns
8. The drug of choice for treatment of anaphylaxis
11. Overgrowth of organisms in the body that are not affected by anti-infective therapy
12. An inhibitor of renal tubule excretion of several antibiotics
14. Organisms frequently responsible for resistant nosocomial infections
15. A substance given orally to reduce the risk of superinfection
16. An antibiotic effective against gram-negative organisms

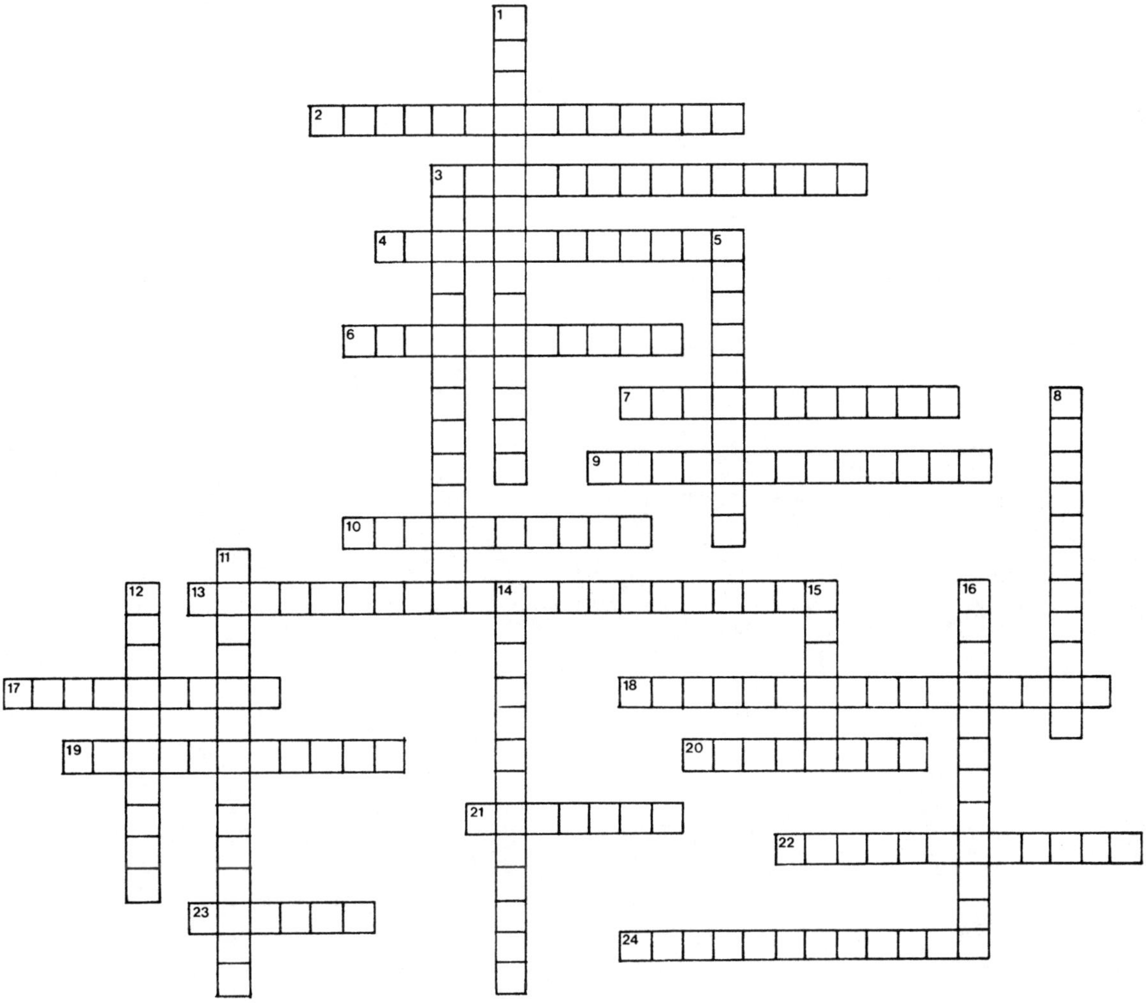
1
2
3
4
5
6
7
8
9
10
11
12
13
14
15
16
17
18
19
20
21
22
23
24

43 ▪ *Other antimicrobial drugs*

The following exercises relate to the material from Chapter 43. A few items review related material from previous chapters on primarily antimicrobials.

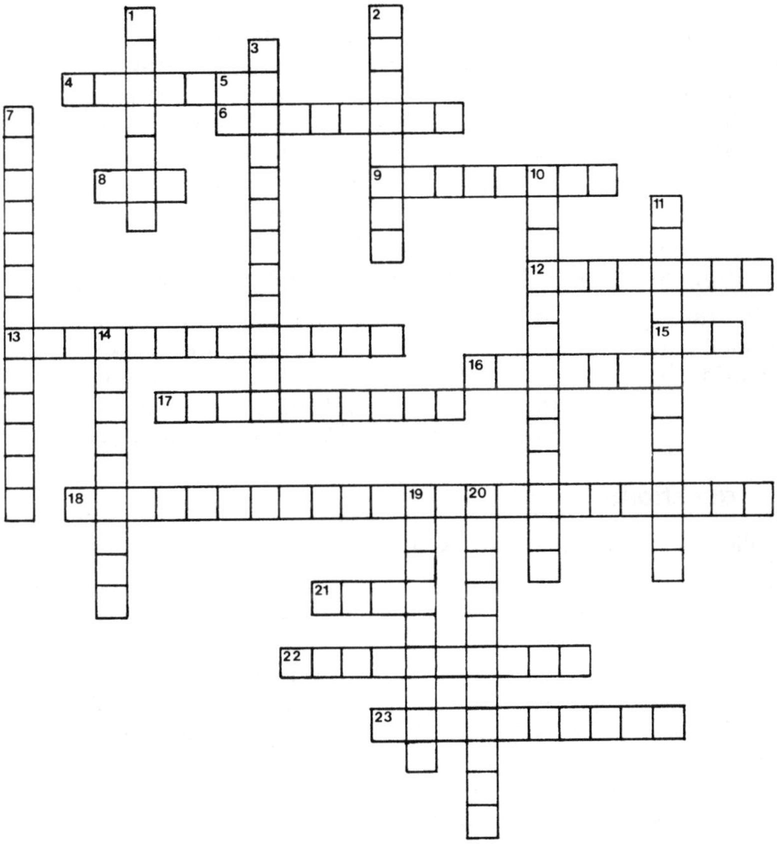

Crossword puzzle

Across

4. Disease caused by a mycobacterium
6. Staining property characteristic of mycobacteria
8. Abbreviated name for drug used alone to prevent active tuberculosis
9. Weak urinary antiseptic used mainly for its analgesic action
12. Color of urine during pyridium therapy
13. Serious adverse reaction to ethambutol
15. Abbreviation for para-aminosalicylic acid

Down

1. Sulfone used to treat leprosy
2. Antimycobacterial drug excreted mainly via the liver in bile
3. Organisms susceptible to rifampin
5. One abbreviation indicating time release
7. Antituberculosis drug that is also effective against gram-negative organisms
10. Route used to administer capreomycin
11. Antituberculosis drug that must be injected parenterally

Across

16. Most frequent adverse reaction to ethionamide
17. Antibiotic that affects only mycobacteria
18. Antituberculosis drug that inhibits folic acid synthesis by the tubercle bacillus
21. Metabolic imbalance that may develop during pyrazinamide therapy
22. The powder form of this antibiotic must be stored in a refrigerator
23. Trade name for colistin

Down

14. Generic name for INH
19. Contraindication for dapsone therapy
20. Antimicrobial that should not be used with neuromuscular agents

Matching

A. For each drug listed at the left, indicate *all* of the appropriate adverse reactions from the list at the right.

_______ 1. Capreomycin
_______ 2. Cycloserine
_______ 3. Ethambutol
_______ 4. Ethionamide
_______ 5. Isoniazid
_______ 6. Pyrazinamide
_______ 7. Rifampin

a. Anaphylaxis
b. Optic neuropathy
c. Peripheral neuropathy
d. Central nervous system toxicity
e. Ototoxicity
f. Hepatotoxicity
g. Nephrotoxicity
h. Arthritis

B. For each of the drugs listed at the left, select the appropriate action(s) from the list at the right.

_______ 1. Cycloserine
_______ 2. Dapsone
_______ 3. Isoniazid
_______ 4. Para-aminosalicylic acid

a. Aminobenzoic-acid antagonism
b. D-alanine antagonism
c. Folic-acid antagonism
d. Pyribenzamine antagonism
e. Vitamin D antagonism

Multiple choice questions

For each of the following, choose the one best answer:

1. When cycloserine is prescribed to treat tuberculosis, clients should avoid use of
   a. alcohol
   b. caffeine
   c. nicotine
   d. all of the above
2. An antimycobacterial drug that is contraindicated for clients who must restrict sodium intake is
   a. streptomycin
   b. ethambutol
   c. isoniazid
   d. *p*-aminosalicylic acid
3. Clients allergic to penicillins or cephalosporins who nevertheless need a beta-lactam antibiotic may receive:
   a. streptomycin
   b. aztreonam
   c. bacitracin
   d. clindamycin
4. Some anti-infectives administered intramuscularly cause pain in the injection site. To alleviate this discomfort, the nurse would
   a. spray the site with a topical anesthetic before injection
   b. add a small amount of procaine to the antibiotic solution
   c. apply heat to the site after injection
   d. apply cold to the site before and after the injection
5. The risk of serious allergic reaction to antibiotic injections is greatest in the client who
   a. has never been exposed to the drug
   b. has previously received the drug by injection
   c. has previously used the drug topically with no allergic reaction
   d. has previously taken the drug orally with no allergic reaction

6. Which fluoroquinolone is used to treat lower urinary tract infections?
   a. ciprofloxacin
   b. nitrofurantoin
   c. spectomycin
7. A client receiving a fluoroquinolone should be advised to
   a. take with food
   b. avoid sunlight to prevent photosensitivity
   c. avoid ingestion of acid-ash foods or liquids
8. The proprietary drug Bactrim (Septra) is a combination of a sulfonamide and
   a. an aminoglycoside
   b. cephalosporin
   c. a penicillin
   d. trimethoprim
   e. vancomycin

Short answer questions

1. Name two diseases caused by mycobacteria.

   ____

2. An aminoglycoside used in the treatment of tuberculosis is ______________________________.

3. Name at least two primary treatment agents for tuberculosis.

   ______________________________.

4. a. Name an antimycobacterial agent that causes body fluids to change color. ______________

   b. What is the color change? ______________________________

   ____

5. List at least four measures the nurse may use to reduce the risk of current urinary tract infections.

   ____

   ____

   ____

6. Why are oral preparations of methenamine enteric-coated?

   ____

   ____

6. Which fluoroquinolone [illegible] used for treat- [illegible] longer in urine [illegible] infections?
a. [illegible]
b. [illegible]
c. [illegible]

7. [illegible] should be [illegible]
a. take with food
b. avoid sunlight to prevent photosensitivity
c. avoid [illegible]

8. [illegible] The proper [illegible] during [illegible] therapy [illegible] a. [illegible] b. [illegible] c. [illegible] d. [illegible]

Short answer questions

1. Name two diseases caused by [illegible].

2. An aminoglycoside used in the treatment of tuberculosis is [illegible].

3. Name at least two of the [illegible] for tuberculosis.

4. [illegible]

5. List at least [illegible] the nurse [illegible] infection.

6. What are [illegible] of [illegible]?

44 ▪ *Drugs that treat viral and fungal infections*

The following exercises relate to material on antiviral and antifungal medications.

Correct the false statement

Indicate whether the following statements are true or false; if false, correct the underlined words or phrases.

_______ 1. The most effective approaches to control virus infections are <u>use of high doses of vitamin C and administration of antiviral anti-infectives</u>.

_______ 2. Viral infections for which we have no effective vaccines include <u>acquired immune deficiency syndrome (AIDS) and herpes simplex</u>.

_______ 3. Acyclovir is administered by <u>intramuscular injection</u>.

_______ 4. Ribavirin is usually administered <u>by inhalation</u>.

Completion exercises

From the choices listed below each table, select the appropriate entries for each section of the table. More than one entry may be needed for each section. Place your answer(s) in the space provided.

1. **Antiviral Compound**	a. **Trade Name(s)**	b. **Therapeutic Use(s)**	c. **Adverse Reaction(s)**
Vidarabine			
Idoxuridine			
Zidovudine			
Acyclovir			
Ribavarin			

a. Trade names: Herplex; Marboran; Stoxil; Vira-A; Virazole; Zovirax; AZT

b. Therapeutic uses: herpes simplex encephalitis; lower respiratory viral infections caused by RSV; complications of cowpox vaccination; herpes simplex keratitis; herpes simplex keratoconjunctivitis; treatment of HIV infection; genital herpes; prevention of smallpox

c. Adverse reactions: bone marrow suppression; vomiting; nephrotoxicity; impaired cardiac and respiratory function; local inflammation; myopathy

2. **Antifungal**	a. **Route(s)**	b. **Mode(s) of Action**	c. **Adverse Reaction(s)**
Amphotericin B			
Clotrimazole			
Griseofulvin			
Ketoconazole			
Miconazole			

a. Routes: oral; topical; intramuscular; intravenous
b. Modes of action: local; systemic
c. Adverse reactions: gastrointestinal upset; hepatotoxicity; local inflammation; nephrotoxicity; skin rash; chills and fever

Short answer questions

1. Identify a characteristic of living organisms shared by viruses.

2. Name at least three common skin conditions caused by fungi.

3. List at least three measures that can reduce the risk of repeated fungal infection.

Multiple choice questions

For each of the following, choose the one best answer:

1. The treatment of infectious illness with drugs has been least effective for diseases caused by
   a. lice
   b. bacteria and protozoa
   c. fungi and viruses
   d. mites
2. The most effective approach to the control of viral infections to date has been the administration of
   a. vaccines
   b. antibacterial antibiotics
   c. viricidal drugs
   d. interferons
3. The effect of zidovudine on a person with AIDS is
   a. rapid improvement and recovery
   b. slow improvement and eventual recovery
   c. delay in the progression of the disease
   d. improvement in the symptoms of opportunistic infections associated with AIDS
4. The antifungal drug griseofulvin is usually administered
   a. topically to suppress fungal infections
   b. topically to eliminate fungal infections
   c. systemically to suppress fungal infections
   d. systemically to eliminate fungal infections
5. A medication ordered to be given as a "swish" should be
   a. used during showering
   b. applied repeatedly to the affected skin as a rinse
   c. sprinkled over the affected area
   d. used to rinse the mouth and then swallowed
6. The nursing care of the client receiving amphotericin B (Fungizone) includes monitoring the client for
   a. hypophosphatemia
   b. hypercalcemia
   c. hypokalemia
   d. hypermagnesemia

Selection of options

For each of the following, select *all* appropriate responses. Circle the correct answers.

1. The antifungal drug nystatin may be administered
   a. topically
   b. orally
   c. parenterally
   d. rectally
2. Substances that should be avoided by those receiving griseofulvin include
   a. alcohol
   b. phenobarbital
   c. warfarin
   d. antacids
3. Fungal infections include those caused by
   a. *Tinea*
   b. *Candida*
   c. gram-positive cocci
   d. mycobacteria

45 ▪ *Drugs that treat parasitic and helminthic infections*

Chapter 45 discusses drugs in the treatment of protozoan infections and helminthiasis. Many of these infections are transmitted by animal or insect vectors. A wide variety of chemical substances are used to prevent and treat contagious diseases caused by these life forms.

Matching

For each drug in the left-hand column, select the appropriate classification(s) from the right-hand column.

_______	1. Niclosamide (Niclocide)	a. Anthelmintic
_______	2. Melarsoprol (Arsobal)	b. Antimalarial
_______	3. Mefloquine (Lariam)	c. Amebicide
_______	4. Metronidazole (Flagyl)	d. Antiprotozoal
_______	5. Quinine (Quinamm)	
_______	6. Primaquine	
_______	7. Quinacrine (Atabrine)	
_______	8. Pyrimethamine (Daraprim)	
_______	9. Praziquantel (Biltricide)	

Short answer questions

1. Name three methods of controlling the tick that causes Lyme disease.

2. Name three rickettsial diseases and their causative organisms.

Correct the false statement

Indicate whether the following statements are true or false; if false, correct the underlined words or phrases.

_______ 1. Clinical signs and symptoms of malaria include <u>chills, fever, and anemia</u>.

_______ 2. Populations likely to experience hemolytic reactions from primaquine include <u>northern Europeans and American Indians</u>.

_______ 3. An important goal of nursing care of those under treatment for amebiasis is <u>the maintenance of nutrition</u>.

_______ 4. Travelers to foreign countries may often avoid infectious illness by <u>eating only hot, thoroughly cooked foods</u>.

_______ 5. Useful measures for the prevention of helminthic infections with hookworm include periodic prophylactic courses of treatment by anthelmintics.

_______ 6. Roundworms caused by <u>Ascaris lumbricoides</u>, are the most common parasite worm infections in the United States.

_______ 7. Cryptosporidiosis is a protozoan infection transmitted to humans from cats.

_______ 8. Ameba, like *Entamoeba histolytica,* can invade extraintestinal tissues, like the liver, and cause abscesses.

Multiple choice questions

For each of the following, choose the one best answer:

1. Which of the following statements by Ms. Y., who is being treated for pinworms, leads you to believe she has understood your teaching related to mebendazole (Vermix)?
   a. I will need to have three negative stool cultures before I will be considered free of the pinworm.
   b. I will not drink alcohol when I am using this medication.
   c. I may continue to expel worms for 3 days after I am through taking the medication.
   d. I need to take a laxative daily to help expel the worms.
2. The client is receiving pentamidine (Pentam 300) for treatment of *Pneumocystis carinii* pneumonia. What will be done to assess the client for adverse effects of the medicine?
   a. serum electrolytes
   b. BUN and serum creatinine
   c. BP and pulse t.i.d.
   d. EKG weekly
3. Which of the following interferes with synthesis of microtubules in a variety of worms?
   a. mefloquine (Lariam)
   b. iodoquinol (Yodoxin)
   c. mebendazole (Vermix)
   d. chloroquine (Aralen)
4. The nurse should explain to the client that a harmless side effect of metronidazole (Flagyl) therapy is
   a. an altered sensation of smell
   b. constipation
   c. a reddish-brown urine color
   d. a tanned appearance to the skin
5. The client is being treated for fish tapeworm. The nurse knows that the evaluation criterion for cure is a negative stool for worm segments or ova for
   a. 2 weeks
   b. 1 month
   c. 6 weeks
   d. 3 months
6. When two or more worm infestations are present concurrently, the first drug ordered is likely to be a drug effective against
   a. pinworms
   b. tapeworms
   c. hookworms
   d. roundworms
7. Medication is likely to be ordered for everyone in a family when infestations are caused by
   a. pinworms
   b. tapeworms
   c. hookworms
   d. roundworms
8. A drug that has been helpful for nocturnal leg cramps is
   a. ascorbic acid (vitamin C)
   b. quinine (Quinamm)
   c. pyrimethamine (Daraprim)
   d. suramin (Bayer 205)
9. Some of the serious complications of Lyme disease are
   a. pediculosis
   b. neurological abnormalities
   c. pulmonary fibrosis
   d. renal dysfunctions
10. An aminoglycoside antibiotic that is useful for treatment of amebiasis is
    a. paromomycin (Humatin)
    b. capreomycin (Capastat)
    c. ethambutol (Myambutol)
    d. pentamidine (Pentam 300)

Selection of options

For each of the following, select *all* appropriate responses. Circle the correct answers.

1. Alternatives to the use of pesticides in the control of vector-borne infectious disease include
   a. screens
   b. composting of wastes in a closed system
   c. encouragement of natural predators
2. Adverse reactions to antimalarial drugs include
   a. ototoxicity
   b. hemolysis
   c. headache
   d. nephrotoxicity
3. The major drugs for prophylaxis or treatment of malaria include
   a. quinine (Quinamm)
   b. praziquantel (Biltricide)
   c. niclosamide (Niclocide)
   d. mefloquine (Lariam)
   e. chloroquine (Aralen)
   f. primaquine
   g. pyrimethamine (Daraprim)

UNIT THIRTEEN
Drugs affecting neoplastic disease

46 ▪ *Chemotherapeutic drugs: Alkylating agents and antimetabolites*

Antineoplastic drug therapy is one of four main ways of treating cancer. Six subgroupings of alkylating agents and three subgroupings of antimetabolites include over 20 active antineoplastic agents. A number of adverse reactions to antineoplastic drugs are very common and often complicate the care of the client receiving this therapy.

Matching

Match the following individual antimetabolites in the left-hand column with their subgrouping in the right-hand column. Place your answers in the space provided.

______	1. Thioguanine	a. Folic acid analogue
______	2. Methotrexate	b. Pyrimidine analogue
______	3. Floxuridine	c. Purine analogue
______	4. Cytarabine	
______	5. Mercaptopurine	
______	6. Fluorouracil	

Short answer questions

1. What drugs are included in the ethylenimine and methylmelamine group of alkylating agents?

2. What alkylating agents are included in the nitrosourea grouping?

3. What does the term *ototoxicity* mean? What are its signs and symptoms? What alkylating agent causes ototoxicity?

4. Define the mechanism of action for each of the following:
   a. Folic acid analogue:

   b. Pyrimidine analogue:

c. Purine analogue:

5. What is topical fluorouracil used for?

6. List some interventions that would help if the client experiences anorexia, taste changes, nausea, and vomiting with antineoplastic therapy.

7. List some interventions that would help to prevent infection with the bone marrow suppression seen with antineoplastic therapy.

Completion exercises

Read each question carefully and place your answer in the space provided.

1. Look up *cyclophosphamide* in the text.
   a. Adverse reactions are ____
   ____.
   b. You are caring for a client receiving this drug. Explain what you would tell the client about the anticipated alopecia. ____
   ____
   ____.
2. Stomatitis is a difficult complication of antineoplastic therapy.
   a. The agents that might be used for general mouth care include ______________________
   ____.
   b. Foods that should be avoided include ____
   ____.
   c. Candidiasis would be treated with ____.
3. Work with the antimetabolite ____________________ led to the development of allopurinol.
4. An alkylating agent used in the treatment of chronic lymphocytic leukemia is ______________.

Essay questions

Read each question carefully and write your answers on a separate sheet of paper.

1. An alkylating agent is usually used in combination with other agents to treat Hodgkin's disease in its more advanced stages. Explain the reasons for combination chemotherapy.
2. Describe five of the factors that affect whether or not antineoplastic drug therapy is used for a client's cancer.
3. Name the five phases of the cell cycle and identify what happens in each phase.
4. What is meant by "rescue therapy"? Describe a clinical application of the concept.

47 ▪ Other anticancer drugs: Natural products, hormones, and antineoplastics

Several natural products, certain antibiotics, and even an enzyme have a role in antineoplastic drug therapy. Adrenocorticosteroids, antiadrenal compounds, androgens and estrogens, antiandrogenic compounds, antiestrogenic compounds, estrogen antimetabolites, progestins, and analogues of luteinizing hormone-releasing hormones are used with cancers of the reproductive system and other defined cancers.

Matching

A. Match the following natural products in the left-hand column with their subgrouping in the right-hand column. Place your answers in the space provided.

_______ 1. Mitomycin
_______ 2. Bleomycin
_______ 3. Vincristine
_______ 4. Plicamycin
_______ 5. Asparaginase
_______ 6. Dactinomycin
_______ 7. Vinblastine
_______ 8. Daunorubicin
_______ 9. Doxorubicin
_______ 10. Etoposide

a. Topoisomerase inhibitor
b. Mitotic inhibitor
c. Antitumor antibiotic
d. Enzyme

B. Match the condition in the left-hand column with the class(es) of drugs used for treatment in the right-hand column.

_______ 1. Inoperable or recurrent endometrial cancer
_______ 2. Remission induction in acute lymphocytic leukemia in children
_______ 3. Advanced breast cancer to control metastatic disease
_______ 4. Vasoactive intestinal peptide-secreting tumors (VIPomas)
_______ 5. Radiation edema
_______ 6. Prostatic cancer
_______ 7. Hypercalcemia

a. Adrenocorticosteroids
b. Estrogens
c. Androgens
d. Progestins
e. Antiestrogens
f. Estrogen-antimetabolites
g. Analogue of luteinizing hormone-releasing hormone
h. Analogue of somatostatin

C. Match the antineoplastic drug in the left-hand column with the appropriate nursing action in the right-hand column.

_______	1. Etopside	a. Observe clients for neurotoxicity
_______	2. Vinblastine	b. Counsel clients regarding body image changes
_______	3. Prednisone	c. Administer over 30–60 min
_______	4. Flutamide	d. Premedicate with diphenhydramine
_______	5. Paclitaxel	e. Following long-term use, taper dose on discontinuation

D. Match the antineoplastic drug in the left-hand column with the adverse reaction in the right-hand column.

_______	1. Vincristine	a. Importance and decreased libido
_______	2. Bleomycin	b. Bone marrow suppression
_______	3. Doxorubicin	c. Cardiotoxic effects
_______	4. Leuprolide	d. Paresthesias
_______	5. Hydroxyurea	

Short answer questions

1. Describe the neurotoxicities that may occur when vincristine is used.

2. How do anthracycline antibiotics produce their antineoplastic effects?

3. Describe the renal toxicities seen with mitomycin.

4. Explain why the hypercalcemia seen with some cancers is of concern. Identify an antibiotic that may be used to treat hypercalcemia.

5. Explain why estrogen receptors are important.

Completion exercises

Read each carefully and place your answer in the space provided.

1. Look up *etoposide* in the text.
   a. Adverse reactions are ______________________________
   ______________________________.
   b. Some of its uses are to treat ______________________________
   ______________________________.
2. Hydroxyurea is used primarily to treat ______________________________.
3. Mitotane acts on the adrenal cortex and causes ______________________________
   ______________________________.
4. Procarbazine does ______________ so it can be used for ______________.
5. Cladribine is used to treat ______________________________.
6. The agent ______________ might be used with inoperable adrenocortical cancer.
7. One unique action of plicamycin is that it ______________________________.

Essay questions

Read each carefully and write your answers on a separate sheet of paper.

1. Describe the pulmonary adverse reaction that can occur with bleomycin.
2. Explain the difference between the two forms of cardiotoxicity that may occur when doxorubicin is used.
3. Describe the mechanism of action of asparaginase.
4. Describe the rationale for the use of estrogens and androgens in antineoplastic drug therapy.

UNIT FOURTEEN
Miscellaneous drug families

48 ▪ *Parenteral supplements*

Parenteral nutritional supplements include clear solutions containing glucose and electrolytes; total parenteral nutrition solutions containing glucose, amino acids, and fats, as well as vitamins and minerals; blood; and blood products. The following exercises relate to these treatment agents.

Matching

Match each characteristic of parenteral fluids in the left-hand column with all appropriate physiologic effects in the right-hand column.

_______ 1. Hypotonic
_______ 2. Isotonic
_______ 3. Hypertonic

a. Crenation of red blood cells
b. Lysis of red blood cells
c. Osmotic diuresis
d. Water diuresis
e. Oliguria
f. Hypervolemia with minimal disturbance of other fluid compartments

Correct the false statement

Indicate whether the following statements are true or false; if false, correct the underlined words or phrases.

_______ 1. <u>Clear parenteral solutions</u> provide all nutrients required by the body.

_______ 2. Plastic tubing used for administration of intravenous lipid solutions should be free of <u>polymers</u>.

_______ 3. Parenteral hyperalimentation <u>is always administered in acute care situations</u>.

_______ 4. Tubing to be used for transfusion may be primed with <u>dextrose solution</u>.

Short answer questions

1. Name the drug administered by hypodermoclysis to facilitate absorption of clear fluids infused subcutaneously or intramuscularly.

2. What effects do dextran solutions have on coagulation?

3. Which of the substances used for parenteral hyperalimentation may be administered in a peripheral intravenous line separate from the central venous line used for the other nutrients?

4. What type of tubing is required for administration of parenteral hyperalimentation mixtures that do not contain fat?

5. If air enters a central venous line, what should be done?

6. How long can blood be stored before being used in transfusions?

7. What is the name of the laboratory test used to determine compatibility of blood for transfusion?

8. How is whole blood stored?

9. Optimum ages for blood donation are considered to be ________ to ________.

Multiple choice questions:

For each of the following, choose the one best answer:

1. Parenteral solutions are most rapidly absorbed and distributed when administered
   a. by hypodermoclysis
   b. intramuscularly
   c. intravenously
   d. subcutaneously
2. An electrolyte likely to cause prolonged diastole, weak heart action, and cardiac arrhythmia when infused rapidly by the parenteral route is
   a. sodium
   b. potassium
   c. calcium
   d. bicarbonate
3. Maximum parenteral dosage of potassium for normal adults is
   a. 20 mEq/hr
   b. 40 mEq/hr
   c. 80 mEq/hr
   d. 100 mEq/hr
4. Parenteral hyperalimentation solutions containing multiple ingredients are usually
   a. isotonic
   b. slightly hypotonic
   c. markedly hypotonic
   d. slightly hypertonic
   e. markedly hypertonic
5. Lipid emulsions may be administered parenterally through
   a. filtered lines inserted into a peripheral vein
   b. filtered lines inserted into a central vein
   c. nonfiltered lines inserted into a peripheral vein
   d. clysis tubing
6. When parenteral hyperalimentation therapy is begun, the recipient is likely to develop a transient
   a. high concentration of trace minerals
   b. hypoglycemia
   c. hyperglycemia
   d. hyperphosphatemia
7. A serious adverse reaction to parenteral hyperalimentation is
   a. glucose deficiency
   b. infection
   c. lysis of red blood cells
   d. metabolic acidosis
8. The hormone administered to recipients of parenteral hyperalimentation solutions to control an adverse reaction is
   a. insulin
   b. glucagon
   c. prednisone
   d. thyroxine
9. The rate of parenteral fluid administration can be controlled most strictly by use of
   a. hand-operated valves
   b. elevation of the container
   c. volume-controlled pumps
10. Clients with fluid volume deficit who respond poorly to intravenous therapy are likely to have the hormone imbalance
    a. hypothyroidism
    b. hypocortism

c. hypoinsulinism
d. antidiuretic hormone deficiency

11. When a central venous line is to be established, the client is placed in
    a. Fowler's position
    b. supine position
    c. Trendelenburg position
    d. reverse Trendelenburg position
12. Because optimum parenteral dosages for these nutrients have not yet been established, the nurse should monitor recipients for parenteral hyperalimentation closely for imbalances of
    a. glucose
    b. minerals
    c. proteins
    d. vitamins
13. A parenteral solution that must be administered through a central venous line is
    a. hyperalimentation mixture
    b. dextrose in water
    c. intralipid
    d. blood
14. At what time are infusions of fat emulsions usually begun?
    a. after early morning blood specimens for laboratory tests have been collected
    b. after the morning hygienic routine
    c. after the midday rest
    d. at bedtime
15. The parenteral fluid that contains all constituents necessary for circulatory homeostasis is
    a. blood
    b. 5% dextrose in water
    c. plasma
    d. Ringer's solution
16. Blood is most likely to produce the electrolyte imbalance
    a. hypercalcemia
    b. hyperkalemia
    c. hyponatremia
    d. hypoglycemia
17. Administration of multiple units of banked blood is likely to cause
    a. hypocalcemic tetany
    b. hypokalemic paralytic ileus
    c. hyponatremic dehydration
    d. iron deficiency anemia
18. The *universal recipient* is someone with blood type
    a. A
    b. B
    c. AB
    d. O
19. Incompatibility reactions are least likely to occur when the blood to be administered is
    a. type AB, Rh+
    b. type AB, Rh–
    c. type O, Rh+
    d. type O, Rh–
    e. the same ABO and Rh type as the recipient's blood
20. Which of these religions proscribe the use of blood transfusions?
    a. Jehovah's Witness
    b. Hindu
    c. Mormon
    d. Seventh Day Adventist

Selection of options

For each of the following, select *all* appropriate responses. Circle the correct answers.

1. The physiologic effects of hypertonic solutions administered intravenously include:
   a. fluid shifts from the interstitial fluid compartment to the intravascular compartment
   b. a tendency toward cellular dehydration
   c. a decrease in urinary output
   d. a tendency to crenate red blood cells
2. Clear parenteral solutions are administered
   a. subcutaneously
   b. intramuscularly
   c. intravenously
   d. by hypodermoclysis
   e. intra-arterially
3. Movement of fluids through the interstitial cellular space is inhibited by the presence of
   a. numerous blood vessels
   b. hyaluronic acid
   c. hypertension
   d. hypotensive shock
4. Rapid infusion of parenteral fluids tends to produce
   a. circulatory overload
   b. left ventricular failure

c. hypervolemia

d. pulmonary edema

5. Rapid infusion of clear solutions by hypodermoclysis tends to produce

a. local tissue swelling

b. hypertension in the interstitial fluid compartment

c. improved local perfusion

6. Adequate hydration and renal function should be established before the following parenteral nutrients are administered

a. dextrans

b. 5% dextrose in water

c. normal saline solutions

d. potassium solutions

7. Plasma extenders include

a. dextrans

b. 5% dextrose in water

c. hetastarch

d. normal saline solution

8. Nutrients administered as solutions for total parenteral hyperalimentation include

a. sugar

b. starches

c. amino acids

d. proteins

e. lipids

f. vitamins

g. minerals

9. Intravenous medications may be administered to clients receiving hyperalimentation solutions through the

a. central venous line while the hyperalimentation solution is infusing

b. central venous line, provided the hyperalimentation solution is not infusing at the time

c. peripheral line while the lipid solution is infusing

d. peripheral line, provided the lipid solution is not infusing at the time

10. Fat emulsions normally appear

a. clear

b. cloudy

c. homogeneous

d. layered

e. colored

11. Adverse effects of blood transfusions include

a. hyperkalemia

b. allergic reactions

c. incompatibility reactions

d. bloodborne infections

12. Signs and symptoms of transfusion reaction include

a. anxiety

b. back pain

c. bradycardia

d. chills and fever

Learning experience

Examine the labels of solutions used for parenteral therapy in the hospital. Note the chemical constituents of the solutions and their concentrations. Which solutions are isotonic? Hypertonic? Hypotonic? How do the concentrations of individual electrolytes compare with their concentrations in normal serum? Which of the solutions has the greatest toxic potential if administered at a rapid rate of infusion?

Enrichment experience

Poll the members of your class to determine how many persons have been tested for blood type and what the ABO and Rh types of these members of the class are. Go to the library and determine the normal proportions of each blood type within the general population. How do the data from your class poll compare with these figures?

49 ▪ *Oral nutritional supplements*

Several therapeutic agents are administered to prevent or correct nutritional deficiencies. Although these agents are normally used in the body, when administered in high dosages they can precipitate adverse reactions. The following exercises relate to nutritional supplements that are usually administered orally.

PART 1: MINERALS AND VITAMINS

Matching

A. Match each deficiency disease in the left-hand column with the nutrient that is lacking in the right-hand column. Place your answer in the space provided.

_______	1. Beriberi	a. Vitamin A
_______	2. Keratomalacia	b. Vitamin B_1
_______	3. Osteomalacia	c. Vitamin B_2
_______	4. Pellagra	d. Vitamin B_{12}
_______	5. Pernicious anemia	e. Niacin
_______	6. Rickets	f. Vitamin B_6
_______	7. Scurvy	g. Vitamin C
_______	8. Xerophthalmia	h. Vitamin D

B. Match each vitamin in the left-hand column with its generic name in the right-hand column.

_______	1. A	a. α-tocopherol
_______	2. B_1	b. Ascorbic acid
_______	3. B_2	c. Cyanocobalamin
_______	4. B_6	d. Dihydrotachysterol
_______	5. B_{12}	e. Pyridoxine
_______	6. C	f. Retinol
_______	7. D	g. Riboflavin
_______	8. E_1	h. Thiamine

C. Match each dietary supplement in the left-hand column with the nutrient(s) it supplies in the right-hand column.

_______	1. Cod liver oil	a. Calcium
_______	2. Dolomite	b. Calcitriol (vitamin D)
_______	3. Kelp	c. Fluoride
_______	4. Powdered oyster shell	d. Iodine
		e. Retinol (vitamin A)

Correct the false statement

Indicate whether the following statements are true or false; if false, correct the underlined words or phrases.

_______ 1. In humans, the conversion of its precursor 7-dehydrocholesterol to vitamin D requires intrinsic factor.

_______ 2. The margin of safety of water-soluble vitamins is much wider than that for fat-soluble vitamins.

_______ 3. The cost of vitamin supplements is usually considerably higher than the cost of foods providing these nutrients.

_______ 4. To minimize vitamin loss, mineral oil should be taken with food.

_______ 5. The mineral magnesium is useful in the treatment of arrhythmias resulting from hypercalcemia or digitalis toxicity.

_______ 6. A mineral used in the treatment of convulsions caused by eclampsia of pregnancy is calcium.

_______ 7. High concentrations of sodium in the intravascular fluid cause smooth muscle contraction and vasospasm.

_______ 8. Calcium deficiency in children causes osteomalacia.

_______ 9. Hard water provides more nutrients than does soft water.

Short answer questions

1. Define the following terms:
   a. Vitamin:

   b. Nutritional minerals:

   c. Minimum daily requirements (MDR):

   d. Recommended daily allowance:

2. Identify and define the two strengths of vitamin preparations marketed in the United States.
   a.
   b.
3. Is iron usually administered with food?

Multiple choice questions

1. Vitamin C, ascorbic acid, is used to
   a. dilate blood vessels
   b. inhibit sebum production
   c. reduce urine pH
   d. stimulate tear production
2. The nutritional deficiency most apt to affect corn-eating populations is
   a. kwashiorkor
   b. pellagra
   c. pernicious anemia
   d. scurvy
3. A chronic lack of vitamin C is likely to cause the deficiency disease
   a. beriberi
   b. kwashiorkor
   c. pellagra
   d. pernicious anemia
   e. scurvy
4. How much vitamin C is recommended daily for routine maintenance?
   a. 50–75 mg
   b. 100–300 mg
   c. 250–500 mg
   d. 1–4 g

5. Water-soluble vitamins include
   a. vitamin A
   b. vitamin C
   c. vitamin D
   d. vitamin K
6. Vitamin B_{12} is needed by the body for
   a. bone metabolism
   b. hemoglobin synthesis
   c. impulse transmission
   d. red blood cell formation
7. The vitamin that is converted by the body to the hormone calcitriol is
   a. vitamin A
   b. niacin
   c. riboflavin
   d. thiamine
   e. vitamin C
   f. vitamin D
8. A vitamin useful as an antidote in warfarin toxicity is vitamin
   a. A
   b. B_1
   c. B_{12}
   d. D
   e. E
   f. K
9. A vitamin that acts as an antioxidant is vitamin
   a. B_1
   b. B_2
   c. B_{12}
   d. D
   e. E
10. Absorption of fat-soluble vitamins is reduced by oral ingestion of
    a. animal fats
    b. mineral oil
    c. starches
    d. vegetable oils
11. Growth in children may be stunted by high dosages of vitamin
    a. A
    b. B complex
    c. C
    d. K
    e. E
12. β-carotene is a precursor that can be converted to vitamin
    a. A
    b. B_{12}
    c. C
    d. D
    e. K
13. The body can convert 7-dehydrocholesterol to vitamin
    a. A
    b. B_1
    c. B_{12}
    d. C
    e. D
    f. K
14. In the United States, the most frequent vitamin toxicity is hypervitaminosis
    a. A
    b. B complex
    c. C
    d. D
    e. E
    f. K
15. Clients who have undergone gastric surgery have a high risk for
    a. hemolytic anemia
    b. osteomalacia
    c. pernicious anemia
    d. xerophthalmia
16. Persons with liver disease may become more seriously ill if they receive treatment with certain forms of vitamin
    a. A
    b. B complex
    c. C
    d. D
    e. K
17. Vasodilation, flushing, and abdominal cramps are caused by taking large doses of
    a. ascorbic acid
    b. α-tocopherol
    c. calcitriol
    d. niacin
    e. riboflavin
18. Physical dependence can develop in persons taking large doses of vitamin
    a. A
    b. B complex
    c. C
    d. D
    e. E
    f. K
19. Which mineral is an electrolyte?
    a. calcium
    b. iodine
    c. iron
    d. zinc

20. People who have gastric disease or who have had gastric surgery are at increased risk for deficiency of vitamin
   a. A
   b. B_1
   c. B_2
   d. B_{12}
   e. C
   f. D
   g. K
21. Intestinal bacteria increase the supply of vitamin
   a. A
   b. B complex
   c. C
   d. D
   e. E
   f. K
22. Persons receiving L-dopa medication should
   a. reduce dietary intake of pyridoxine
   b. maintain a steady dietary intake of pyridoxine
   c. decrease dietary intake of vitamin K
   d. maintain a steady dietary intake of vitamin K
23. A regimen of gradually decreasing dosages (weaning) is desirable when persons are planning to discontinue large doses of vitamin
   a. A
   b. B complex
   c. C
   d. D
   e. E
   f. K
24. The tissue or organ most involved in the storage of metallic elements is
   a. bone
   b. fat
   c. the liver
   d. the thyroid gland
25. The thyroid gland traps and stores the mineral
   a. calcium
   b. iodine
   c. magnesium
   d. sodium
26. A mineral found to be helpful in the treatment of some decubiti is
   a. calcium
   b. iodine
   c. iron
   d. zinc
27. The most common mineral toxicity in the United States is excess intake of
   a. calcium
   b. iron
   c. potassium
   d. sodium
28. Hypercalcemia tends to cause
   a. hypertension
   b. prolongation of cardiac systole
   c. weak heart contraction
   d. a widening of the QRS complex on the ECG
29. The mineral most likely to precipitate allergic reaction is
   a. calcium
   b. iodine
   c. iron
   d. potassium
   e. sodium
30. Osteosclerosis and mottling of tooth enamel is likely to result from chronic toxicity of
   a. calcium
   b. fluoride
   c. iodine
   d. iron
   e. magnesium
31. A mineral used to treat digitalis toxicity is
   a. calcium
   b. iron
   c. sodium
   d. potassium
32. For most clients with delutional hyponatremia, the safest way to administer sodium supplements is by giving
   a. oral salt tablets
   b. oral table salt
   c. intravenous infusions of 2% sodium chloride solution
   d. intravenous infusions of normal saline solution
   e. subcutaneous infusions of 10% sodium chloride solution
33. Whether potassium is administered orally or parenterally, it is important that
   a. the chloride salt rather than the iodide salt be used
   b. adequate calcium is administered with it
   c. it be well diluted by fluids
   d. the client is on a cardiac monitor

34. Sodium deficit is most likely to develop in
    a. sedentary persons in cool, dry environments
    b. sedentary persons in hot, humid environments
    c. physically active persons in cool, dry environments
    d. physically active persons in hot, humid environments
35. A factor that predisposes to sodium deficit is
    a. hypocortism
    b. hypothyroidism
    c. oliguria
    d. potassium therapy
36. A factor predisposing to hypokalemia is
    a. hypocortism
    b. increased stress
    c. therapy with potassium
    d. therapy with spironolactone
37. A mineral that tends to cause constipation is
    a. calcium
    b. iodine
    c. magnesium
    d. sodium
38. The metal found in high concentrations in brain lesions of some persons with Alzheimer's disease is
    a. aluminum
    b. calcium
    c. iron
    d. magnesium
39. Which of the following materials is likely to be safest for cooking pots?
    a. aluminum
    b. ceramics with lead glazes
    c. lead-free glass
    d. stainless steel
40. A mineral known to be teratogenic is
    a. calcium
    b. iron
    c. zinc
    d. magnesium
41. The best way to supplement dietary intake of iodine is to
    a. take a drop of tincture of iodine diluted in water daily
    b. supplement the diet with dolomite
    c. increase intake of soybeans and cabbage
    d. use iodized table salt
42. Are vitamin and mineral supplements controlled by the Food and Drug Administration?
    a. no
    b. vitamins are but minerals are not
    c. minerals are but vitamins are not
    d. yes

Selection of options

For each of the following, select *all* appropriate responses. Circle the correct answers.

1. Vitamins that require fat and bile salts for absorption in the small intestine include vitamin(s)
    a. A
    b. B complex
    c. C
    d. D
    e. E
    f. K
2. The liver serves as a tissue storage depot for vitamin(s)
    a. A
    b. B complex
    c. C
    d. D
3. Which vitamins are teratogenic?
    a. A
    b. B complex
    c. C
    d. D
    e. E
4. Signs and symptoms of excesses of vitamins A and D include
    a. fatigue and lethargy
    b. abnormal bone changes
    c. bone tenderness
    d. headache
    e. constipation
    f. oliguria
    g. soft tissue calcification

5. Intrinsic factor greatly enhances intestinal absorption of vitamin(s)
   a. A
   b. B_1
   c. B_2
   d. B_{12}
   e. C
   f. D
   g. K
6. Ingredients often used in multivitamin preparations include
   a. citrus pulp
   b. fish liver oils
   c. meat extracts
   d. vegetable oils
   e. yeast
7. Vitamin C breakdown in food can be minimized by
   a. pasteurization
   b. refrigeration
   c. reduction
   d. use of copper storage containers
8. During pregnancy, serious adverse reactions can be caused by taking mega-vitamin doses of vitamin(s)
   a. A
   b. B_1
   c. B_2
   d. B_{12}
   e. C
   f. K
9. Mineral elements involved in the proper physiologic function of nerves and muscles include:
   a. aluminum
   b. calcium
   c. magnesium
   d. potassium
   e. sodium
10. Substances that play important roles in the tissue distribution of calcium include
    a. ascorbic acid
    b. calcitonin
    c. calcitriol
    d. parathormone
    e. thyroxine
11. Clients with renal failure are likely to develop high serum concentrations of
    a. calcium
    b. iodine
    c. magnesium
    d. potassium
    e. sodium
12. Goiter (thyroid gland enlargement) is apt to develop as a result of
    a. calcium deficiency
    b. calcium toxicity
    c. iodine deficiency
    d. iodine toxicity
    e. iron deficiency
    f. iron toxicity
13. Substances useful in the correction of calcium deficits include
    a. Amphojel antacid
    b. dolomite
    c. kelp
    d. milk
    e. Tums antacid
14. Foods rich in potassium include
    a. bananas
    b. cabbage
    c. green leafy vegetables
    d. meat
    e. orange juice
15. To add helpful minerals to the diet, the nurse may recommend the use of cooking pots made of
    a. aluminum
    b. enameled steel
    c. glass
    d. iron
    e. stainless steel
16. To prevent the migration of undesirable metals into food, the nurse may recommend the use of cooking utensils made of
    a. aluminum
    b. enameled steel
    c. glass
    d. iron
    e. stainless steel
17. General measures used in the treatment of metal toxicity include
    a. fever therapy to promote diaphoresis
    b. administration of ion exchange resins
    c. administration of chelating agents
    d. diuretic therapy
18. Fruits that are good sources of potassium include
    a. apples
    b. bananas
    c. cranberries
    d. oranges

PART 2: HEALTH FOOD PRODUCTS

Correct the false statement

Indicate whether the following statements are true or false; if false, correct the underlined words or phrases.

_______ 1. The labels on health food products <u>must adhere</u> to the standards set for over-the-counter drugs.

_______ 2. The labels on health food products <u>usually recommend</u> safe dosages.

_______ 3. Information on health food supplements is readily available from the <u>medical literature</u>.

_______ 4. Health food publications <u>are allowed</u> to accept advertisements of nutritional supplements produced by the health food business.

_______ 5. Health food products <u>do not</u> exert drug effects.

_______ 6. Linoleic acid is considered to be <u>an essential fatty acid</u>.

_______ 7. When nurses are not expert in the area of health food products, they should advise clients to <u>avoid use of all proprietary health food products</u>.

50 ▪ *Diagnostic drugs*

Pharmacologic agents are frequently used to carry out diagnostic procedures. Because of side effects and toxic effects these procedures must be conducted as carefully as any therapeutic measure to ensure that reliable diagnostic data will be obtained with the least risk to the client.

Multiple choice questions

For each of the following, choose the one best answer:

1. A substance administered orally and rectally to facilitate radiographic examination of the gastrointestinal tract is barium
   a. sulfate
   b. sulfite
   c. sulfide
   d. chloride
2. Screens that shield body parts from x-radiation are uncomfortable because they
   a. feel cold to the touch
   b. feel heavy
   c. must be applied snugly
   d. all of the above
3. The most common side effect of barium used for radiograms is
   a. diarrhea
   b. constipation
   c. nausea and vomiting
   d. inflammation of the gastrointestinal tract
4. A contraindication for the use of barium sulfate is
   a. abdominal pain
   b. intestinal fistulas
   c. peptic ulcer disease
   d. ulcerative colitis
5. Preparation of a client for gastrointestinal x-rays using barium sulfate is likely to include administration of a(n)
   a. laxative
   b. sedative
   c. analgesic
   d. antiemetic
6. Protocols for aftercare of clients undergoing diagnostic x-rays employing barium sulfate are likely to call for administering to the client
   a. an analgesic
   b. intravenous fluids
   c. an antidiarrheal
   d. a laxative
7. Following an upper gastrointestinal series (diagnostic x-rays using barium), clients should be monitored for
   a. cardiac arrhythmias
   b. allergic reaction
   c. constipation
   d. blood in the stool
8. Clients at high risk for complication from gastrointestinal x-ray studies are those with a history of
   a. a tendency toward diarrhea
   b. a tendency toward constipation
   c. hypotension and frequent fainting
   d. peptic ulcer disease
9. A serious adverse reaction to iodinated contrast media is
   a. subclinical pulmonary embolism
   b. inflammation of the urinary tract
   c. anaphylaxis
   d. intestinal obstruction
10. Iodine compounds with radiopaque properties are not administered to clients
    a. with hyperthyroidism
    b. undergoing computed tomography procedures
    c. with gastrointestinal upsets
    d. with allergic hypersensitivity to iodine

11. When oral iodinated contrast media are administered in preparation for a gallbladder series, they are most likely to be given
   a. immediately before the x-rays are taken
   b. 30–60 minutes before the x-rays are taken
   c. several hours before the x-rays are taken
   d. several days before the x-rays are taken
12. Following a serious adverse reaction to iodinated contrast media, clients should be advised to
   a. apply iodine to the skin regularly at least once a week to minimize allergic sensitivity
   b. avoid exposure to all halogens
   c. avoid all radiographic diagnostic tests
   d. wear a medical identification device
13. The most common adverse reaction(s) to radiopaque iodine are
   a. allergic reactions
   b. nausea, vomiting, and flushing
   c. hypotension
   d. persistent impairment of thyroid function
14. A nursing measure that reduces the risk of adverse reaction to barium or radiopaque iodine compounds in clients undergoing radiograms is
   a. administering an antihistamine prior to the test
   b. ensuring adequate hydration prior to the test
   c. ensuring adequate nutrition prior to the test
   d. draping the client with a lead apron to reduce exposure of the target area to ionizing radiation
15. Most nonradioactive compounds used for volumetric diagnostic studies are administered
   a. orally
   b. subcutaneously
   c. intramuscularly
   d. intravenously
16. Clients receiving indigotindisulfonate for diagnostic testing should be reassured that
   a. the red discoloration of the stools is not harmful, and will disappear within a few days
   b. the blue discoloration of the skin is not harmful, and will subside gradually
   c. the red discoloration of the urine is not harmful, and will disappear within a few hours
   d. green-colored stools may occur for a few days following the test, but are not harmful
17. The client at highest risk for adverse reaction to polysaccharides and dyes for volumetric testing is the person with a history of
   a. allergic sensitivity to iodine
   b. atopic asthma
   c. frequent exposure to ionizing radiation
   d. adverse reaction to barium sulfate
18. Clients who have received polysaccharides or aminohippurate for assessment of kidney function should be monitored for
   a. hypotension
   b. increased venous pressure
   c. fever
   d. hematuria
19. Dosage of radionuclides is measured in
   a. units
   b. micrograms
   c. rads
   d. curies
20. Radioactive emissions by radionuclides cause a decline in potency of the drug. This process can be controlled by
   a. storing the drugs in lead-lined containers
   b. storing the drugs in opaque containers
   c. freezing the drugs
   d. none of the above; at present, the rate of disintegration cannot be controlled by any method
21. As radioactive drugs age, the volume required for a given dose
   a. increases
   b. decreases
   c. stays the same
22. Following the diagnostic tests using radionuclides, what precautions are necessary to limit exposures of vulnerable persons to ionizing radiation?
   a. Urine must be diluted and dispersed by disposing of it in a central sewage system.
   b. Feces must be diluted and dispersed by disposing them in a central sewage system.
   c. Recipients must be isolated from vulnerable persons for about 1 week.
   d. All of the above
   e. None of the above
23. A physiologic antagonist of edrophonium is
   a. atropine
   b. muscarine
   c. propranolol
   d. neostigmine

24. All radionuclides should be stored in
   a. opaque containers
   b a refrigerator
   c. a freezer
   d. lead-lined containers

25. Autocoids used as provocative agents are usually stored in
   a. an opaque container
   b. a refrigerator
   c. a freezer
   d. a lead-lined container

Answer Section

1 ▪ Orientation to pharmacology

Sequences

__2__ Ebers Medical Papyrus (Egypt)
__6__ Injection techniques
__5__ Use of foxglove by William Withering
__7__ Drug production as a major technical industry
__1__ Chinese codification of mixtures for medicine
__3__ Roman Materia Medica
__4__ Sophisticated Arabian pharmacology

Matching

1. a 2. a 3. b 4. a 5. a 6. b 7. a 8. a 9. b 10. a 11. c 12. c 13. b 14. b 15. c 16. d 17. c 18. b 19. d 20. a

Completion exercise

1. The following are examples of answers that might be given:

Substance Used	Who Prescribed	Reason for Use	Type of Approach Represented
Aspirin	Self	Headache	Empiric-rational
Tetracycline	Physician	Acne	Rational
Saline gargle	Self	Sore throat	Empiric

2. 19th century
3. Markedly diluted preparations
4. Avoided harmful heroic measures
5. The *United States Pharmacopeia* and the *National Formulary*

Personal exercise: History of pharmacologically active substances

The following are examples of entries that may be included:

Drug Name	Response	Desirable	Undesirable
Prescription Drugs		(Check one)	
Penicillin	Decrease in pain and	x	
	soreness of throat		
	(tonsillitis)		
	Itchy skin rash		x
Erythromycin	Decrease in pain and	x	
	soreness of throat		
Patent Medicines			
Hydrocortisone	Relief of skin itching	x	
ointment			
Tylenol	Lowering of fever	x	
Folk Remedies			
Tea (applied to skin for	None		
relief of itching)			
Herbs			
Chamomile tea	Relaxation	x	
Mint tea	Relaxation	x	
Foods			
Prunes	Relief of constipation	x	
Social Drugs			
Nicotine (cigarettes)	Elevated mood	x	
	Relaxation	x	
	Stimulation	x	
	Cough		x
	Bad breath		x
	Stained teeth and		x
	fingers		
Alcohol	Relaxation	x	
	Silliness	Undecided	
	Irritability		x
Poisons			
HCI (spilled in lab)	Pain in burned area		x
Pollutants			
Exhaust fumes (e.g., in	Headache		x
underpass in traffic			
jam)			

Short answer questions

1. Large drug industry with advanced technology; large numbers of medicinal drugs; growing problems of drug abuse; growing problems of chemical pollution; renewed interest in herbal and traditional medicines; and increased concern about overuse of chemicals

2. a. The dose-effect relationship of a drug
   b. Time and chemical factors involved in absorption, distribution, chemical transformation, and removal of a drug into and out of living material
   c. Localization of the site of action of a drug
   d. Scientific mechanism of action of a drug

e. Relationship between the chemical constitution of a drug and its biologic activity

3. The pharmacist (or pharmacy) who dispensed the drug

Multiple choice questions

1. a 2. d 3. a 4. c 5. b 6. a 7. d 8. c 9. b 10. a 11. a 12. c 13. a 14. c 15. d 16. c

Essay question

List drug name(s), drug family(ies), mechanism of action, side effects, adverse reactions, toxic effects and antidotes, drug interactions, precautions and contraindications, dosage range, routes of administration and elimination, and nursing implications.

Personal experience: Attitude toward drugs

There is no right or wrong answer to this question. It is important to know what your personal bias is, so as to guard against it influencing your judgment unduly in clinical situations.

2 ▪ Drug preparations, controls, and standards

Matching

1. c 2. g 3. a 4. e 5. b 6. d 7. f 8. d 9. a 10. a 11. e 12. d 13. b 14. b 15. b 16. a 17. c

True and false

1. T 2. F 3. T 4. F 5. F 6. T 7. F 8. F 9. T 10. F 11. F 12. T

Multiple choice questions

1. b 2. a 3. a 4. b 5. d 6. d 7. a 8. c 9. a 10. c 11. c 12. b 13. a 14. c 15. d 16. b 17. c 18. c 19. c 20. d 21. b 22. c 23. d 24. a 25. b 26. b 27. b 28. a 29. b 30. a 31. d 32. a 33. a 34. a 35. b 36. d 37. d 38. d 39. c

Selection of options

1. a,b,c,d,e 2. c,d,e 3. a,c,d,e 4. a,c,d,e 5. e,f,h 6. d,f 7. b only 8. a,g 9. c only 10. d,f 11. d,f 12. b,d,e 13. b,c,d,e 14. c,d 15. d only

Rank-order question

c, f, e, d, a, b

Correct the false statement

1. F; trade, brand, or proprietary
2. T
3. T
4. T
5. F; are
6. F; prevent them from sticking to the machines used to press the tablets
7. F; volatile
8. F; an emulsion
9. F; Drug Enforcement Agency of the Department of Justice
10. F; more severe
11. T
12. F; was never enforced in relation to drug efficacy
13. F; the Harrison Narcotic Act of 1914
14. T
15. F; nonprescription or over-the-counter
16. F; any healthcare practitioner
17. F; only physicians, dentists, and pharmacists

Short answer

1. The degree to which a preparation is free of substances other than the intended (desired) ingredients
2. The strength of a drug's effect, relative to that of other drugs
3. The degree to which a drug can be absorbed and transported by the body to its site of action
4. Effectiveness of a drug in treatment
5. The nonproprietary name of a compound used medicinally (e.g., digitalis)

6. Name of a drug adapted by an authority designated by a governing body (e.g., aspirin)
7. A chemical that produces a drug effect (e.g., thyroxine, aspirin)
8. A substance added to an active ingredient to impart desired characteristics to a drug preparation (e.g., vehicles, diluents, fillers, dyes, flavorings, disintegrators, lubricants)
9. Organic compounds containing nitrogen, and having a basic *p*H (e.g., atropine, morphine)
10. Plant derivatives containing a sugar and one or more additional chemical components in their molecules (e.g., digitalis)
11. Compounds containing amino acids joined by a peptide linkage (e.g., insulin)
12. Compounds containing a structure composed of three hexagonal carbon rings, and one pentagonal ring (e.g., digitalis, cortisone, testosterone, estrogen)
13. Substances that give form and substance to a drug preparation (e.g., oil, water, syrup, cocoa butter, petroleum)
14. Relatively inert substances added to a preparation to provide bulk (e.g., lactose, dextrose, starch)
15. Substances used to reduce the concentration of the active ingredient in a preparation (e.g., vehicles, fillers)
16. Substances added to increase the cohesiveness of dry ingredients in a drug preparation (e.g., dextrose, lactose)
17. Substances added to drug preparations to facilitate disaggregation and dissolution (e.g., starch)
18. Substances added to drug preparations to prevent adhesion of the dry ingredients to compression machinery used to form tablets and caplets (e.g., talc, stearate, vegetable oil)
19. Substances added to drug preparations to improve their flavor (e.g., cherry, chocolate, licorice, raspberry)
20. Coloring agents added to drug preparations to improve their appearance and facilitate their identification (e.g., tartrazine)
21. Emulsions
22. Tablets, pills, or capsules
23. Suppositories
24. Liniments
25. Aromatic waters
26. Fluid extracts
27. Elixirs
28. Alkaloids
29. It is used to test substances for mutagenicity, a property believed to reflect carcinogenicity.
30. Examples of some family practices and attitudes include the following: religious beliefs that the use of alcohol is sinful (leading to pressure toward total abstinence); cultural patterns regarding the use of wine as a table beverage, even for children; permissiveness in relation to the use of marijuana; either strictures against or permissiveness toward the use of tobacco; avoidance of local anesthetics, for example, because (1) the numbing of gums is believed to promote careless drilling on the part of the dentist, or (2) the drugs are totally ineffective in some family members; avoidance of drugs to which many family members develop allergies (e.g., aspirin, penicillin); avoidance of drugs to which many family members develop unpleasant side effects (e.g., depression following the use of diazepam); reliance on the use of health food products such as kelp; a tendency to discontinue dosing with a prescription drug as soon as the symptoms subside because the use of drugs is feared and distrusted; persistence in seeking medical help from different physicians until a drug is prescribed because of belief that medication is required to treat most illnesses.
31. Potency
32. Safety margin
33. Efficacy
34. Purity
35. Bioavailability
36. Unlike the drug-dependent person, the drug addict either endangers the public or has lost the power to control the addiction.
37. Among the possible answers are the following: prohibition of alcohol in the 1920s and severe penalties for the use of marijuana in the mid-20th century. In both cases, there was widespread noncompliance with the law.
38. Unsafe drugs cannot be sold; labels on drugs must be accurate; information required on labels is delineated; drugs must meet official standards; the manufacturing processes for producing certain drugs are subject to approval; the safety of drug batches is subject to approval; the sale of certain drugs may be forbidden; some drugs are limited to prescription use; refills of prescriptions for controlled drugs are limited; prescriptions for designated drugs must indicate the condition to be treated; sale of hallucinogens is forbidden; distribution of sample drugs is limited to physicians, dentists, and pharmacists; prescription and controlled drugs may not be advertised to the general public; specific regulations may control the use of certain drugs. Canadian law forbids the use of thalidomide. A *controlled* drug is one (such as amphetamines) that must be prescribed for a limited time with specific directions for its use. A prescription for a *designated* drug must indicate the condition for which it is prescribed. *Pr* is the symbol placed on the labels of drugs that are limited to prescription use.

Completion exercises

1. Thalidomide
2. Salk polio vaccine
3. Effective
4. Kefauver-Harris Amendment of 1962
5. Personal choice

3 ▪ Nursing process: Management of clients with drug-related problems

Personal exercise: Nursing care plan

The personal nursing care plan is a learning experience that can influence the student's self-care practices. Even when substances not commonly considered to be true "drugs" such as nutritional supplements (vitamins and minerals) or aspirin are involved, the student will find that the use of the substance involves some risk, the effects of the medicine may be enhanced by nondrug measures, and the properties of the chemicals involved must be considered if optimal health care is to result.

Correct the false statement

1. F; involves many independent, as well as dependent, nursing functions
2. T
3. F; clients in the community; treatment of acute or chronic health problems
4. F; use judgment in deciding whether to encourage or discourage drug use by individual clients
5. F; each time goals are established or revised

Short answer questions

1. Promotion of optimal response to drugs; decreasing the risk of adverse reactions to drugs; assisting clients to achieve optimal health through proper use of drugs
2. Assessment; diagnosis; planning; intervention; evaluation
3. Drugs prescribed by physicians; self-prescribed medicines; nonmedicinal drugs used; chemical exposure in the recent past
4. Minimization of side effects; prevention of drug dependence; prompt detection of adverse reactions; withdrawal from a dependency-producing chemical; reduction (or promotion) of drug use
5. Therapeutic response; adverse reactions; unusual reactions; allergic reactions; tolerance; dependence
6. Because unusual reactions are often associated with inherited (genetic) factors that may be shared by the client
7. The quality of the desired change; the magnitude of the change desired; a method for measuring the magnitude of change; a time limit for achieving the desired change

Multiple choice questions

1. a 2. a 3. c 4. d 5. c 6. b 7. c 8. b 9. b

Selection of options

1. a,b 2. c,d 3. a,b,c,d

4 ▪ *Pharmacodynamics and pharmacokinetics*

Matching

A. 1. b 2. a 3. a 4. c 5. a 6. b 7. c 8. c
B. 1. b 2. d 3. a 4. c
C. 1. b 2. a 3. a 4. d 5. c 6. a 7. b,c,d 8. a

Checklist

2, 5, 6, 7, 9

Correct the false statement

1. F; a decrease
2. T
3. F; wider
4. F; higher
5. F; very narrow to nonexistent (because it is as likely to harm as to produce a therapeutic effect)
6. F; lipid-soluble
7. T
8. F; for both local and systemic effects
9. T
10. F; acidic
11. F; retards and may reduce
12. F; acidic
13. F; duodenum or small intestine
14. F; gradual absorption
15. F; lesser
16. T
17. F; decrease
18. F; only when a prompt therapeutic response to a drug is critical
19. T
20. F; liver
21. T
22. F; is sometimes
23. T

Completion exercises

1. Intra-arterial infusion; extracorporeal perfusion; topical application for local effect; injection for local effect (e.g., regional anesthesia, joint injections)
2. Hyaluronidase (Wydase)
3. Epinephrine (Adrenalin)
4. Less than 100
5. Liver by way of the biliary tract
6. Constant rate intravenous infusion

Draw a drug map*

1. penicillin G procaine

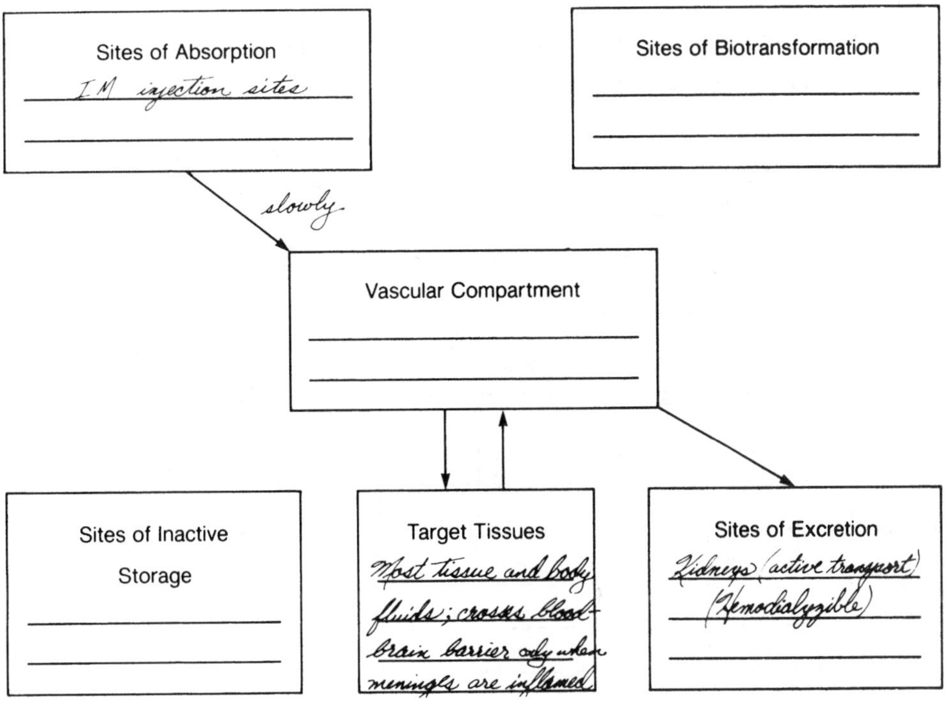

2. prednisone

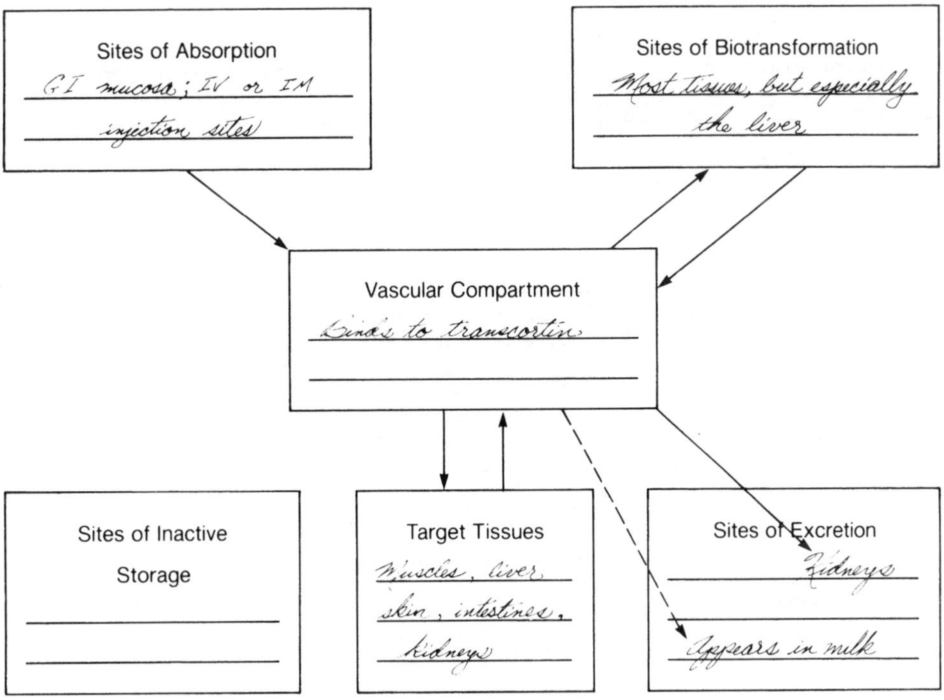

*Information in this section has been taken from the American Society of Hospital Pharmacists. (1991). *Drug Information.* Bethesda, American Society of Hospitals.
Key: → = major pathways; and
- → = minor pathways.

3. insulin

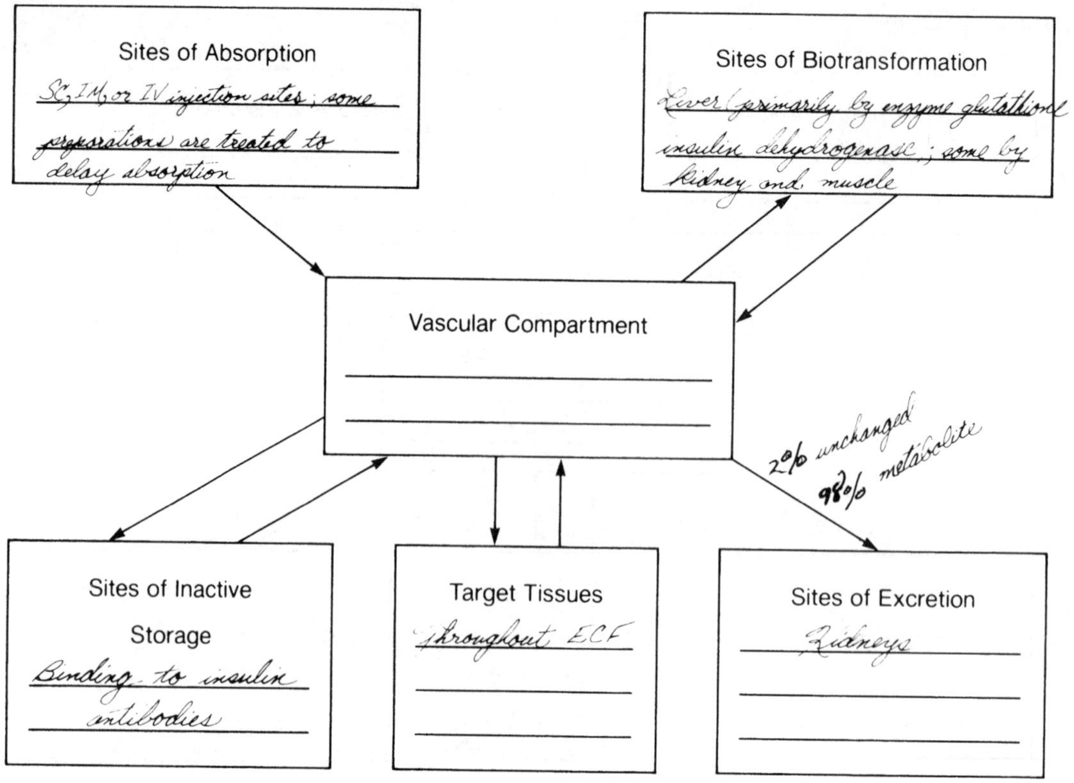

Sites of Absorption
SC, IM, or IV injection sites; some preparations are treated to delay absorption
Sites of Biotransformation
Liver (primarily by enzyme glutathione insulin dehydrogenase; some by kidney and muscle
Vascular Compartment
2% unchanged
98% metabolite
Sites of Inactive Storage
Binding to insulin antibodies
Target Tissues
Throughout ECF
Sites of Excretion
Kidneys

4. milk of magnesia

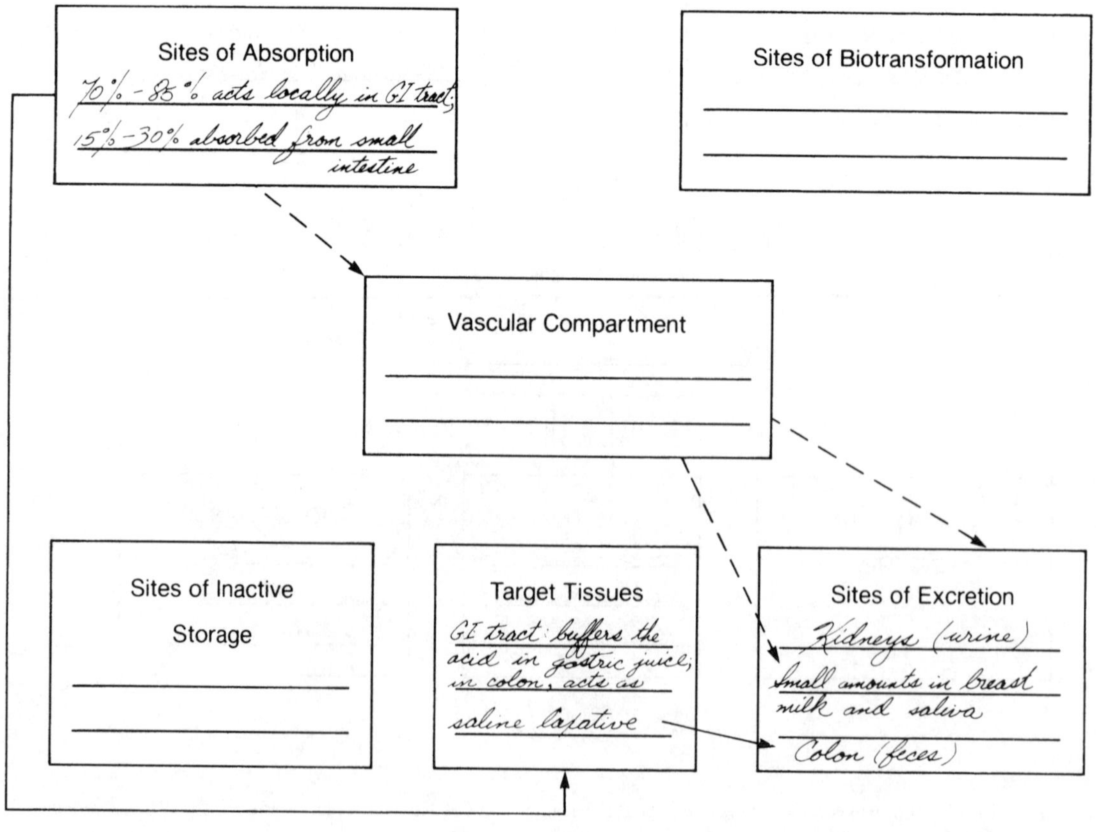

Sites of Absorption
70%–85% acts locally in GI tract; 15%–30% absorbed from small intestine
Sites of Biotransformation
Vascular Compartment
Sites of Inactive Storage
Target Tissues
GI tract: buffers the acid in gastric juice; in colon, acts as saline laxative
Sites of Excretion
Kidneys (urine)
Small amounts in breast milk and saliva
Colon (feces)

5. morphine sulfate

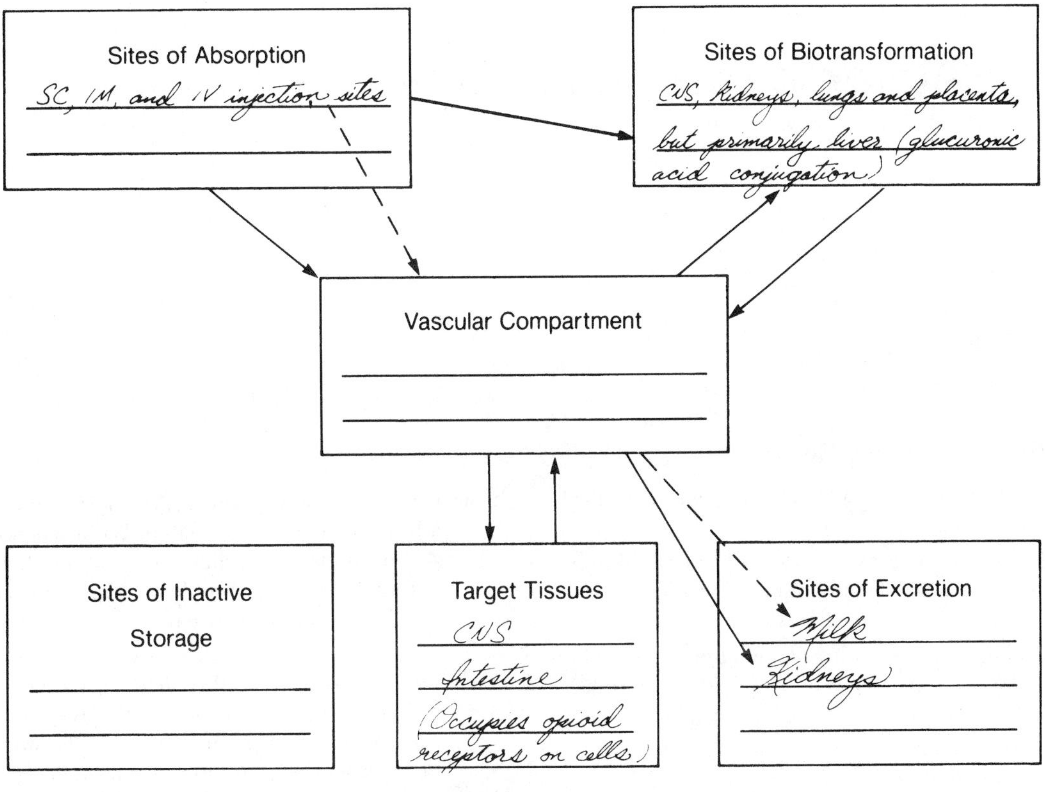
Sites of Absorption
SC, IM, and IV injection sites
Sites of Biotransformation
CNS, kidneys, lungs and placenta, but primarily liver (glucuronic acid conjugation)
Vascular Compartment
Sites of Inactive Storage
Target Tissues
CNS
Intestine
(Occupies opioid receptors on cells)
Sites of Excretion
Milk
Kidneys

6. methotrexate sodium

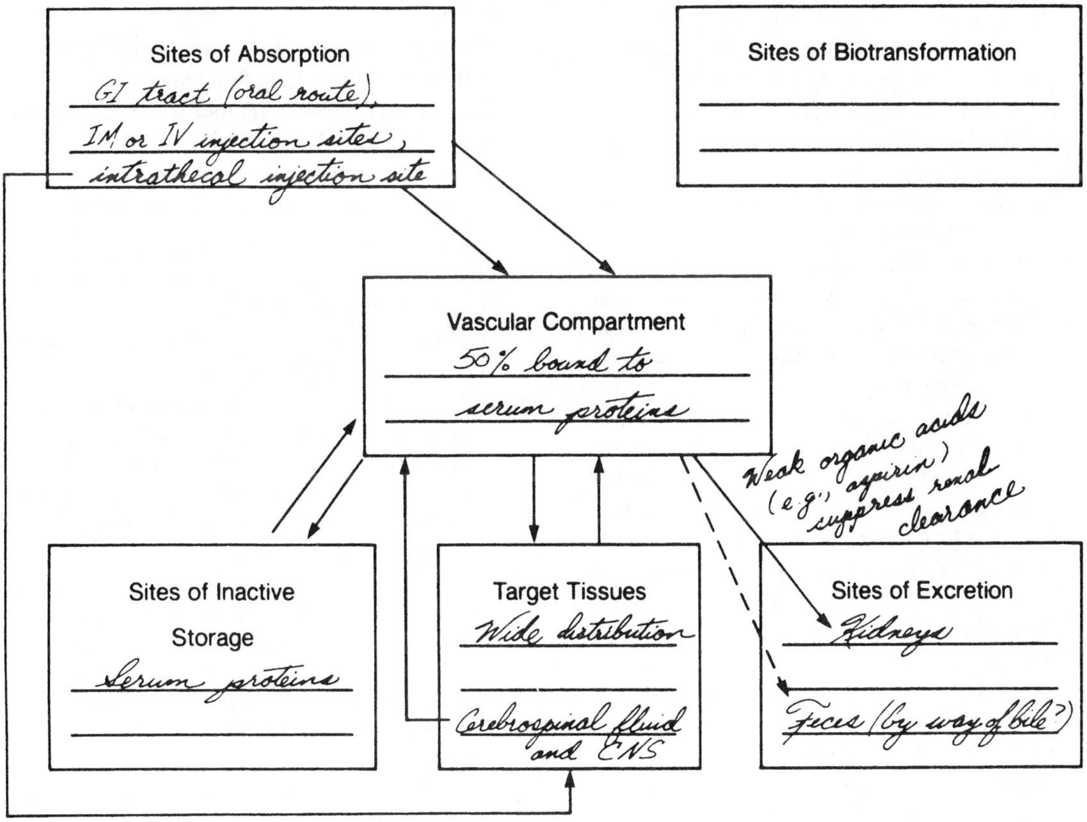
Sites of Absorption
GI tract (oral route),
IM or IV injection sites,
intrathecal injection site
Sites of Biotransformation
Vascular Compartment
50% bound to
serum proteins
Weak organic acids (e.g., aspirin) suppress renal clearance
Sites of Inactive Storage
Serum proteins
Target Tissues
Wide distribution
Cerebrospinal fluid and CNS
Sites of Excretion
Kidneys
Feces (by way of bile?)

5 ▪ *Adverse drug reactions*

Matching

A. 1. b 2. a 3. d 4. c 5. a 6. b 7. c 8. d 9. b 10. d 11. c 12. a

Short answer questions

1. a. Iatrogenic: arising from or caused by medical treatment
   b. Adverse drug reaction: any of several undesirable reactions that can occur when a drug is taken
   c. Side effect: any physiologic effect other than that for which a given drug is administered
   d. Toxic effect: a drug effect that is deleterious to the organism, especially an effect characteristic of high doses
   e. Allergic reaction: an adverse response to a chemical caused by the presence in an organism of immune bodies whose production was stimulated by previous exposure to that chemical
   f. Carcinogenic: capable of causing cancer
   g. Chain reaction: a response that occurs when the use of one drug necessitates the use of multiple additional drugs to control side effects of the first drug
   h. Cumulative reaction: toxicity caused by the accumulation of a drug in the body that occurs when the dosage absorbed exceeds the amount the body can degrade through metabolism or excretion
   i. Idiosyncratic reaction: an abnormal response to a drug that may take the form of extreme sensitivity to low doses, extreme insensitivity to high doses, or a response that is qualitatively different from the usual response
   j. Teratogenic: property of developing abnormal structures in an embryo resulting in fetal deformities
   k. Tolerance: a condition of decreased responsiveness that is acquired after a single or repeated exposure to a given drug or to one closely allied in pharmacologic activity
   l. Dependence: a condition in which the user of a drug has a compelling desire to continue taking the drug, either to experience its effects or to avoid the discomfort of its absence
2. a. Generalized skin rash is the most common adverse reaction to penicillin. Local reactions to injections are characterized by erythema and itching. Skin problems often precede more serious allergic reactions.
   b. Anaphylaxis is the most serious allergic reaction to penicillin. In this life-threatening condition, swelling of tissues of the respiratory tract, bronchospasm, and generalized vasospasm cause cardiorespiratory collapse.
3. Factors that suggest that the client may experience an adverse drug reaction include the following:

   The client is undergoing treatment by two or more physicians at the same time.

   The client has other temporary or permanent medical or dental problems.

   The client uses prescription drugs.

   The client uses over-the-counter preparations.

   The client has a history of allergies.

   The client has experienced adverse drug reactions to medications previously.

   Other factors include age, body size, hepatic function, and renal function.
4. a. Advise the client to change position slowly, especially when arising from a lying position. Promote ample fluid intake to maintain hydration and blood volume. Assist client with ambulation. Consult with physician about a change in medication.
   b. Consult with physician about a change in medication. Keep client comfortably cool; apply cold compresses to affected areas. Teach client to exert pressure on affected area rather than scratching it; encourage engrossing activities to divert client's attention from the problem.
   c. Eliminate noxious stimuli. Serve frequent small feedings. Offer food favored by the client. Present food attractively. Offer between-meal snacks. Administer antiemetics,

when ordered, before meal time. Consult with physician about a change in medication.

Encourage client to consume foods with laxative properties. Encourage ample fluids. Encourage exercise. Promote a regular habit of defecation. Consult with physician about a change in medication.

Encourage foods and fluids to replace intestinal losses of fluid and electrolytes. Advise client to avoid foods with laxative properties. Consult with physician about a change in medication.

Completion exercise

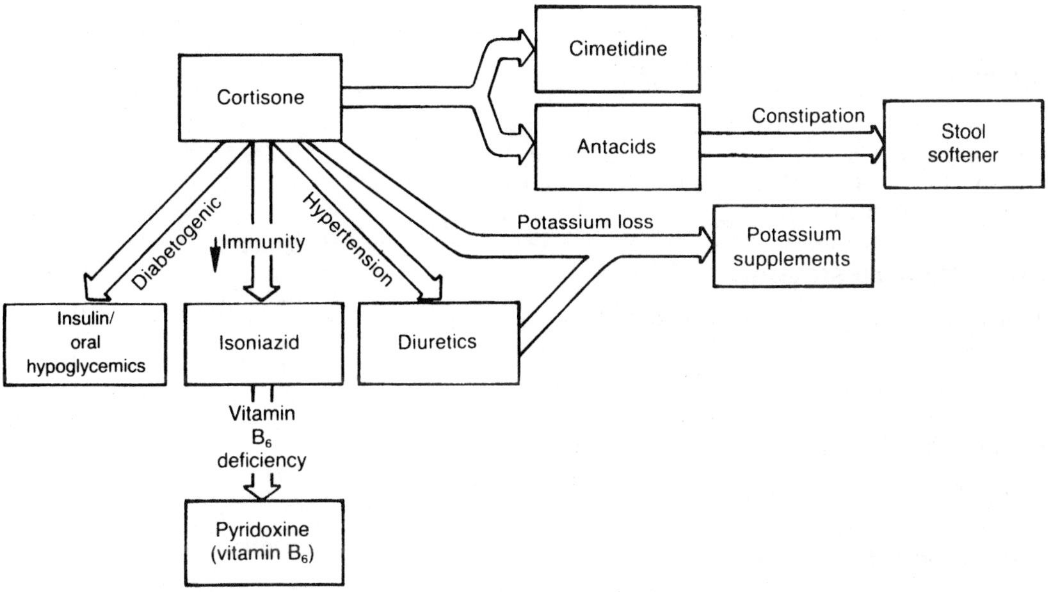

6 ▪ Drug interactions

Matching

A. 1. h 2. b 3. c
B. 4. e 5. a,b,h 6. a,h 7. h 8. h 9. g 10. d 11. f
C. 12. d 13. c 14. a 15. a 16. b 17. d 18. c 19. a
D. 20. d 21. f 22. c

Correct the false statement

1. F; only those foods to which the client reacts adversely
2. F; reduce absorption of drugs by absorbing them
3. T
4. F; liquids that will not raise stomach *p*H

Selection of options

1. b,c,e,f 2. c,e 3. b,d 4. d,e 5. a,d 6. d,e

Short answer questions

1. Dyes (as tartrazine), sulfites, parabens, monosodium glutamate, aspartame, butylated hydroxyanisole and butylated hydroxytoluene, nitrates
2. Aged cheeses, red wine, fava beans, broad bean pods
3. Poverty, preexisting malnutrition, long-term dietary restriction, anorexia, pregnancy, lactation, rapid growth, certain chronic diseases, prolonged or severe stress, chronic dialysis, certain long-term medication regimens
4. a. Detrimental drug interaction: a drug interaction that is hazardous or deleterious to the client
   b. Clinically desirable interaction: a beneficial drug effect that is enhanced by the concomitant use of another drug or a detrimental drug effect that is mitigated by the concomitant use of another drug
5. Client is under treatment by two or more physicians at the same time; client has other temporary or permanent medical or dental problems; client uses over-the-counter preparations; client's diet includes components that will conflict with medications that are to be prescribed
6.

Drug with Decreased Absorption	Interactant Drug
Tetracycline	Aluminum and magnesium antacids and laxatives; food products containing calcium; ferrous sulfate
Phenytoin	Sucralfate
Griseofulvin	Phenobarbital

7. Do not give the drugs simultaneously. Separate the doses of the two interactant drugs by 3 or 4 hours.
8. a. Phenylbutazone and warfarin
   b. Sodium valproate and phenytoin
   c. Methotrexate and acetylsalicylic acid
9. a. Drug inhibitor: a drug that reduces the metabolism of others, such as allopurinol, erythromycin, or cimetidine

b. Drug inducer: a drug that can induce the synthesis of hepatic drug-metabolizing enzymes, such as rifampin, griseofulvin, or nicotine

10. Theophylline, ethanol
11. Uric acid is formed by xanthine-oxidase-catalyzed oxidation of hypoxanthine and xanthine. Allopurinol inhibits the xanthine oxidase. This inhibition reduces plasma concentration and urinary excretion of uric acid and increases plasma concentration and renal excretion of uric acid precursors.
12. Benzodiazepines, warfarin, theophylline, phenytoin, quinidine
13. When tyramine is not oxidized, it is freely absorbed and can reach the adrenergic nerve endings through the circulating blood. Here there is an accumulation of norepinephrine as a result of the preceding effect of the MAO inhibitor. Tyramine causes the release of this surplus norepinephrine, resulting in an accentuated hypertensive effect. Fatal cerebral hemorrhages have occurred.
14. The acceleration of metabolism caused by smoking can result in a reduction of blood levels and reduction of therapeutic effects of the interactant drug.
15. Kidney, hepatobiliary route, lung, skin, saliva, milk, sweat
16. By alkalinizing the urine through the use of antacids in large doses

7 ▪ Principles of medication

Matching

A. 1. g 2. c 3. a,d 4. f 5. b 6. h
B. 1. a,b,c 2. c 3. a,b 4. c 5. a,b,c

Correct the false statement

1. F; until the first dose is drawn from it, after which it is stored at room temperature
2. F; to place the container in a pocket near the body until the container no longer feels cool to the touch
3. F; in a locked cabinet in a cool, dry room
4. T
5. F; a stock bottle
6. F; the physician must be consulted to determine the route to be used
7. F; the nurse should not administer the dose unless he or she no longer considers the dose likely to harm the client
8. T
9. T
10. F; water
11. F; the physician should be consulted to determine the route desired
12. F; physicians, nurses, and respiratory therapists
13. F; refuse to carry out drug orders that are likely to cause harm to the client (other answers, such as questioning inappropriate order, would also be correct)
14. T

Multiple choice questions

1. a. A remaining half-tablet should be given the next time the drug is administered to even out any discrepancy of dose as soon as possible.
2. d. For most drugs, accuracy within 10 percent of the dose ordered is acceptable. The physician is responsible for informing the client, initially, about the benefits and risks of the treatment.
3. b. In community and hospital settings nurses need to consult with physicians, but the degree of influence exercised by nurses over drug regimens is usually less than in skilled nursing facilities in which physicians rely on nurses to manage most aspects of care of the chronically or terminally ill. In some states, nurses in independent practice cannot diagnose illness or prescribe medication, although they are allowed to counsel clients regarding the use of over-the-counter preparations and measures to optimize response to prescription drugs.
4. a. In institutional settings vocational-technical nurses practice under the supervision of professional nurses.
5. a. Enteric-coated tablets should not be broken, because the drug would be released prematurely in the stomach. Solutions made from tablets are usually unpalatable.
6. b
7. c
8. b
9. a

Selection of options

1. a, d. Only in selected situations would b or c be appropriate.
2. d. Most medicine glasses do not have scales containing markings for 18 ml or its factors. Whereas 4 drams would be approximately equal to 18 ml (1 dram is 4 to 5 ml), a syringe would be more accurate. Fill the 6-ml syringe three times and eject the drug into a medicine glass.
3. b, c. The nurse would also be responsible if the client were harmed by the drug.

4. a, b, c. Although a large dose might alert the nurse to an increased risk of toxicity, individual responses to a given dose of drug vary greatly, and absolute level of dosage does not predict client response.
5. b, c, e
6. c, e, f, h
7. b, c, e

Sequence

__3__ Notify the physician of the client's failure to improve.

__2__ Check the chart to see how many doses of antibiotic the client has received.

__1__ Interview the client to determine whether the oral antibiotic has been retained.

Completion exercises

1. Standing orders accompanied by criteria for their use
2. Superscription, inscription, and subscription
3. Household, apothecary, and metric
4. Metric
5. Dispensing
6. Prescribing
7. Compounding

Short answer questions

1. (In any order) the right drug, the right client (patient), the right dose, the right route, the right time
2. 7. Drug levels decline as follows: after 1 half-life, 50%; after 2, 25%; after 3, 12 1/2%; after 4, 6 1/4%; after 5, 3 1/8%; after 6, 1 9/16%; after 7, 25/32%.
3. 7 half-lives, or 7 full days
4. Intravenous
5. Right eye
6. Once a day
7. Before meals
8. At bedtime
9. One drop
10. One ounce
11. One dram
12. Milligram
13. Gram
14. Milliliter
15. Once when necessary
16. After meals
17. Once a day
18. Once an hour
19. Immediately
20. Intramuscular
21. Hypodermic
22. Five
23. One-half
24. Saturated solution of potassium permanganate
25. Soap suds enema
26. Morphine sulfate
27. Milk of magnesia
28. Mineral oil
29. Tap water enema
30. Gram
31. Microgram
32. Kilogram
33. Cubic centimeter
34. Liter
35. Aspirin

Situational exercises

1. When the nurse asked the physician to spell the name of the drug, it was recognized as Evacugen (E-vac-u-jen), a common laxative preparation.
2. Determine whether or not food interferes with the absorption of the drug. In this case it does not. Remove the drug and store it in a secure place until tray time, when you would again offer it to the client. It would be wise to change the time assigned for administration of the drug so that in the future it will be given at mealtime. If the drug had been ordered more than once a day (b.i.d. or t.i.d.), the times for subsequent administration on this day might need adjusting to prevent dosage at too-short intervals.

Personal exercise: Drug history

Of particular importance in this situation would be foods or other chemicals that might be toxic and therefore be the cause of the pain. Also of concern would be exposure to antibiotics, because use of such drugs could alter the intestinal flora, resulting in superinfection or in predisposition to antibiotic-resistant infections (and, in this situation, surgery might be required). All chemicals to which you have been exposed within the last 14 days should be listed, as should all drugs that produce an adverse reaction in you.

8 ▪ Strategies to promote therapeutic alliance

Short answer questions

1. a. Enhancement: the drug is more effective than expected
   b. Negation: the drug is not, or is only minimally, effective
   c. Adverse reaction: an allergic or undesirable effect that is unwanted is experienced
2. Feelings of dependency, anger, hostility, resentment; feelings of security and well-being; anxiety
3. Alleviating pain and anxiety; inducing sleep; decreasing or minimizing allergic reactions
4. Refusing to take the medication; taking enough of the medication to feel better without having to give up the sick role; taking the medication but developing other symptoms
5. Taking a larger dosage than prescribed; taking the drug more often than indicated; taking the drug longer than indicated; taking several drugs concurrently in spite of drug-drug interactions

Matching

1. c 2. d 3. a 4. f 5. e 6. b

Multiple choice questions

1. a 2. b 3. b 4. b 5. d 6. a

9 ▪ Cultural aspects of drug therapy

Matching

A. 1. f 2. e 3. d 4. b 5. a 6. c
B. 1. d 2. b 3. a 4. c

Short answer questions

1. Doctrine of signatures is the belief that "like cures like." Ex.: Red plants used to treat blood-related problems. Moxibustion—Application of heat to traditional acupuncture points using burning herb. It is a hot treatment while acupuncture is a "cold treatment."
2. Part of plant collected; amount of processing required to render it useful; time of day; life cycle of plant at time of harvest; season of harvest.
3. Degree of cross-cultural influences; socioeconomic status; language facility; strength and significance of kinship ties; degree of acceptance of dominant culture's values.
4. Alcohol—Asian and American Indians do not metabolize alcohol as effectively as white or African Americans. Psychotropic/neuroleptics—Asians require lower doses and metabolize more slowly than white and African Americans.

Completion exercises

Group	Common Illness	Remedy
African Americans	open wound	salt pork, sour milk and stale bread
	congestion/cold	Hot lemon, water, honey; hot toddy
	boil	Raw egg shell skin
Hispanic Americans	menstrual disturbances	Borage, spearmint, orange leaf tea
	stomach aches	Purple sage, rue, anise
	whooping cough	Purple sage
Native Americans	headache	Skunk cabbage in form of snuff, rhubarb, buttercup teas
	constipation	Buttercup tea
European Americans	sore throat	saltwater gargle
	burns	cold, wet tea bags

Chemical Component	Effect on the Body
Vitamins	healing and overall health
Alkaloids	act on vascular and central nervous system
Antibiotics	attack microorganisms
Heterosides (sugars)	interact with body elements to produce various effects on body systems, such as diuretics, irritants, antispasmodics, laxatives

Medicinal Plant	Active Ingredient(s)	Medicinal Use
American hellebore *(Veratrum viride)*	alkaloids, glycosides	hypotensive action
Periwinkle *(Catharanthus roseus)*	vinblastine, vincristine	treatment of cancer
American mandrake *(Atropa mandragora)*	irritating resin	purgative, emetic or for treatment of condyloma acuminatum
Rauwolfia *(Rauwolfia serpentina)*	reserpine	hypotension, sedative
Purple foxglove *(Digitalis purpurea)*	digitalin, digitoxin	acts on cardiac muscle
Cocaine *(Erythroxylon coca)*	cocaine	pain reduction, local anesthetic
Opium poppy *(Papaver somniferum)*	morphine alkaloid, narcotine alkaloid	sedation, pain relief

Checklist

1. a 2. b 3. d 4. c

10 ▪ *Drug therapy in maternal care*

Matching

A. 1. b 2. c 3. a,d 4. d
B. 1. d 2. c 3. a 4. e 5. b
C. 1. b 2. c 3. d 4. a 5. e 6. f

Correct the false statement

1. T
2. F; antiemetic drugs may cause birth defects when taken during pregnancy
3. T
4. F; they should gain at least 15 lb
5. F; intervention is contraindicated in the presence of fetal demise, diabetic mother, or in some cases of PIH
6. T
7. T
8. T
9. F; fluid intake should be limited to between 9 and 100 mL/hr
10. F; some drugs used late in labor may cause respiratory depression in the neonate

Short answer questions

1. a. Slower
   b. Faster
   c. Faster
2. a. 8–100 g
   b. 2.5–6 g
   c. 6–8 glasses
3. Beta sympathomimetics, magnesium sulfate, calcium antagonists, and prostaglandin inhibitors
4. Cardiac arrhythmias, pulmonary hypertension, bronchial asthma, hyperthyroidism, or pheochromocytoma
5. 3 to 5
6. a. This drug may lead to premature labor and/or neonatal problems (e.g., hyperbilirubinemia, respiratory depression).
   b. Oxytocic effects may precipitate labor.
   c. Anticoagulation abnormalities of the fetus increase the risk of cerebrovascular accidents and central nervous system abnormalities.
   d. Maternal hypovolemia and reduced placental perfusion may result in low birth weight infants.

Completion exercises

1. Oxytocin
2. Ergonovine maleate
3. Erythromycin or tetracycline ophthalmic
4.

Drug	Possible Maternal Side Effects
Meperidine (Demerol)	Nausea, vomiting; respiratory depression
Hydroxyzine (Atarax, Vistaril)	Hypotension; vertigo; drowsiness
Diazepam (Valium)	Hypotension; vertigo; drowsiness

Possible Fetal Side Effects

Respiratory depression

CNS depression

Hypothermia; CNS depression; may remain active in fetus for 10 days

Situational exercises

A. 1. a. Check fetal viability; observe frequency and intensity of uterine contractions; observe effect of contractions on fetus

b. Check fetal age; note cervical dilation and effacement; look for fetal membranes in lower canal

c. Complications; baseline blood studies; information on labor (e.g., ruptured membranes, bloody show)

d. Mother in lateral recumbent position; 150 mg ritodrine in 500 ml 5% dextrose in sterile water to be used continuously up to 12–14 hours after contractions stop; microdip and infusion pump for administration.

2. Check maternal pulse and blood pressure q15min during increases of drug, and q30min during maintenance; monitor fluid intake and output; observe for side effects (dyspnea, chest pain, pulse above 120 beats/min, blood pressure below 90 mm Hg, or decrease from baseline)

3. Report pulse over 120 beats/min; report agitation, nervousness; report palpitations, tremors

B. Maternal glucose goes through the placenta, while maternal insulin does not. Insulin is produced by the fetus by the 28th week. B cells hypertrophy to produce additional insulin needed to handle excess glucose. Hyperinsulinemia produces a fetus with excessive growth and storage of excess glycogen, causing fetal obesity. Hyperinsulinemia continues after birth, causing hypoglycemia.

11 ▪ *Drug therapy in pediatric nursing*

Matching

A. 1. a 2. c 3. b
B. 1. b and c 2. a only 3. b and c

Short answer questions

1. a. Calculate drug dosage using an appropriate source for reference. Consider the toxic effects of any medication on a client with an immature body system.
   b. Ensure safe administration by assessing correct client, drug, dose, route, and time.
2. Knowledge of a preschooler's growth and development would include attention to a child's concrete thinking, occasional resistant behavior, response to clear explanations and expectations, preference for liquid or chewable medications, response to praise and rewards, and comfort measures following painful experiences.
3. a. Play may be used to allow the child an opportunity to vent feelings and concerns about an invasive procedure.
   b. The nurse may use play to instruct a child about health care and to assist the child in understanding the procedure.
4. Pharmacokinetic responses, immature body systems, cumulative toxicity, genetic endowment, age, psychological and cognitive development, environmental factors, and underlying chronic conditions.
5. Fewer numbers of glomeruli, underdeveloped active transport system, slow rate of drug filtration, and potential for toxicity.
6. Because dehydrogenation of alcohol is depressed in neonates, administration of elixirs with high alcohol contents should be avoided in this age group. Immature liver function significantly alters the infant's drug metabolism capacity of preservative additives.
7. Body surface area formula
8. .5 mls can be administered to infants in each injection site
9. a. 6.136 kg × 40 mg = 245.4 mgs per day
   b. 245.4/3 = 81.8 mgs per dose
   c. No, Amoxicillin 55 mg po is too low.
10. a. Low range 30.9 kg × 5 mg = 154.5 mg
    High range 30.9 kg × 7 mg = 216.3 mg
    b. 30.9 kg × 6 mg = 185.4/2 = 93 mg per dose

Case example

Assessment Data

A. 1. Postoperative child
Ambulation ordered

B. 1. Fear of needles

Diagnosis

1. Altered comfort related to surgical site and ambulation
1. Anxiety related to needles and medical procedures

Goal

1. Alleviation of pain and anxiety
1. Alleviation and expression of anxiety

Intervention

A. 1. Administer analgesia after teaching child about necessity of intramuscular injection.

Outcome Criteria for Evaluation

1. The child will tolerate intramuscular injections and be comfortable during ambulation as evidenced by normal vital signs, verbalization of decreased pain, and ability to ambulate.
2. Teach child alternative comfort measures such as correct positioning, relaxation techniques, breathing exercises, visual imagery

Intervention

B. 1. Provide an opportunity for play using hospital equipment; play may be structured or occur spontaneously so the nurse may assess feelings, concerns, and fears.
2. Information is supplied with concrete explanations; dolls or models with anatomic parts may be used.
3. Parental participation is encouraged to alleviate parents' anxiety and increase their knowledge.
4. Monitor vital signs.
5. Monitor intravenous infusion.
6. Monitor amount, pH, guaiac of nasogastric secretions.
7. Assess mucus membranes.
8. Monitor urinary output, specific gravity, and pH.

Outcome Criteria for Evaluation

3. Use analgesia prior to severe pain.
4. Allow child to express or play out concerns about intramuscular injections.

1. The child and parents will relax and be less anxious.
2. The child will play with medical equipment and exhibit his or her fears.
3. The child will be adequately hydrated as evidenced by moist mucus membranes, urinary output and specific gravity, normal electrolyte values, and vital signs.

12 · *Drug therapy in gerontological nursing*

Short answer question

1. Changing pharmacokinetic parameters; polypharmacy; chronic disease; diminishing physical, emotional, social, and economic resources
2. Physical resources such as weakened motor function, decreased hearing, decreased vision, alterations in taste and smell, loss of natural teeth, changed nutritional requirements; mental resources such as decreased memory; material resources such as limited finances
3. Monitor drug use; suggest use of generic drugs; monitor use of over-the-counter products; interpret physicians' orders; provide counseling on drug interactions; dispense smaller portions of prescriptions as necessary; give discounts; extend credit; provide delivery service
4. a. Depressed respiratory function
   b. Angina from increased metabolic rate, enhanced effect of digoxin, palpitations
   c. Syncope from cerebral ischemia secondary to lowered blood pressure, confusion, dizziness
5. Confusion, depression, excitation, dizziness, loss of memory, slurred speech
6. Most drugs are eliminated by the kidney. In the elderly you would expect an accumulation of drugs because of decreased kidney function. The accumulation could lead to toxicity.

Correct the false statement

1. F; healthcare professionals are too quick to prescribe medication for every ache and pain
2. T
3. F; to request regular caps from their pharmacists
4. F; of altered pharmacokinetic parameters
5. F; lack of assessment and teaching by healthcare professionals
6. T

Matching

1. d 2. g 3. a 4. e 5. b 6. f 7. c 8. h

Personal exercise

1. 7 A.M.: ranitidine (do not take milk of magnesia within 1 hour)
   1 P.M. after lunch: docusate sodium
   hydrochlorothiazide (if given in morning, diuresis would occur during her therapy)
   KCL (after meals prevents gastric irritation)
   digoxin (after meals prevents gastric irritation)
   warfarin (give at same time each day to assure stable levels)
   multivitamin
2. Dry mouth, blurred vision, constipation, difficulty with urination, fever or feeling very hot, red face

13 ▪ *Drug therapy in the home and community*

Matching

1. c 2. d 3. a 4. c 5. b

Multiple choice questions

1. d 2. b 3. b 4. c 5. b 6. a 7. c 8. b 9. a 10. c

Short answer questions (part 1)

1. Use for relief of minor symptoms or self-limiting conditions; low dosage and decreased risk of adverse reactions; decreased demand on healthcare system
2. Fosters delay in seeking professional care for potentially serious illness and promotes avoidance of professional health care; use of multiple preparations with same ingredients increases risk of adverse reactions; increases potential for adverse reactions when used in combination with prescription drugs.
3. The greater the number of active ingredients, the greater the chances of adverse reactions to the preparation and interaction with other drugs; long-acting preparations should not be used when a product is being tried for the first time because if an adverse reaction occurs, it will be difficult to treat due to continued absorption of the drug; self-medication with OTC preparations could mask symptoms of serious illness
4. Aspirin should not be taken by consumers who concurrently are taking prescription drugs for arthritis because of the increased risk of gastric irritation and bleeding; aspirin should be avoided by diabetics who are taking oral hypoglycemics because this and other salicylates increase the hypoglycemic effect of the drugs; acetaminophen may increase the blood levels of zidovudine in consumers who are human immunodeficiency virus positive; for clients who are taking prescription drugs for hypertension, decongestants may block effects of these drugs; alcohol in liquid OTC preparations may produce severe vomiting in consumers who are taking disulfiram

Completion exercise

Type of Drug	Advantages	Disadvantages
Prescription	Effective for relief of serious and self-limiting conditions; prescribed and monitored by a healthcare professional; drug and dosage chosen to meet individual client needs	Relatively expensive; increased risk of adverse reactions due to use of more dangerous drugs; increased burden on healthcare system in terms of time and resources of healthcare professionals
Nonprescription	Effective for relief of self-limiting and nonprogressive conditions; relatively safe for consumers; increased client control over health care; less expensive than prescription drugs	Lack of professional diagnosis and monitoring; risk of delay in treatment for serious illness; inadequate dosage for some consumers

Personal exercise: OTC drug history

This answer will be different for each student. It should reflect knowledge about the use of nonprescription drug products, benefits and risks to their use, and an understanding of the potential interaction between nonprescription and prescription drugs.

Correct the false statement

1. T 2. T 3. T 4. F; drug

Short answer questions (part 2)

1. Administration; regimen; action and effects; side effects; contraindications
2. Client's name and address; physician's name; pharmacy's name; prescription number
3. a. For client: dosage is fixed for both or all drugs and difficult to alter, may have potentiating or contraindicating effects; for nurse: difficult to assess the intended action, effects, and adverse reactions of each drug
   b. Variability of the drug's effects because of ingestion of food, physical status (e.g., stomach problems), use of alcohol or other drugs that interfere with the sustained-release drug's effects.
4. Various answers may be given, including tea: tends toward constipation; yogurt: replaces intestinal flora; pears and prunes: tend to loosen stool; bananas and oranges: increase blood potassium; green leafy vegetables: increase body stores of folate
5. Various answers might be given. For example, use of an iron supplement, with or without a vitamin compound, could result in constipation, irregular bowel regimen, and possible decreased appetite and weight loss.

Situational exercises

1. c 2. d 3. c

Jumbled words

KNOWLEDGE + MOTIVATION + CAPABILITY = COMPLIANCE

14 ▪ *Substance abuse*

Matching

1. a or c 2. d 3. f 4. b 5. e

Correct the false statement

1. F; stimulants, depressants
2. F; agonists
3. F; impair

Multiple choice questions

1. c 2. a 3. a 4. b 5. c 6. c 7. b 8. b 9. d 10. d 11. d 12. b 13. b 14. a 15. d 16. d 17. b 18. d 19. d 20. d 21. b 22. c 23. d 24. d 25. b 26. c 27. d 28. a 29. c 30. a 31. d 32. a

Selection of options

1. a,b,d 2. a,c,e,f 3. b,c,d,e,f 4. c only 5. a,c,d 6. a,c 7. a,b,c,d 8. a,c 9. a,b,d 10. a,b,d 11. a,c,d 12. a,b,c,d,e,f,g,h,i,j 13. a,b,d,e 14. a,b 15. c,d

Short answer questions

1. a. The self-directed use of chemical substances for nontherapeutic reasons, in conflict with generally accepted norms and cultural values
   b. The state of behavior characterized by the inability to control a craving or drive for a substance
   c. A state that exists when an increasing amount of substance is required to produce the desired effect experienced with the original dose
   d. The altered state (physical or psychological) that results from continuous use of a psychoactive substance
2. a. Tolerance and physicial dependence→metabolic changes similar to withdrawal symptoms→attempt to mediate symptoms→ tolerance and physical dependence
   b. Abuse→ central nervous system damage → mental capacity reduction→ inability to make judgments→ abuse
   c. Abuse→ social disapproval→ need to find like-minded companions → abuse
   d. Abuse → guilt and shame→ attempt to resolve these feelings→ abuse
3. a. Barbs, blue devils, downers, green dragons, goofballs, yellow jackets, nimbles, pink ladies, rainbows, red devils, reds, stumblers
   b. Scag, smack, junk, horse, H, brown sugar
   c. Snow, big C, coke, flake, gold dust, nose candy, rock, white
   d. Acapulco Gold, gold, gage, grass, hay, hemp, J.Jane, Mary Jane, Panama Red, pot, reefer, smoke, weed
   e. Hash, kif, black Russian, quarter moon, soles
   f. Acid, beast, blue heaven , brown dots, California sunshine, chocolate chips, haze, mellow yellows, orange mushrooms, orange wedges, paper acid, sugar, sunshine, white lightning, yellows
   g. Cube, hocus, first line, morf
   h. Quads, soapers, sopes
   i. Angel dust, peace pill, surfer, killer weed, hog, DOA, rocket fuel, elephant tranquilizer
4. Nausea, vomiting, weight loss, nasal septum perforation
5. Topical
6. A temporary return of signs and symptoms of drug effects although drug use has been discontinued
7. Decrease stimuli; therapeutic communication ("talking down")

15 · *Toxicology*

Multiple choice questions

1. d 2. b 3. d 4. c 5. b; the liver degrades them 6. c; inhalation is a close second 7. d; the poison goes directly into the blood 8. d; they cause more instances of poisoning than any other class of substances 9. b; statistically, the most frequent environmental cause of poisoning 10. d; since lead has been removed from gasoline 11. d 12. a; degradation by the liver requires an enzyme that can be depleted by large dosages; intermediate metabolites damage the liver 13. d; though present in the body in very low quantities, arsenic is actually a component of a body enzyme 14. d 15. c 16. d; fresh, acidic water does add to the pollution but this is more diluted 17. c; burning destroys many poisons; it does, however, vaporize others without destroying them 18. b; ether may cause some drowsiness but not poisioning, halogens are not usually present in poisonous concentrations 19. d; so as to reestablish communication if the call is disrupted 20. a; to keep the victim alive 21. d 22. b

Selection of options

1. a,c,d

Short answer questions

1. a. Antidote: an agent that counteracts the action of a poison
   b. Toxicology: the study of the effects of chemicals on biologic systems that focuses on the harmful effects of the substance
   c. FEP: free erythrocyte protoporphyrin, an essential element in the composition of hemoglobin
   d. Chelate: to combine an element at the receptor site of a metal in a weakly dissociated complex, allowing the metal to be excreted from the body
2.

Toxin Route	**Example**
Percutaneous	DDT; hexachlorophene
Gastrointestinal	Lead, drugs
Inhalational	Carbon monoxide
Parenteral	Medications

3. a. With gag reflex present, and in a conscious victim, give milk or water to dilute the poison. Induce emesis if not contraindicated.
   b. Remove victim to fresh air.
   c. Flood the skin with water for 2–3 minutes. Remove affected apparel when patient is under the stream of water; after flooding the skin, gently wash with soap and water.
   d. Irrigate the eyes copiously with lukewarm water for 15 minutes. Do not use eye drops.
4. Skin decontamination; emesis; lavage; charcoal; cathartic
5. Forced diuresis; peritoneal dialysis; hemodialysis; exchange transfusions; hemoperfusion
6. a. Two successive venous Pb levels ≥70 μg/dl with or without symptoms
   b. FEP ≥250 μg/dl and venous Pb level of ≥50 μg/dl, with or without symptoms
   c. FEP ≥109 μg/dl and elevated venous Pb level of ≥30 μg/dl with symptoms
   d. Venous Pb level > 49 μg/dl with symptoms and evidence of toxicity, such as abnormal FEP and positive results from provocative chelation

16 ▪ *Drugs that affect the autonomic nervous system*

Matching

A. 1. b 2. d 3. b 4. b 5. a 6. b 7. c
B. 1. b 2. b 3. a 4. b 5. a 6. b 7. a 8. a
C. 1. b,e,h,j 2. c,i 3. a,k 4. b,f 5. b,j 6. b,g

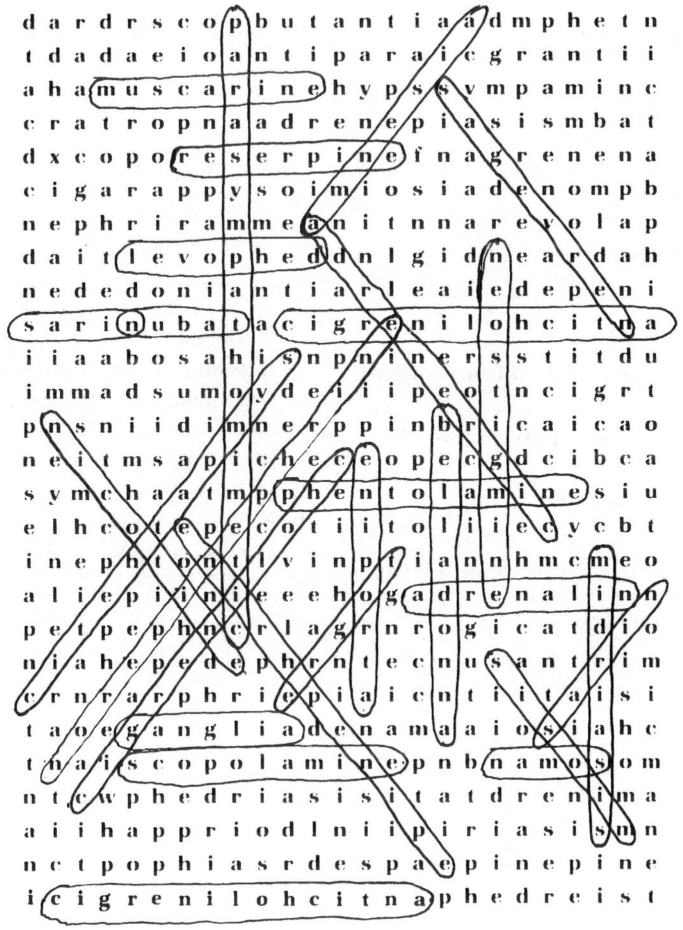

Correct the false statement

1. F; longer
2. T
3. F; is not dependent on
4. T
5. F; discontinued 2 to 3 weeks prior to the surgery
6. F; anticholinesterases
7. T
8. F; muscarinic

Completion exercise

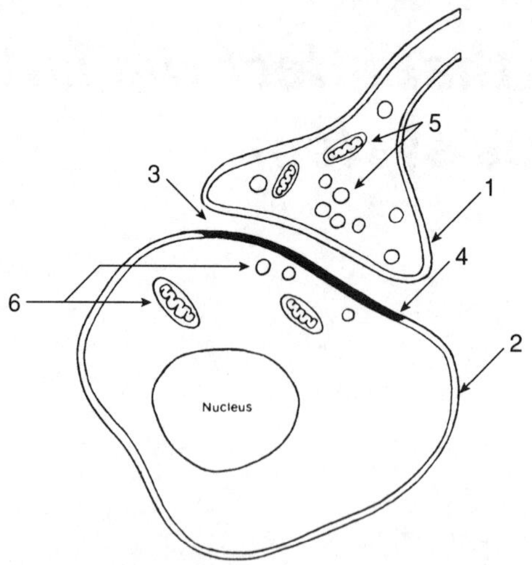

Multiple choice questions

1. b 2. d 3. c 4. d 5. b 6. d 7. c 8. c 9. a 10. c 11. b 12. a 13. a 14. b 15. e 16. c 17. d 18. a 19. a 20. d 21. d

Selection of options

1. b,c 2. a,b,c,e 3. b,c 4. a,b,d,e 5. b,c 6. b,c 7. b,d,e 8. d only 9. b,c 10. a,b,d 11. a,b,c 12. a,b 13. a,c,d 14. b,c 15. a,c 16. b,c 17. a,b,d 18. a,b

Short answer questions

1. Brain; spinal cord
2. Cortex; brain stem
3. Respiratory; cardiac; vasomotor; appetite; vomiting
4. α_1-receptors, α_2-receptors, β_1-receptors, β_2-receptors
5. Nicotinic receptors; muscarinic receptors
6. Sympathomimetic (adrenergic) ; parasympathomimetic (cholinergic); sympatholytic (antiadrenergic, sympathetic blocking agents); parasympatholytic (anticholinergic)
7. Treatment of myasthenia gravis, glaucoma (as a miotic), intestinal atony, atony of the urinary bladder
8. The cranial nerves are part of the parasympathetic system.
9. Duration of effect in the person: mealtime; sleep-wake cycle (drugs are best taken before meals and before and after sleeping, but must be scheduled frequently enough to prevent respiratory arrest)
10. Failure to respond to a drug that develops rapidly on repeated administration of the drug

17 ▪ *Central nervous system stimulants*

Matching

1. d 2. c 3. a

Short answer questions

1. Theophylline
2. Reduce stimuli; use cool colors (blue, green); keep client warm; give sedative massage
3. Nervousness, irritability, restlessness, agitation, tremor, insomnia
4. Wave the broken ampule before the client's face; administer only whiffs
5. Increased mental alertness; increased capacity for work; improved motor performance (particularly of skills that have been mastered); euphoria; stimulation of respirations, heart function, and metabolism
6. Tremor, restlessness, insomnia, impaired motor performance, hypertension, seizures, and exhaustion
7. Treatment of narcolepsy; treatment of hyperkinesis, learning disabilities, and behavioral problems stemming from minimal brain dysfunction in children; treatment of catalepsy; initiation of weight reduction regimens

Correct the false statement

1. F; stimulating release of endogenous neurotransmitters in the nervous system
2. T
3. T
4. F; impair
5. F; from an inactive substance to an active drug
6. F; it cannot cross the blood–brain barrier
7. F; a relatively high dose of levodopa to maintain brain tissue concentrations
8. F; 6–8 weeks
9. T
10. F; stimulations; depressants

Multiple choice questions

1. a 2. d 3. d 4. c 5. b 6. d 7. d 8. c 9. d 10. d 11. b 12. a 13. b 14. a 15. b 16. b 17. b 18. b 19. b 20. b

Selection of options

1. a,b,d 2. a,c,e,f 3. a,b,d,e 4. b,c 5. a,b,c,d

18 · *Central nervous system depressants*

Short answer questions

1. Lethargy, coma, cardiovascular collapse, respiratory arrest, death
2. Hypnotics the night before surgery; narcotic analgesics, tranquilizers, and anticholinergics preoperatively; rapid-acting induction agent; one or more inhalant anesthetics; oxygen; skeletal muscle relaxants
3. Schedule IV
4. Yes, in some people
5. a. Eliminate stimuli; promote muscle relaxation; alleviate stress and anxiety; promote comfort; follow the client's personal bedtime ritual
   b. Relaxation techniques, heat, cold, positioning, duration, imagery
6. Advantages: decrease in the client's anxiety, better control of pain, general decrease in overall quantity of drugs required for pain control, greater autonomy for the client, decreased risk of development of habit of pain, decrease in conditioned response to use drugs, decrease in the level of stress in the client. Disadvantages: difficulty in maintaining security over controlled drugs, (possibly) an increased risk of tolerance and dependence in some clients.
7. Local anesthetic, amnesia-producing drug, antiolytic, and sometimes subanesthetic doses of IV anesthetics
8. The need for expensive equipment, including infusion-control devices; increased risk of infection; inconvenience of the cumbersome equipment
9. 300 mg
10. Client's description and rating of pain, objective evidence of pain (e.g., vital signs, muscle rigidity, facial expression), nature of the pain (type, location, severity), physician's orders for medication, time interval since last dose of analgesic drugs, client's history of pain experience, client's usual response to pain (including coping behaviors)

Sequences

Provided that the priorities are consistent with those of the client, the order would be 4, 3, 1, 2.

Situational exercises

1. 10 mg
2. 1.25 mg/hr
3. Greater than that dosage

Personal exercise

Neither the nature of the biases nor their strengths are of great importance in this exercise. What matters is how well the student has analyzed and clarified these personal factors, and has prepared to counteract their influence on nursing actions.

m	o	r	p	r	o	p	o	x	e	h	e	r	o	e	t	h	e	r	e	r	h	t	e	i	r	b
m	e	p	e	n	e	h	p	q	a	n	a	n	i	t	v	s	l	e	e	a	n	a	l	i	g	a
a	n	e	s	t	h	e	t	i	c	m	o	r	t	i	n	i	l	c	l	x	j	u	p	s	e	r
p	i	n	t	w	i	l	m	o	r	p	h	x	a	n	o	p	t	o	p	i	u	s	e	d	a	b
e	d	i	i	i	x	w	r	a	n	g	e	r	o	u	t	i	t	a	s	h	e	r	o	d	s	i
r	i	t	r	l	o	c	n	o	c	t	r	a	i	l	e	h	e	r	i	e	a	n	a	v	a	s
i	r	i	p	i	d	a	i	l	i	w	t	h	e	m	a	r	c	o	v	c	r	e	h	p	r	o
d	e	m	a	h	l	s	e	d	a	p	y	t	o	n	o	n	s	i	c	r	o	s	p	o	r	p
e	p	s	r	g	a	j	e	n	e	p	a	r	e	r	p	a	t	i	i	a	h	s	e	d	a	e
p	e	r	e	t	i	c	u	l	a	r	a	c	t	i	v	a	t	i	n	g	s	y	s	t	e	m
r	m	s	i	s	i	c	o	m	u	l	e	n	a	i	d	o	n	e	a	l	c	i	p	i	n	e
e	i	v	r	l	n	r	i	t	c	i	n	m	o	e	n	i	t	r	o	u	s	o	x	i	d	e
c	c	g	u	e	u	a	i	o	r	a	i	l	s	p	o	m	a	s	p	o	t	o	n	p	y	h
o	i	l	e	e	a	b	h	n	p	y	h	a	y	l	p	n	t	a	i	p	e	l	o	r	a	l
d	t	a	n	p	r	o	p	o	x	y	p	h	e	n	e	h	i	m	o	e	h	t	e	l	o	h
e	e	n	m	a	l	e	p	t	w	i	r	e	h	t	h	e	r	o	i	n	u	h	o	c	l	a
i	r	a	b	a	r	b	i	t	w	i	o	p	i	a	n	a	p	c	d	i	t	t	r	o	m	l
t	e	r	e	t	i	c	u	a	c	t	m	e	p	e	r	i	d	i	n	e	h	s	e	d	a	f

Correct the false statement

1. T
2. F; only fractional parts
3. T
4. F; hyperthyroidism
5. T
6. F; double-locked cabinets
7. F; benzodiazepines
8. F; active metabolites
9. F; quiet activities
10. F; outside the bedroom or in the care of another person
11. F; central nervous system depressants
12. T
13. T
14. F; may develop
15. T
16. F; sometimes helpful, but can be a very misleading indicator of subjective pain
17. T
18. F; lower
19. F; may vary greatly
20. F; more severe
21. F; may be very helpful when given (e.g., if a pain-producing activity is to be carried out)

Multiple choice questions

1. a 2. a 3. d 4. b 5. b 6. d 7. b 8. b 9. d 10. b 11. d 12. a 13. d 14. d 15. d 16. d 17. a 18. b 19. b 20. c 21. b 22. c 23. c 24. c 25. c 26. d 27. c 28. c 29. d 30. d 31. b 32. a 33. c 34. c 35. d 36. b 37. c 38. c 39. b 40. b 41. c 42. c 43. c

19 ▪ *Drugs that control seizures*

Correct the false statement

1. F; occipital lobe
2. F; is not influenced when
3. F; whether or not
4. T
5. F; central nervous system depressants
6. T
7. T
8. F; phenobarbital and phenytoin
9. F; ethosuximide
10. T
11. F; impair
12. F; other weak acids
13. F; slow; 12–15 hours
14. T
15. F; binds highly
16. F; more
17. T
18. F; still carries a stigma
19. T
20. F; decreased

Short answer questions

1. Epilepsy is the name of a syndrome characterized by seizure disorder.
2. Seizure threshold is the relative level of excitation at which seizure activity is initiated in the brain.
3. Level of the basal seizure threshold; presence of foci that initiate abnormal stimuli; irritation of nerve cells as a result of biochemical changes in the body
4. Eating regular meals; limiting salt intake; getting adequate rest and sleep; engaging in physical exercise; avoiding exhaustion; practicing good mental hygiene; avoiding alcoholic beverages; avoiding stimulant drugs; prevention or early treatment of infections
5. Shaving, bleaching the hair; electrolysis of hair follicles

Matching

1. a,b,c,f,g,h,i,j,n,o,p 2. c,e,i,j,k,l,m 3. a,i,n,q 4. c,d,h,i,r 5. c,e,h,i 6. e,h,k,s 7. b,h,e 8. h,n

Multiple choice questions

1. d 2. c 3. b 4. b 5. c 6. a 7. b 8. d 9. d 10. a 11. b 12. c 13. a 14. d 15. d 16. b 17. a 18. c 19. c 20. b 21. b 22. c 23. c 24. d 25. d 26. d 27. c 28. b 29. a 30. b 31. d 32. a 33. b 34. e

Selection of options

1. a,b,c,e 2. a,d 3. a,c,d 4. a,b,d,e 5. a,c 6. a,c,d 7. c,d 8. a,b,d 9. b,c

20 ▪ Drugs that affect emotional and psychological functions

Multiple choice

1. b 2. d 3. d 4. a 5. b 6. a 7. a 8. c 9. a 10. b 11. b 12. d 13. b 14. b 15. d 16. d 17. d 18. a 19. a 20. c 21. c 22. a 23. a

Matching

A. 1. d 2. a 3. c 4. b 5. e 6. f
B. 1. c 2. a 3. d 4. e 5. b
C. 1. b 2. c 3. d 4. e 5. a
D. 1. d 2. e 3. b 4. a 5. d
E. 1. e 2. c 3. c 4. a 5. d 6. c 7. c 8. e

Correct the false statement

1. T
2. T
3. T
4. T
5. T
6. F; are highly protein bound
7. T
8. T
9. F; 800 mg/day
10. T
11. T
12. T
13. T
14. T
15. T

Short answer questions

1. Avocados, aged cheese, chicken liver, chocolate, cocoa, fava beans, figs, licorice, raisins, sauerkraut, soy sauce, yeast products, coffee, red wine, beer, sherry, chianti, liquors
2. a. Lithium has an inverse relationship with sodium, thus making it necessary to have an adequate salt and water intake to avoid drug toxicity.
   b. MAOIs and tyramine interact to increase amine levels in the blood and subsequently in the CNS. This contributes to the further release of CNS neurotransmitters resulting in a hypertensive crisis.
3. Many drugs are highly bound to proteins. When two or more drugs are administered, they will compete with each other for binding to a protein. If one particular agent has a greater capacity for binding, the other agent will be displaced resulting in increased unbound levels in the blood. Increased blood levels of an agent can result in drug toxicity. Most psychoactive agents are highly bound to proteins. Thus, co-administration of other drugs with psychoactive medications warrants close attention for drug interactions including toxicity. Concurrent administration of such drugs may necessitate lower dosage adjustments of one of the displacing agents.
4. Alcohol acts to further depress the CNS. Concurrent use of alcohol and psychoactive medications can increase the risk for seizures, as both decrease the seizure threshold.
5. The need for intermittent dosing for individuals having difficulty complying to a more frequent medication regimen; considering when to initiate a new drug regimen following discontinuation of the original agent; and calculating necessary time intervals between incompatible drugs

21 · *Drugs that manage heart failure*

Correct the false statement

1. T
2. T
3. F; enhancing tissue perfusion in the kidney
4. F; will not
5. F; will not
6. F; congestive heart failure
7. F; palliative
8. F; a relative
9. T

Crossword puzzle

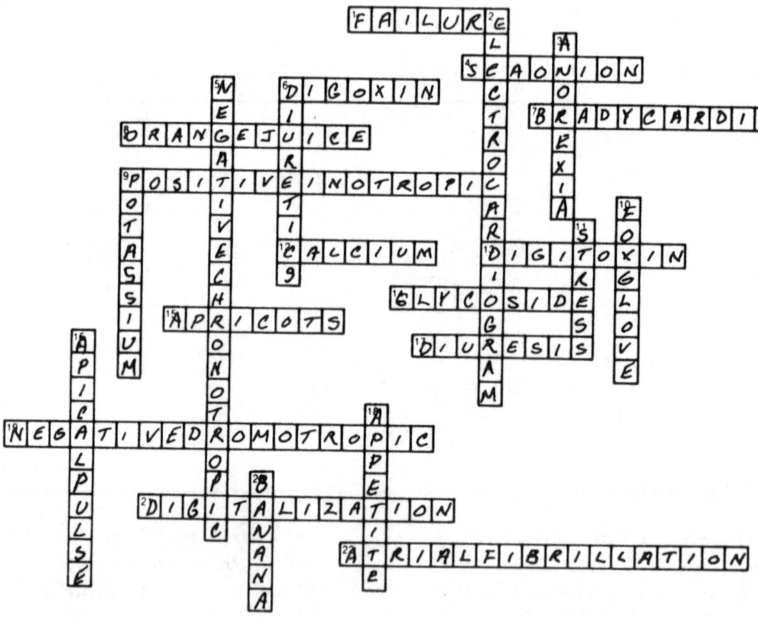

Matching

A. 1. c 2. a 3. d

B. 1. a 2. c 3. e 4. d 5. f

Selection of options

1. b,c,d,e 2. a,c 3. a,b,c 4. a,c,d,e,f 5. a,b,c 6. a,b,d 7. a,b 8. a,b,d,f,g 9. a,c,d 10. a,b,c,d,e 11. a,c,e 12. a,c 13. a,b,c,e,f,g

22 ▪ Drugs that regulate cardiac rhythm

Correct the false statement

1. T
2. F; procainamide
3. T
4. F; arterial embolism
5. T
6. F; prolongation of repolarization
7. F; verapamil
8. F; SA NODE
9. T
10. F; torsades de pointes

Crossword puzzle

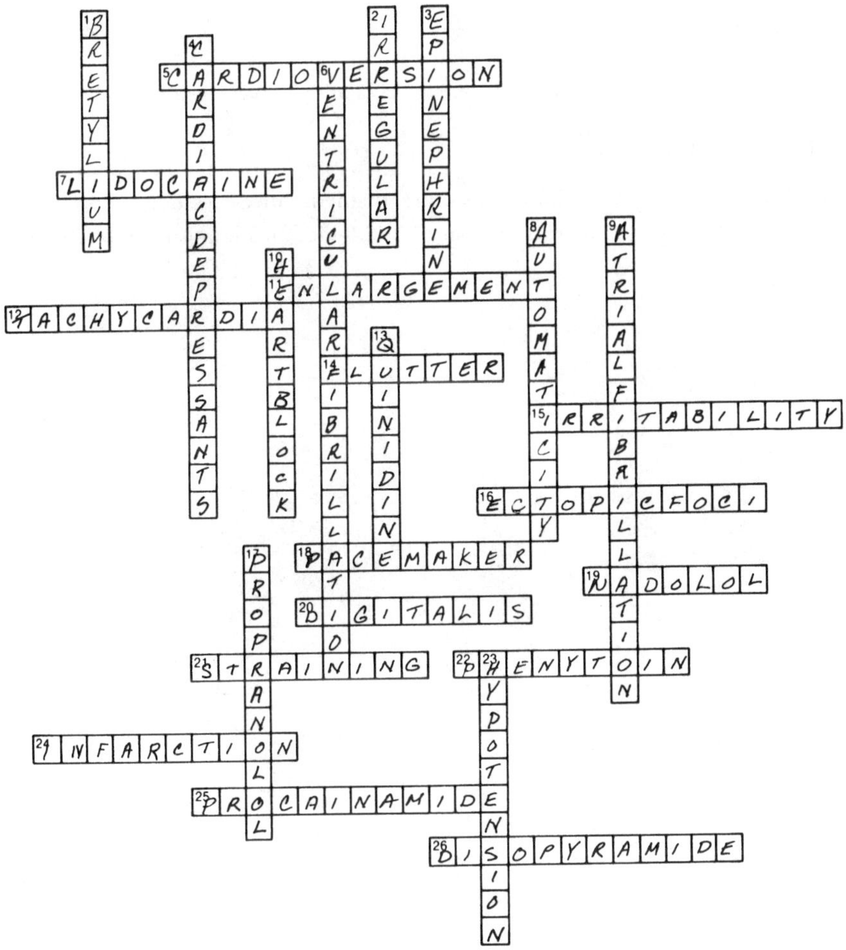

1 BRETYLIUM
2 IRREGULAR
3 EPINEPHRINE
5 CARDIOVERSION
6 VENTRICULAR FIBRILLATION
7 LIDOCAINE
8 AUTOMATICITY
9 ATRIAL FIBRILLATION
10 HEART BLOCK
11 ENLARGEMENT
12 TACHYCARDIA
13 QUINIDINE
14 FLUTTER
15 IRRITABILITY
16 ECTOPIC FOCI
17 PROPRANOLOL
18 PACEMAKER
19 NADOLOL
20 DIGITALIS
21 STRAINING
22 PHENYTOIN
23 HYPOTENSION
24 INFARCTION
25 PROCAINAMIDE
26 DISOPYRAMIDE

Selection of options

1. a,b,c,d 2. a,b,c,d,e,f,g 3. a,d 4. a,b,d 5. b,d 6. a,b,f,g,h

23 ▪ *Drugs that regulate lipid levels*

Correct the false statement

1. F; liver enzymes
2. F; fluvastatin
3. T
4. F; are not; locally in the gastrointestinal tract
5. T
6. T
7. F; must be well diluted in fluids prior to ingestion
8. F; bile acid-sequestering resins
9. F; HMG CoA reductase inhibitor
10. T
11. F; cutaneous flushing and pruritus
12. T
13. F; does not include
14. T

Selection of options

1. b,d 2. a,b,c,d 3. b,c,e 4. a,b 5. a,b,e 6. a,b,d,e 7. a,c 8. b,e 9. a,b,e 10. a,b,c,d

Short answer questions

1. They are used when more conventional methods of treatment are unsuccessful.
2. Avoid inhaling the powder; mix the powder with ample fluids; do not administer with other drugs; advise an increased intake of fluid and fiber.

24 ▪ *Drugs that affect circulation*

Anagram

1.

HYPOTENSION
THROMBI
POOLING
FIBROSIS
ARTERIOSCLEROSIS
CALCIFICATION
PRESSURE
ATHEROSCLEROSIS
OBSTRUCTION
PLAQUE
VASOSPASM
DECREASED PATENCY
LOSS OF ELASTICITY
SHOCK
HYPERTENSION

(POOR CIRCULATION)

2.

STRESS
INACTIVITY
EXCESS LDLS
SMOKING

HIGH FAT DIET
DIABETES
HIGH BLOOD CHOLESTEROL
HYPOTHYROIDISM
LOW HDLS
HYPERTENSION
OBESITY

(RISK FACTORS)

Multiple choice questions

1. c 2. c 3. b 4. d 5. d 6. a 7. d 8. a 9. e 10. b

Selection of options

1. c,d 2. a,b,c,d,f,h 3. b,c

Short answer questions

1. Antiplatelet agents, anticoagulants, beta-adrenergic blocking agents, calcium channel antagonists, angiotensin-converting enzyme inhibitors, thrombolytic agents
2. Doing active exercises; avoiding prolonged sitting or standing; avoiding use of constricting bands on the legs; avoiding obesity; the limiting the number of pregnancies; using supportive hose

25 ▪ *Drugs that regulate blood pressure*

Multiple choice questions

1. b 2. d 3. c 4. c 5. c 6. d 7. a 8. c 9. b 10. b 11. d 12. b

Selection of options

1. a,c,d,e 2. c,d 3. b,c 4. c,d

Short answer questions

1. Increase attention to client and client's concerns, encourage client's active participation in resolving barriers to compliance, reinforce explicit treatment goals, set realistic short-term objectives, concentrate first on the compliance behavior that will make the greatest contribution to the treatment goals, assist client to tailor regimen to personal habits and daily routines, consult physician to see if dosing frequency may be decreased or therapy may be simplified in any other ways, teach client to monitor own blood pressure and keep ongoing record of its values, reinforce information about regimen's efficacy, give continuous positive reinforcement, include family members and/or significant others in planning sessions.
2. Teach client to recognize that dizziness or lightheadedness with position change may be symptoms of an adverse reaction to the antihypertensive agent; encourage to report to healthcare provider dizziness, lightheadedness, or fainting that perseveres; teach client to rise from lying to standing position by sitting up slowly first, teach to then sit quietly for a few minutes to allow time for body to adjust to change in position, teach to then stand slowly; teach to avoid activities that contribute significantly to vasodilation that might worsen orthostatic hypotension like hot baths and showers and use of saunas.

26 ▪ *Drugs that regulate hemostasis*

PART 1: HEMOSTATICS

Correct the false statement

1. F; a markedly reduced or absent response
2. T
3. F; concentrates of vitamin-K dependent clotting factors (e.g., Proplex T, Proplex SX-T)
4. T
5. F; phytonadione (vitamin K, Aquamephyton)
6. T
7. F; fibrinolytic agents
8. F; impede
9. F; about ten times more
10. F; acute hypotension

Multiple choice questions

1. a 2. b 3. a 4. b 5. b 6. d 7. c 8. a 9. c 10. a

Short answer questions

1. Vessel vasoconstriction

   Platelet adhesion, activation, aggregation

   Platelets release an enzyme that activates thromboplastin.

   Thromboplastin catalyzes conversion of prothrombin to thrombin.

   Thrombin catalyzes formation of fibrin from fibrinogen.

   Clot retraction

2. 10 foods

Frozen broccoli	1 cup, 332 mg
Raw shredded cabbage	1 cup, 221 mg
Fresh asparagus	1 cup, 288 mg
Frozen chopped spinach	1 cup, 611 mg
Brussels sprouts	1 cup, 494 mg
Turnip greens	1 cup, 368 mg
Kale	1 cup, 417 mg
Liver	3 oz, 309 mg
Frozen lima beans	1 cup, 694 mg
Beet greens	1 cup, 1308 mg

Figures from: Davis, J. and Sherer, K. (1994). *Applied Nutrition and Diet Therapy for Nurses.* 2nd ed. Philadelphia: W. B. Saunders Co.

PART 2: ANTICOAGULANTS

Correct the false statement

1. F; but will not dissolve clots already formed in the blood vessels
2. F; 1.5 to 2.5 times
3. F; prothrombin time
4. F; heparin
5. T
6. F; heparin
7. T
8. F; not increase or decrease significantly
9. F; warfarin sodium
10. F; thrombin action

Multiple choice questions

1. d 2. b 3. b 4. c 5. c 6. b 7. d

Short answer questions

1. No. It is destroyed by digestive enzymes.
2. It results in large ecchymoses.
3. Aspiration is omitted; massage is omitted; abdominal site is used.
4. No. They increase the risk of hemorrhage in the infant.
5. No. Intake should be kept stable.
6. It combines chemically with the acidic heparin to form a stable salt that has no anticoagulant properties.

Completion exercise

	Coumadin	Heparin
Mechanism of action	Competitively inhibits vitamin K's role in production of clotting factors	Forms a complex with antithrombin III and inhibits factor Xa and conversion of prothrombin
Route(s) of administration	PO, IV	IV, SC
Unit of measurement of doses	mg	Units
Frequency of dosage	Once daily	Twice a day SC, continuous infusion
Onset of action	Peak 1.5–3 days	IV peak 5–10 min, SC 30–60 min
Antidote(s)	Vitamin K	Protamine sulfate
Laboratory test(s) for monitoring	PT, INR	APTT
Adverse reactions	Hemorrhage, purple toe syndrome, alopecia	Hemorrhage, allergic reactions, thrombocytopenia

PART 3: DRUGS THAT AFFECT PLATELET AGGREGATION

Correct the false statement

1. F; promotes
2. F; antiplatelet drug
3. T
4. T

PART 4: FIBRINOLYTIC AGENTS

Correct the false statement

1. F; enzymes
2. T
3. F; intravenously
4. F; tissue plasminogen activator/t-PA (alteplase/Activase)
5. F; streptokinase or anisoylated plasminogen streptokinase activator complex
6. F; heparin

Multiple choice questions

1. b 2. c

Short answer questions

1. Listen to client and family expressing their concerns.

   Follow through and take appropriate action regarding client and family concerns.

   Perform procedures competently and efficiently.

   Respond quickly to client requests for assistance.

   Express a warm personal concern for the client and family.

PART 5: CHAPTERWIDE EXERCISES

Selection of options

1. a, b, d 2. a, b, d, e 3. a, c, d, e 4. a, b, c, f 5. a, c, d 6. a, b 7. a, b, c

27 ▪ *Drugs that affect the kidneys*

Correct the false statement

1. F; hydrostatic pressure
2. F; similar in concentration to
3. T
4. T
5. T
6. F; intestinal atony and constipation
7. T
8. F; hot humid
9. F; loop diuretics
10. T
11. F; electrolyte imbalance
12. T
13. F; chronic conditions associated with edema
14. F; promotes sodium reabsorption and potassium loss

Matching

A. 1. a,b,c,d,e,f,g,h 2. a 3. m 4. g,j,k 5. a,i

B. 1. a 2. c 3. b 4. c 5. b 6. b 7. c 8. c 9. c 10. a

Find the hidden words

c e e e r u i d o s a l i m a c e t a z o l a m i d e r i

a a l d a s i l u e c a r b l a s i n t u b u l i i d e p

a r e i u r e a b s o a a i d i a w b u t r i c n a e n o

b s c l e d i r o l i m a l a n d e n o t c a d l a s o s

d o t a a i n t a m e i b o c t r i n t a c i m a i r t o

s r r s m n t i e d r l s r h a m g i d i a m o x n e c m

m p o u o t e l e c t r o l y t e h p n o a e s a t a a s

o t l d i a a m i u r e r d d a y t y h n u r e a m b l d

s h y p o k a l e m i a p e r k a r h n k a t n i a s o b

e y t s r e a b s o r p t i o n c l i s a l a p m s o n r

c p e e a l d a o s e d i h c a g t u r l d n r u a c o a

r i p i b a i r d m a a o y h r o t m e e a o e p t a r c

e y r t s s e c i f b r n t l l d i u r i l p a i g d i e

h t e c i t e r u i d b e d o a m n e p h r y b l e l p d

y n a t r g d r m a n o c a r b o n i c a n h y d r a s e

s i s o m s o a r p e n r e o s m a n a o e c r e o s m o

e e e d e s i u e d r e a b t u b m t i r e o v r s n e p

c a r s e c r e t i o n e p h r o n s o r p p i e b a m i

a d i m d r r d e e d e d e i r i u u o n h y d i a m a n

r e i n t t e e n i e a e n a t f a l a s y h e n o t c a

b d s a n e a l t n l d m a z f t a m i l p r e a c e t a

e n b n b a b s i n t i i n i l u i d t d e l v c t r i a

t a a l a e s h o e u u a d d r b a i r e d e c r i n e p

h m l a i r t o n p g l o m e r u l u s k r e p i e e d o

a e d s a n e e y h y f c n e p l e r e a b e o m i d e n

c d d i a l d a s i n d o l i n e d e c a r b n a t n i a

r e a x a c e t o o s m o s e c r e d e c a r b e d e m o

Multiple choice questions

1. d 2. d 3. d 4. d 5. d 6. a 7. b 8. d 9. a 10. a 11. b 12. d 13. a 14. c 15. a 16. b 17. c 18. d

Selection of options

1. b, d, e 2. b, c, d 3. b, c, e 4. a, b, d, e 5. b, d 6. a, b,c,d 7. a, b 8. a, c, d, e

Short answer questions

1. Heart disease, nephrosis, hepatic cirrhosis
2. Glaucoma, seizure disorders
3. Freely filterable by their glomerulus; not readily reabsorbed by the tubule; lacking in other pharmacologic action
4. Diabetes mellitus, gout
5. 2.2 pounds or 1 kilogram

28 ▪ *Drugs that affect the upper gastrointestinal tract*

Matching

A. 1. a,b 2. a,b,d,e 3. a,e,f 4. b,d,f
B. 1. a,c,g 2. b,e,f 3. a,e,f 4. b,d,f

Crossword puzzle

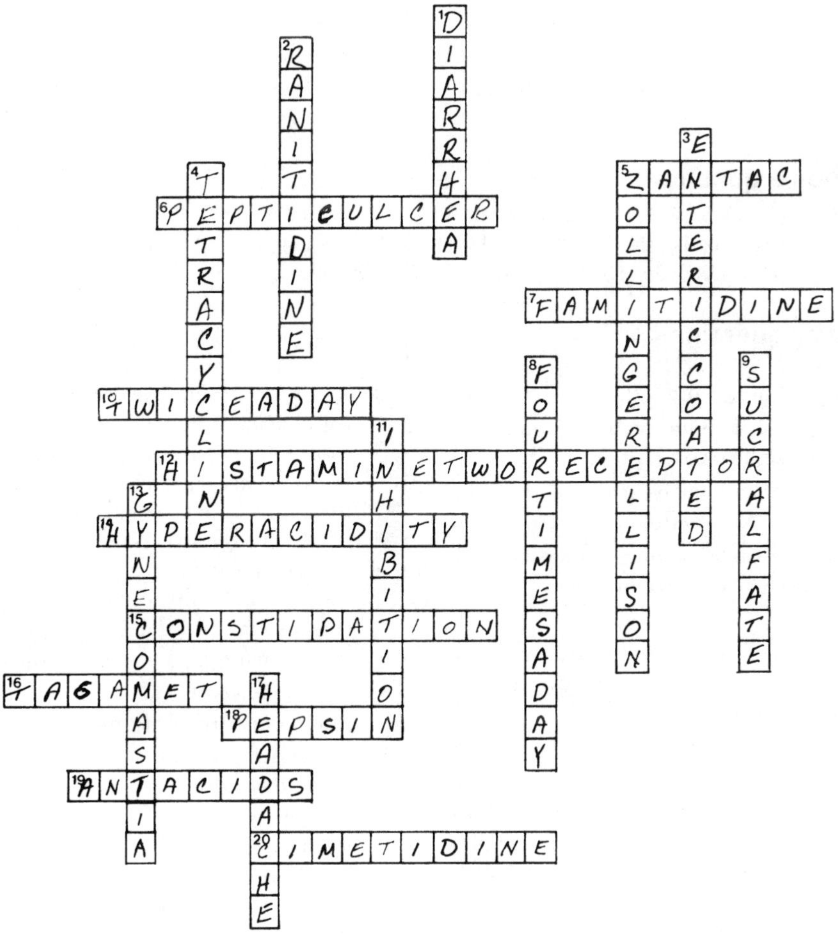

1 DIARRHEA
2 RANITIDINE
3 ENTERICCOATED
4 TETRACYCLINE
5 ZANTAC
5 ZOLLINGERELLISON
6 PEPTICULCER
7 FAMITIDINE
8 FOURTIMESADAY
9 SUCRALFATE
10 TWICEADAY
11 INHIBITION
12 HISTAMINETWORECEPTOR
13 GYNECOMASTIA
14 HYPERACIDITY
15 CONSTIPATION
16 TAGAMET
17 HEADACHE
18 PEPSIN
19 ANTACIDS
20 CIMETIDINE

Correct the false statement

1. T
2. F; whether they are applied topically or are ingested for systemic effect
3. F; age 6 years and older
4. F; sugars and starches
5. F; 15–30 minutes
6. F; not to exceed the dosage recommended on the label
7. F; soluble
8. T
9. T
10. F; with meals
11. T
12. T
13. F; acidic
14. F; liver
15. T
16. F; fat-soluble
17. T
18. F; histamine
19. F; act on different receptors than do the antihistamines
20. F; less than
21. T
22. F; do not readily cross
23. T
24. T
25. T
26. T
27. F; does not rule out
28. F; have not been established as safe
29. F; are free from adverse side effects
30. T
31. T
32. F; both a comfort and therapeutic measure; adequate use of antacids may prevent or delay the development of esophageal peptic ulcers or strictures
33. F; local rather than systemic
34. F; water should be given by mouth
35. T
36. T
37. F; stimulates upper GI tract
38. F; replaces prostaglandin

Multiple choice questions

1. e 2. d 3. c 4. d 5. b 6. c 7. b 8. b 9. e 10. c 11. b 12. a 13. c 14. c 15. d 16. c 17. d 18. d 19. b 20. b 21. a 22. b 23. d 24. d 25. b 26. d 27. d 28. d 29. a 30. b 31. b 32. b 33. b 34. b 35. a 36. c 37. d 38. a 39. c

Short answer questions

1. Mix equal parts of salt and sodium bicarbonate.
2. a. Take ½ tsp of sodium perborate and add water to make 3⅓ oz of solution.
   b. Take ¼ tsp of sodium bicarbonate and add water to make 3⅓ oz of solution.
   c. Take a scant ¼ tsp of sodium chloride and add water to make 3⅓ oz of solution.
3. 0.9%
4. A drug preparation that contains small amounts of substances essential for breakdown of food into soluble, absorbable particles.
5. Acids, bile, enzymes, choleretics
6. Dilute the solution 10–20 times; sip it through a glass straw; rinse mouth with a mild alkaline solution after taking the medicine; practice proper oral hygiene; consume food immediately after taking HCI solution.
7. Excessive hydrochloric acid production; inadequate pancreatic secretions, inadequate mucus secretion; impaired mucosal resistance to acid; inadequacy of cardiac sphincter; hypermotility of the stomach
8. An excessive number of acid-secreting parietal cells; inadequate mucus production; mucosal susceptibility to acid penetration; metabolism favoring excess production of chemicals such as histamine that stimulate acid secretion; diaphragmatic structure susceptible to development of a hiatal hernia; stress response patterns with a predominance of parasympathetic nervous system activity; undue sensitivity to external stimuli that trigger acid secretion
9. A resurgence of acid secretion that follows elevation of gastric *p*H from the use of antacids
10. These are relatively new drugs, and there are likely to be adverse reactions that have not been recognized as yet.
11. Smoking; ingestion of gastric irritants; high levels of stress; overeating; increased intra-abdominal pressure (e.g., from girdles)
12. Only in small amounts (less than 4 oz) because large amounts stimulate gastric emptying
13. From hourly to four times a day (after meals and at bedtime)

14. No, the daily costs of each are roughly comparable.
15. Assuming institutional policy allows it, yes, provided amounts used are monitored and the client is taught how to use the medication
16. Usually not—side effects of and adverse reactions to various preparations are usually different
17. Mostly (unabsorbed) in the feces; the small amount that is absorbed systemically is eliminated by the kidneys
18. They should be chewed thoroughly or dissolved by sucking them before swallowing
19. An emetic is a substance that induces vomiting.
20. An antiemetic is a substance that reduces nausea and vomiting.
21. Scopolamine
22. Hallucinations, disorientation, confusion
23. Vomiting involves the forceful expulsion of stomach contents and usually results in larger volumes of emesis than does regurgitation.
24. No, because many antiemetics have adverse effects on the fetus

Personal exercise: Self-medication

The consumer needs to distinguish the various signs and symptoms of upper gastrointestinal problems: heartburn, pain (sharp, burning, gnawing), distention, nausea, vomiting, regurgitation. For short-term treatment, it is necessary to match these signs and symptoms with those described by the medication label as appropriate for use of the drug. Some trial and error is required to determine the best agents for an individual. The consumer needs to know that severe or persistent problems require the attention of a physician. If more than one drug is effective, the consumer should compare the prices for comparable doses and choose the most economical preparation.

29 ▪ Agents affecting the lower gastrointestinal tract

Correct the false statement

1. T
2. F; are contraindicated for
3. F; the bulk-forming laxatives
4. T
5. T
6. F;1–2 minutes
7. F; increases sympathetic nervous activity
8. F; bulk-forming laxatives
9. T
10. F; too toxic
11. F; are not effective
12. F; removing irritants and toxins from the intestines

Crossword puzzle

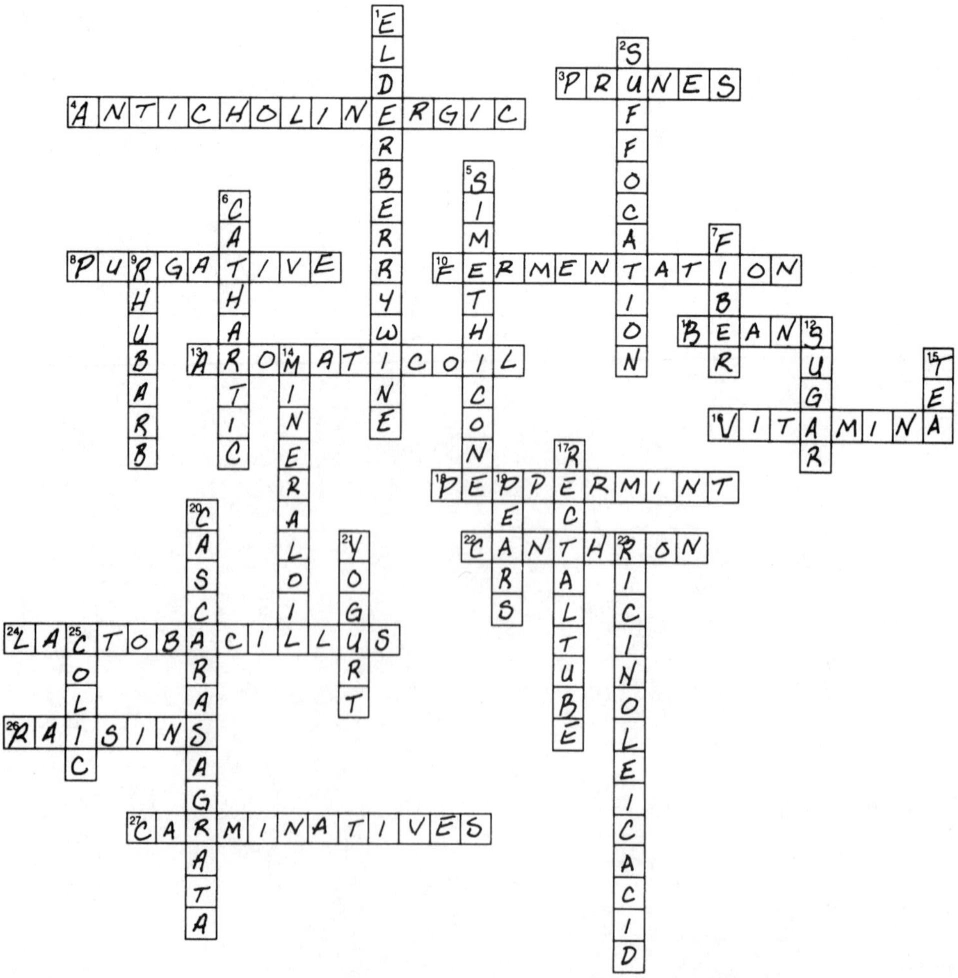

1 ELDERBERRY WINE
2 SUFFOCATION
3 PRUNES
4 ANTICHOLINERGIC
5 SIMETHICONE
6 CATHARTIC
7 FIBER
8 PURGATIVE
9 RHUBARB
10 FERMENTATION
11 BEANS
12 SUGAR
13 AROMATIC OIL
14 MINERAL OIL
15 TEA
16 VITAMIN A
17 RECTAL TUBE
18 PEPPERMINT
19 PEARS
20 CASCARA SAGRADA
21 YOGURT
22 CANTHRON
23 RICINOLEIC ACID
24 LACTOBACILLUS
25 COLIC
26 RAISINS
27 CARMINATIVES

Multiple choice questions

1. a 2. c 3. c 4. b 5. a 6. b 7. c 8. d 9. d 10. b 11. c 12. c 13. d 14. b 15. c 16. a 17. d 18. b 19. c 20. d 21. a 22. b 23. a

Short answer questions

1. Increase exercise, advise patient to decrease intake of gas forming foods, increase dietary fiber
2. a. The passage of frequent, semiliquid, or liquid stools

   b. The passage of infrequent, hard stools

   c. A drug that stimulates defecation

   d. A chemical able to hold other chemicals on the surface of its molecules
3. They are relative terms denoting the strength of action of the agents; purgatives are the strongest, cathartics are intermediate, while laxatives are the most gentle. (Laxative is also used as a class title to refer to all agents that induce defecation.)
4. Effectiveness in producing defecation; inability to affect the stomach; inability to produce a systemic effect if absorbed; inability to produce discomfort such as nausea or cramping
5. Undiagnosed abdominal pain, perforation of bowel, obstruction of bowel, suspected appendicitis, fecal impaction. Caution use in third trimester of pregnancy.
6. Figs, prunes, pears, raisins, rhubarb, coffee
7. Bile and pancreatic enzymes convert castor oil to the irritant ricinoleic acid.
8. Glycerin, lactulose, magnesium hydroxide, magnesium sulfate, sodium phosphate, sorbitol
9. Increased fiber in the diet; ample hydration; exercise; regular habits of defecation
10. Lack of exercise; lack of privacy; disruption of usual defecation patterns; fasting; fluid restriction; use of depressant drugs
11. Tea, blackberries, blueberries, elderberries; beta block is anticholinergics, psychotropic drugs, calcium channel blockers, diuretics
12. Charcoal, chalk, kaolin, pectin
13. They inhibit intestinal absorption of beneficial nutrients and drugs
14. Irritation
15. Gas-forming foods (cabbage, onions, beans); artificial sweeteners (saccharin or cyclamates); laxative foods (prunes, raisins, figs, rhubarb, pears, bran); coffee

30 ▪ Drugs that regulate steroidal hormone levels

Matching

1. a 2. c 3. b 4. a 5. a

Correct the false statement

1. T
2. F; do occur even though
3. T
4. F; on arising
5. T
6. F; live vaccines such as oral polio vaccine
7. F; insomnia
8. F; high concentrations of drug are not legal in over-the-counter preparations
9. T
10. F; altering enzyme function in the renal tubule
11. F; sodium reabsorption and potassium excretion
12. T
13. F; glucose tolerance test
14. T
15. F; hypertensive crisis
16. F; a 20-gauge or larger needle
17. F; fluorocortisone
18. T
19. F; by adrenals as well as by gonads
20. T
21. T
22. F; anabolism
23. T
24. F; exert some masculinizing effects
25. F; increased
26. F; estrogens
27. F; less
28. T
29. F; less markedly
30. T
31. T
32. F; chlorotrianisene
33. F; do
34. F; considerably lower than
35. T
36. T
37. F; less soap (or more oils)
38. T
39. T
40. F; increase

Short answer questions

1. General debility; hypovolemia, weak heart action ; hypotension; tendency toward shock; intestinal colic; increased skin pigmentation
2. Yes, and they may produce systemic effects.
3. Hyperglycemia and increased risk of diabetes mellitus; osteoporosis and increased risk of bone fracture; hypertension; hypernatremia, hypokalemia, decreased resistance to infection; increased risk of abnormal clotting; insomnia; signs and symptoms of peptic ulcer or hyperacidity, abnormal hirsutism; menstrual disturbances; infertility; striae; delayed healing
4. Complete blood count (especially red blood count); electrocardiogram; blood glucose, sodium, potassium, and cholesterol; chest and spinal x-ray; glucose tolerance test; height, weight; growth status in children; signs and symptoms of infection; intraocular pressure
5. Because response to these medications fluctuates with stress levels
6. They produce a marked increase in sodium retention and potassium excretion, a secondary increase in water retention and extracellular

fluid volume, and decreases in body fluid concentrations of potassium and hydrogen ions.

7. Edema, hypernatremia, hypervolemia, hypokalemia, alkalosis, increased blood pressure, cardiac enlargement, cardiac arrhythmias, headache, arthralgia, tendon contractures, congestive heart failure, cerebrovascular accident, weakness, intestinal atony or paralytic ileus
8. Tissue turgor, blood pressure, body weight, serum electrolyte concentrations, muscle strength, cardiovascular function, intestinal function, emotional status
9. Premature cessation of growth; permanent impairment of fertility; cancer of the liver
10. They are sometimes helpful, but their use should be avoided or delayed because of the risk of permanent impairment of fertility or short stature caused by early closure of the epiphyses.
11. No, they can impair sexual response, produce permanent infertility, and increase the risk of cancer of the liver.
12. A diet abundant in fluids, high in protein, adequate for calcium and calories, high in minerals and vitamins
13. Androgens
14. Estrogens, progesterone
15. Yes, unless a penile prosthesis is implanted.
16. Not until growth is complete, because estrogens can cause premature closure of epiphyses.
17. Surgical castration prior to the age of menopause; acute symptoms of menopause such as severe hot flashes or dyspareunia; family history of dowager's hump or brittle bones
18. Cancer of the body of the uterus, hypertension, diabetes mellitus
19. Bleaching of dark hairs, electrolysis of hair roots
20. Tamoxifen

Multiple choice questions

1. c 2. d 3. d 4. d 5. a 6. d 7. a 8. b 9. d 10. b 11. b 12. d 13. d 14. c 15. d 16. b 17. b 18. a 19. c 20. a 21. c 22. b 23. d

Selection of options

1. a,b 2. a,d,e,f,h 3. a,b,e 4. c,e 5. a,b,c,f,g 6. a,b,d,e 7. a,b,c,d 8. a,b,c,d,e,f,g,h,i,j,k,m,n 9. a,only 10. b,d 11. a,c,d 12. a,b,c 13. a,b,c 14. a,b,c,e 15. b,d 16. a,b,d,e 17. b,c 18. a,c,d 19. b,c 20. a,b,c,d 21. a,c 22. b,c,e,g,h 23. b,c 24. b,c 25. b,d,e

31 ▪ *Drugs that affect sexual behavior and reproduction*

Multiple choice questions

1. b 2. d 3. a 4. b 5. b 6. a 7. a 8. b

Sequences

1, 7, 2, 5, 3, 4, 6 or 7, 6, 1, 4, 2, 3, 5

Completion exercises

1. Estrogen; epiphyseal closure and completion of transformation of cartilage into bone
2. Follicle-stimulating hormone (FSH), luteinizing hormone (LH); the latter is also known as interstitial cell-stimulating hormone (ICSH)
3.

Hormone	Action	Time of Highest Level
FSH	Initiates development of the graafian follicle in the ovary	Follicular phase
LH	Stimulates graafian follicle to mature and produce estrogen	Ovulation and luteal phase

Correct the false statement

1. F; decreases sexual desire
2. T
3. F; may decrease sexual desire, excitement, or both

Matching

1. d 2. e 3. a 4. b 5. c

Short answer questions

1. a. Impotence, male infertility, high-risk pregnancies
   b. Anginal pain during intercourse
   c. Impotence
   d. Infertility
2. Nutrition, health status, age, medications, drugs, toxins, testicular temperature, body development, endocrine factors
3. Acetylsalicylic acid (aspirin): pain relief, mild inhibition of prostaglandin production; ibuprofen (Motrin), mefenamic acid (Ponstel): inhibit prostaglandin production; progesterone (with or without estrogen):raises progesterone level
4. Alter diet to limit salt and carbohydrate intake; eliminate caffeine
5. High calcium diet (1,500 mg); estrogen replacement therapy; weight-bearing exercise

32 · *Drugs that regulate blood glucose levels*

Correct the false statement

1. T
2. T
3. T
4. F; never (because it is destroyed by intestinal peptidases)
5. F; do not require
6. T
7. T
8. F; more slowly than
9. F; discarded as unfit for use
10. F; generally opposite to
11. F; does not differ from
12. T

Short answer questions

1. Insulin, glucagon, somatotropin, thyrotropin
2. In urine by the kidneys
3. Increased blood sugar level
4. Interrupted insulin therapy; family or personal history of allergy
5. To decrease the risk of lipodystrophy
6. No, not until therapy has stabilized the diabetic condition
7. Reduced blood sugar, increased adiposity; accelerated cardiovascular degeneration; stimulation of production of insulin antibodies; (in toxic doses) hypoglycemia, sympathoadrenal discharge, headache, stroke, coma
8. Temperature of 60–70 degrees F; darkness; protection from agitation; protection from freezing
9. Sugar (candy, sweetened orange juice), glucagon
10. The regular insulin
11. Every 20 minutes
12. Less than 30 minutes
13. 1–2 hours

Multiple choice

1. c 2. a 3. b 4. c 5. b 6. e 7. d 8. d 9. a 10. c 11. a 12. d 13. c 14. a 15. d 16. b 17. d 18. b 19. b 20. d 21. b 22. a 23. d 24. a 25. b 26. b 27. d 28. a 29. b 30. a 31. d 32. b 33. b 34. c 35. b 36. c 37. a 38. d 39. b 40. b

Selection of options

1. a,b,d 2. e,f 3. a,d,e 4. a,b,e,f 5. a,b,d 6. a,e 7. a,b,c,d 8. b,c 9. a,b,c,e,f 10. a,c 11. b,d 12. b,c 13. b,d 14. a,b,c 15. b,d 16. b,c 17. b,c,d 18. a,b,d 19. a,d 20. a,c,d 21. a,b,d 22. b only 23. a,c

33 ▪ *Drugs that affect the thyroid, parathyroid, pituitary, and hypothalamic glands*

Matching

1. d 2. b 3. c 4. a 5. e 6. h 7. g

Correct the false statement

1. F; Usually multiple and global, producing many effects.
2. F; Protein hormones
3. F; Often

Short answer questions

1. Steroid, polypeptide
2. Cholesterol
3. A condition in adults characterized by deficient glucocorticoids (and sometimes mineralocorticoids)
4. To verify a therapeutic response and to detect early hormone excess

Multiple choice questions

1. a 2. b 3. c

Crossword puzzle

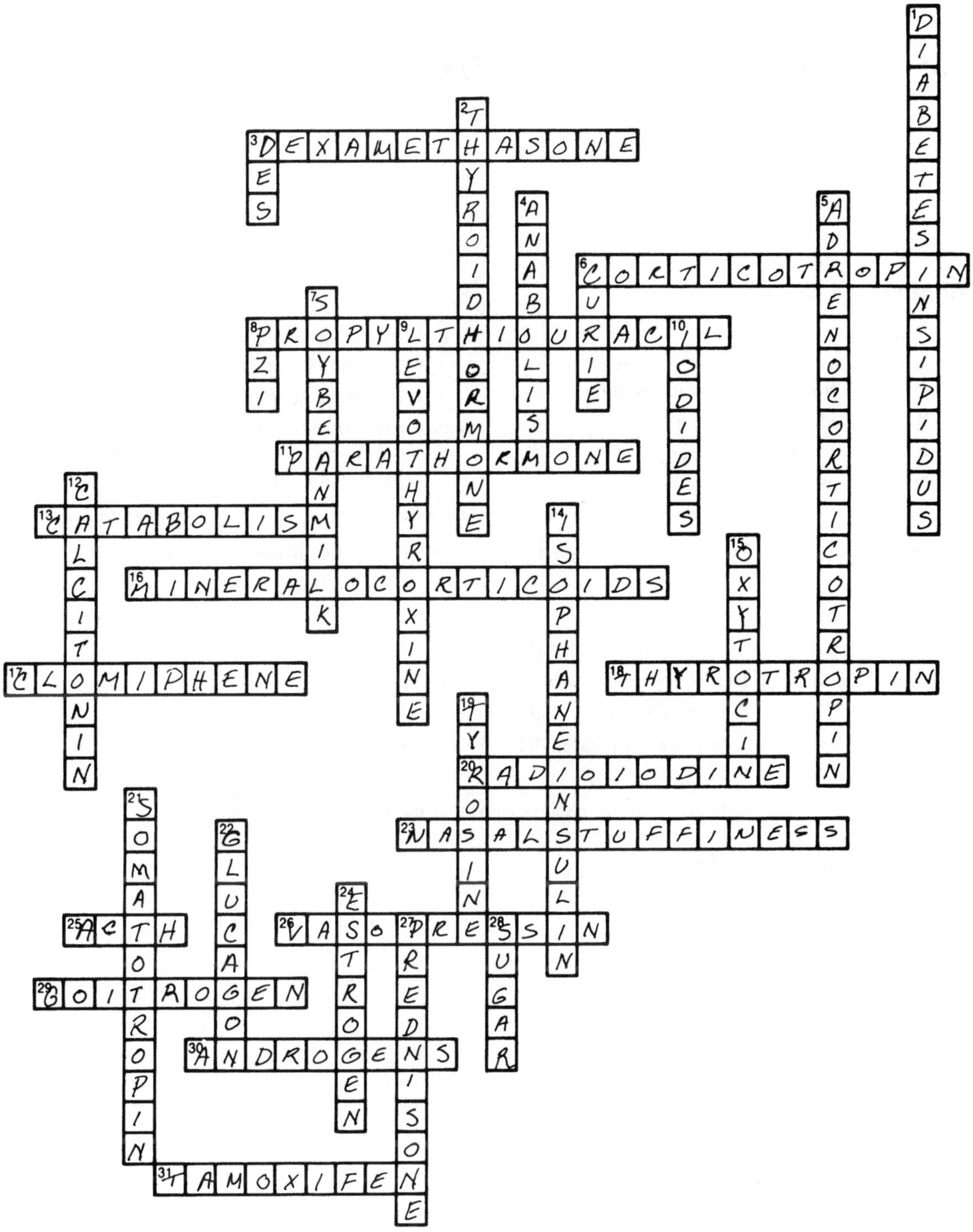

Selection of options

1. a,e,f,g,h 2. b,d,e 3. a,b,c 4. b,c,d,f 5. b,c,e 6. b,c,e,f

34 · *Drugs that control allergies*

Completion exercises

1. History; observation
2. Description of symptoms; documentation of possible factors (e.g., medications, food)
3. Reaction may be severe, even fatal
4. Milk, wheat, seafood
5. Penicillin, aspirin, local anesthetics
6. Dust, pollen, industrial chemicals
7. Cheeks, antecubital fossae, popliteal fossae
8. Preventing future contact with the allergen
9. Medication (epinephrine IM, inhalant IV); life-support system (administer IV fluids, perform CPR, establish airway)
10.

Drug	**Possible Side Effects or Secondary Effects**	**Possible Idiosyncrasy**
Penicillin	Hemolytic anemia; vasculitis; elevated fever level; malaise; vertigo; nausea; vomiting; urticaria; itching; diffuse erythema	Anaphylaxis
Anticonvulsants	Agranulocytosis; elevated fever level	Anaphylaxis
Chloramphenicol	Hematologic manifestations (thrombocytopenia, agranulocytosis, aplastic anemia); arthralgia; elevated fever level; urticaria, delayed skin allergy	Anaphylaxis
Mercurial diuretics	Elevated fever level	
Aspirin	Urticaria; rhinitis; nasal polyposis; asthma; tinnitus	

Multiple choice questions

1. b 2. e 3. c 4. b

35 ▪ Drugs that moderate the immune system

Short answer questions

1. a. 2 months, 4 months, 6 months, 12 months, 4–6 years
   b. 11–12 years, every 10 years thereafter
   c. 2 months, 4 months, 6 months, 4–6 years
   d. 12 months
2. a. Very few cases worldwide; risks outweigh benefits
   b. Of the children infected with hepatitis B at birth, 90 percent will become chronic carriers and up to 50 percent of those infected before their fifth birthday will become chronic carriers.
   c. To prevent mumps orchitis that might lead to sterility
   d. Possibility of a systemic reaction
   e. Healthcare workers are at high risk because of possible contact with contaminated specimens from HBV carriers.
   f. Mutations may occur in some viruses, making vaccine ineffective; risk-to-benefit factors may eliminate or increase the need for a particular vaccine.

Correct the false statement

1. F; several deficiencies of immune function can occur that are congenital or genetic
2. T
3. F; through the placenta, in colostrum, by immunization with appropriate materials, or by having the disease

Completion exercises

1. Placenta
2. Breastfeeding
3. Specific antigen
4. siblings
5. An acute febrile infection or illness
6. It could cause autoinoculation
7. granulocyte colony-stimulating factor
8. chronic renal failure
9. interferons

Multiple choice questions

1. c 2. d

36 ▪ *Drugs that treat inflammation*

Find the hidden words

l a n t k r a b w o l l i w c h d t o r a b d e l e
y s c l y s i n n a s a l i c y l a t e s a c l y n
s p h e n a c e t i n l l n p p c p n h p r o w s o
i i n d t l g l u i y g l u c o c o r t i c o i d s
r r i n d a e e m m p m p r d t h e r m r h n l a a
c i s e r d m r u y o y i n d h t l y s e o y l i c
a n l y e e c i i d h s r e f e v y s a o e l o h r
n d p h e r r n n d e l e e c r i s i s f d e e y i
t o y a i e d i e o y a v h t m c i n e a t u b n n
i m r s l t h e r h p e c r i i a s d e h e c a y e
f e v e r e t h e r p h h e c a c h i l l h r r e o
e t d e l m u u h y p o e a l b y y n y p z o k t m
t h e r m o b d d h p h e n y l b u t a z o n e h r
t a t s o m r e h t c i m a l a h t o p y h a t p e
a c e t o r l p y r r c c e s n h y p e r e s y w h
w i h h y e y h y p i h l a n k e t h y p y r o p t
a n t i y h n i p s p y r o g e n h y y n n s h y n
p h e n l t h e i n d o l l i t w o l l i s a l i c

Matching

1. b 2. g 3. k 4. j 5. e 6. c

Multiple choice

1. b 2. d 3. c 4. d 5. b 6. a 7. d 8. b 9. a

Selection of options

1. c,f,g 2. a,c 3. b,c,d

Short answer questions

1. Dehydration, nutritional depletion; stress on the heart; breakdown of enzyme systems; tissue damage (including brain damage)
2. Immersion in tepid water; use of hypothermia blankets
3. Prostaglandins exist in increased concentrations in inflammatory exudates. The inflammatory process damages cell membranes and arachidonic acid is released. Arachidonic acid is a precursor of prostaglandins, and prostaglandin synthetase catalyzes the conversion of arachidonic acid to intermediary substances. Certain prostaglandins promote the inflammatory process.
4. Many drugs inhibit the release of prostaglandin synthetase; thus, prostaglandin production will be decreased and, hence, pain will be decreased.

5. Give the anti-inflammatory medications with meals or during meals. Give the anti-inflammatory medications with milk or with antacids.
6. Para-aminophenol derivatives (phenacetin and acetaminophen) have the analgesic and antipyretic properties but not the anti-inflammatory or uricosuric properties of aspirin.
7. Acetaminophen normally is detoxified by glutathione in the liver. Toxic doses of acetaminophen exhaust glutathione stores, allowing a toxic acetaminophen metabolite to accumulate and damage liver cells. Acetylcysteine (Mucomyst) is used in its management.
8. Primary gout represents a group of inborn metabolic disorders causing hyperuricemia and deposition of sodium urate crystals in joints. Secondary gout occurs in certain diseases in which there is an increased breakdown of nucleic acids, producing hyperuricemia, or in clients who have an interference with renal excretion.
9. Uric acid is formed by the xanthine oxidase-catalyzed oxidation of hypoxanthine and xanthine. Allopurinol inhibits the xanthine oxidase. This inhibition reduces plasma concentration and urinary excretion of uric acid and increases plasma concentration and renal excretion of uric acid precursors.
10. If penicillin and probenecid were given simultaneously, the effect of the probenecid would be to decrease the excretion of penicillin by inhibition of its tubular secretion. If the two drugs are given together, there are higher (double) concentrations and more prolonged concentrations of the penicillin in the plasma than when the penicillin is given alone.
11. Alkalinization may be accomplished through the use of 3–7.5 g of sodium bicarbonate daily or 7.5 g of potassium citrate daily. Alkalinization might be recommended because uric acid tends to crystallize out of an acidic urine. Therefore, there is the possibility that renal calculi will be formed from the uric crystals.

37 ▪ *Drugs that affect the respiratory tract*

Short answer questions

1. a. P refers to partial pressure—tension. A gas contains molecules and can collide with those of other gases. We breathe air that is a mixture of gases which vary as to concentration. Each gas exerts its own pressure, independently of others, on the molecules of other gases. This pressure is called partial pressure and is expressed as P. The amount of pressure created by any one gas is referred to as its partial pressure.
   b. PO_2 is the partial pressure of oxygen.
   c. PCO_2 refers to the partial pressure of carbon dioxide.
   d. PaO_2 refers to the partial pressure of oxygen in the arteries.
   e. $PaCO_2$ refers to the partial pressure of the arterial carbon dioxide level. (Note: $PACO_2$ refers to alveolar carbon dioxide partial pressure.)
2. a. Refers to the amount of oxygen dissolved in plasma. Expressed as the partial pressure, it is the force that the oxygen molecules exert trying to escape from the solution.
   b. Refers to the percent of saturation of hemoglobin with oxygen content of the blood. Blood leaving the lung usually has a pressure of 100 mm Hg.
   c. Force is required to move air along the airways because resistance is encountered to the airflow. This resistance comes from the bronchi and smaller airways. Compliance refers to the elastic properties of the lungs and wall of the chest. Compliance may change as a result of disease and this affects airway resistance. Infection, mucus, and change in surfactant can also affect airway resistance. Asthma, bronchitis, and emphysema all affect airway resistance.
   d. Refers to constriction of the bronchi
   e. Carbon dioxide narcosis is a condition where, because of disease, the person has high blood levels of carbon dioxide, which he or she is unable to remove. The $PaCO_2$ levels are high. As a result, the person may be in a coma and the driving force for breathing is no longer carbon dioxide but rather low levels of oxygen.
   f. A lipoprotein that decreases the surface tension of fluids in the alveoli and prevents alveolar collapse
   g. Decreased level of oxygen in the body cells and tissue
   h. Increased ventilation; deep, rapid, or labored respiration; increased respiratory rate (normal after exercise)
   i. Decreased levels of carbon dioxide in tissue
   j. Capacity of oxygen in carbon dioxide to diffuse across pressure gradients; ability of the gases to interpenetrate
   k. Bluish coloration of the skin and mucous membranes as a result of reduced or deoxygenated hemoglobin in the blood
   l. Lack of oxygen; may be local or systemic; may be mild to total lack of oxygen (not specific in terms of amount)
   m. Cardiac disease as a result of long-standing pulmonary disease with pulmonary hypertension. Right ventricular hypertrophy results from the obstruction of airways, leading to pulmonary vasoconstriction as a result of hypoxia and acidosis.
3. It filters, warms, and moistens inspired air.
4. The air is no longer warmed and humidified and that injures the respiratory tree.
5. It carries sputum and debris up out of the alveoli and lungs whereby it can be coughed out. It also protects against infection and keeps the respiratory tract moist.
6. Smoking, emphysema, pollutants
7. Respiration is the process by which oxygen and carbon dioxide are changed between the atmosphere and cells of the body. Movement of air into the lung is inspiration and movement of air out of the lung is expiration. Usually, this occurs passively, though we can control it to make it active, or voluntary. The body senses peripherally and in the brain the need for oxygen and alveolar ventilation adjusts to needs. The respiratory center in the brain is sensitive to changes in acidity and the level of carbon dioxide. Oxygen sensors in the carotid and aortic bodies monitor the oxygen level.

8. Allergic response leading to bronchospasm and constriction:

Stimulus	*Extrinsic*
(Inhaled allergen)	Antigenic Dust Pollen Mold Dander ↓
Interact with specific IgE antibodies fixed to mast cells lining tracheobronchial tree	IgE (in mast cells) ↓
Response	*Triggers release of mediators* Histamine Eosinophilic factors of anaphylaxis (ECF-A) Slow-reacting substance of anaphylaxis (SRS-A) Serotonin Prostaglandins Possibly kinins ↓
Response in bronchi	Smooth muscle contraction Vasodilation → Edema → Mucous secretion Eosinophils

9. a. Sympathomimetics mimic the action of the sympathetic nervous system and thus stimulate the conversion of ATP to cyclic AMP which then leads to bronchodilation.
   b. Anticholinergics block the effects of acetylcholine, resulting in stabilization of most cells and bronchodilation.
10. Sputum becomes very thick if a person is dehydrated. Increased hydration leads to thinning of the secretions.
11. Expectorants can increase the secretion of mucus. Expectorants can reduce the viscosity of secretions. Some liquefy secretions.
12. Anxiety will decrease the attention span and decrease learning. Fatigue will prevent learning but most important are the changes that occur in consciousness with a decrease in oxygen and an increase in carbon dioxide.
13. Relieve anxiety; improve respiratory function (deep breathing techniques, coughing); improve hydration; preserve energy through rescheduled rest; prevent infections and other complications; instruct the person to live with the disease to improve his or her level of functioning.
14. Young children, older adults, and any client who has difficulty holding and coordinating metered-dose inhalations.
15. Surfactants replace natural surfactants that may be deficient in premature infants. Surfactants reduce surface tension in alveoli, allowing them to reexpand more fully and more evenly.

Sequences

4,1,2,7,5,6,3

Completion exercises

1.

Drug	Receptor	Action	Adverse Reactions
Epinephrine	Acts on alpha and beta receptors	Relieves bronchospasm and vasoconstriction	Arrhythmias
			Anxiety
			Tension headache
Albuterol	Acts on beta receptors	Bronchodilation and decreased bronchospasm	Increased pulse
			Tremor
			Palpitation
Metaproterenol	More selective to stimulate beta-2 receptors	Bronchodilation	Increased pulse
			Headache
			Nervousness
Terbutaline	Beta-2 stimulation	Bronchodilation	Increased pulse
			Tension
			Anxiety
			Nausea
			Vomiting

2. a. Paranasal sinuses
   b. Nasal concha
   c. Pharynx
   d. Epiglottis
   e. Larynx
   f. Glottis

3. a. Trachea
   b. Bronchus
   c. Bronchiole
   d. Alveolus

4.

Drug	Effect on Theophylline
Cimetidine	Increases concentration and effect
Furosemide	Increases or decreases concentration and effect
Propranolol	Increases concentration and effect
Phenobarbital	Decreases concentration and effect
Phenytoin	Decreases concentration and effect
Smoking	Decreases concentration and effect

Situational exercises

1. a. Low oxygen
   b. Abnormal. Most people respond to hydrogen levels and *p*H of blood and increases in carbon dioxide.
   c. Change in mentation, cyanosis, apnea or coma, reddish skin color, drowsiness, headache
2. Tachycardia, anorexia, vomiting, abdominal cramps, headache, irritability, palpitations, arrhythmia. This is above the therapeutic level.
3. This drug is not used in emergencies. It is not used after the onset of the asthmatic attack, but rather is used to prevent an attack.
4. If you give oxygen, it removes the person's mechanism to breathe; which in this case is low oxygen and not the high carbon dioxide. The person may become apneic and go into respiratory arrest.

38 ▪ Drugs that affect the musculoskeletal system

Matching

A. 1. d 2. g 3. f 4. h 5. e 6. a 7. b 8. c
B. 1. f 2. b 3. a 4. c 5. d 6. e

Completion exercises

1. Carisoprodol and aspirin
2. Methocarbamol and aspirin
3. Orphenadrine, aspirin, and caffeine

Short answer questions

1. Multiple sclerosis; spinal cord tumors; cerebral palsy; "whiplash"; spinal cord injury; herniated disc; tetanus
2. The client should be advised to avoid potentially hazardous tasks, such as the operation of motor vehicles and machinery. The client should be told to avoid the use of alcohol and over-the-counter sleep-inducing agents.
3. a. Allergic-type reactions because of its content of FD&C Yellow No. 5
   b. Liver damage, hepatitis
   c. Nephrotoxicity (related to polyethylene glycol 300 vehicle) when given IV
   d. Anticholinergic effects such as dryness of the mouth
   e. Cardiotoxic complications
4. Bedrest for acute injury; massage; moist heat; relaxation techniques; correct techniques for lifting; correct posture; prescribed exercises

39 ▪ *Drugs that affect the eyes and ears*

Short answer questions

1. Activation of the sympathetic (alpha-adrenergic) receptors causes mydriasis.
2. Blocking the parasympathetic (cholinergic) receptors of the iris causes mydriasis.
3. Paralysis of accommodation is called cycloplegia.
4. Aqueous humor is the fluid found in the anterior chamber of the eye. It is generated by the ciliary processes, and normally drains through the canal of Schlemm.
5. Sympathomimetics, Beta-blockers, Carbonic anhydrase inhibitors, Osmotic diuretics
6. Anti-infectives, Cerumenolytics

40 ▪ *Drugs that affect the integumentary system*

Matching

A. 1. a 2. d 3. g 4. i 5. e 6. f 7. c
B. 1. d 2. a 3. i 4. e 5. f 6. h 7. g
C. 1. h 2. e 3. i 4. c 5. j 6. d 7. f 8. a

Short answer questions

1. Acts as barrier; serves as sensory organ; plays role in vitamin D synthesis; stores glycogen; regulates body temperature; can express emotions; serves as barometer of individual's health
2. Apply to dry skin 30 minutes after washing skin; do not use abrasive soaps for washing; apply at bedtime; do not use concurrently with agent such as benzoyl peroxide; use birth control measures
3. a. Scabies, pediculosis, psoriasis, atopic dermatitis, xerosis, dermatitis herpetiformis, prurigo nodularis, papular urticaria/arthropod bite reactions, pemphigoid, varicella, mastocytosis
   b. Hyperthyroidism, pregnancy, chronic renal failure, cholestatic/obstructive liver disease, polycythemia vera, paraproteinemia, iron deficiency, parasitic infestation, drug reaction, Hodgkin's disease, cutaneous T cell lymphoma/mycosis fungoides, central nervous system tumors, psychogenic pruritus, senile pruritus

41 ▪ *Antimicrobial drugs that affect bacterial cell wall synthesis*

Personal exercise: Antimicrobials

Most students will probably have received antimicrobial drugs in the fairly recent past. Evaluating this experience will promote a sensitivity to the needs of clients who are placed on anti-infective therapy.

Short answer questions

1. a. Effectiveness
   b. Broadness of spectrum
   c. Inability to induce resistance in microbial populations
   d. Retention of potency in presence of tissue materials and other drugs
   e. Penetration to all tissues and fluids in therapeutic concentrations
   f. Lack of toxicity to host cells and organs
2. Cell wall; cell wall synthesis; protein synthesis; metabolism; nucleic acid synthesis
3. Selected reproduction; transduction; transformation; conjunction
4. The spectrum of an anti-infective is the number and type of organisms vulnerable to its action
5. Adrenalin or epinephrine
6. First-generation cephalosporins exert good action against gram = positive organisms, but only moderate action against gram = negative organisms.

   Second-generation cephalosporins are more effective against gram = negative organisms than are first-generation cephalosporins.

   Third-generation cephalosporins are most effective of all against gram = negative organisms but have less activity against gram = positive organisms than do first-generation cephalosporins.

Multiple choice questions

1. b 2. a 3. d 4. c 5. a 6. c 7. b 8. b 9. d 10. c 11. c 12. b 13. d

Selection of options

1. a, b 2. a, b, c 3. c only 4. b, c, d

42 ▪ *Antimicrobial drugs that affect protein synthesis*

Multiple choice

1. b 2. b 3. c 4. a 5. b

Selection of options

1. a,c,d,e 2. a,b 3. a,c 4. b,c,d

Crossword puzzle

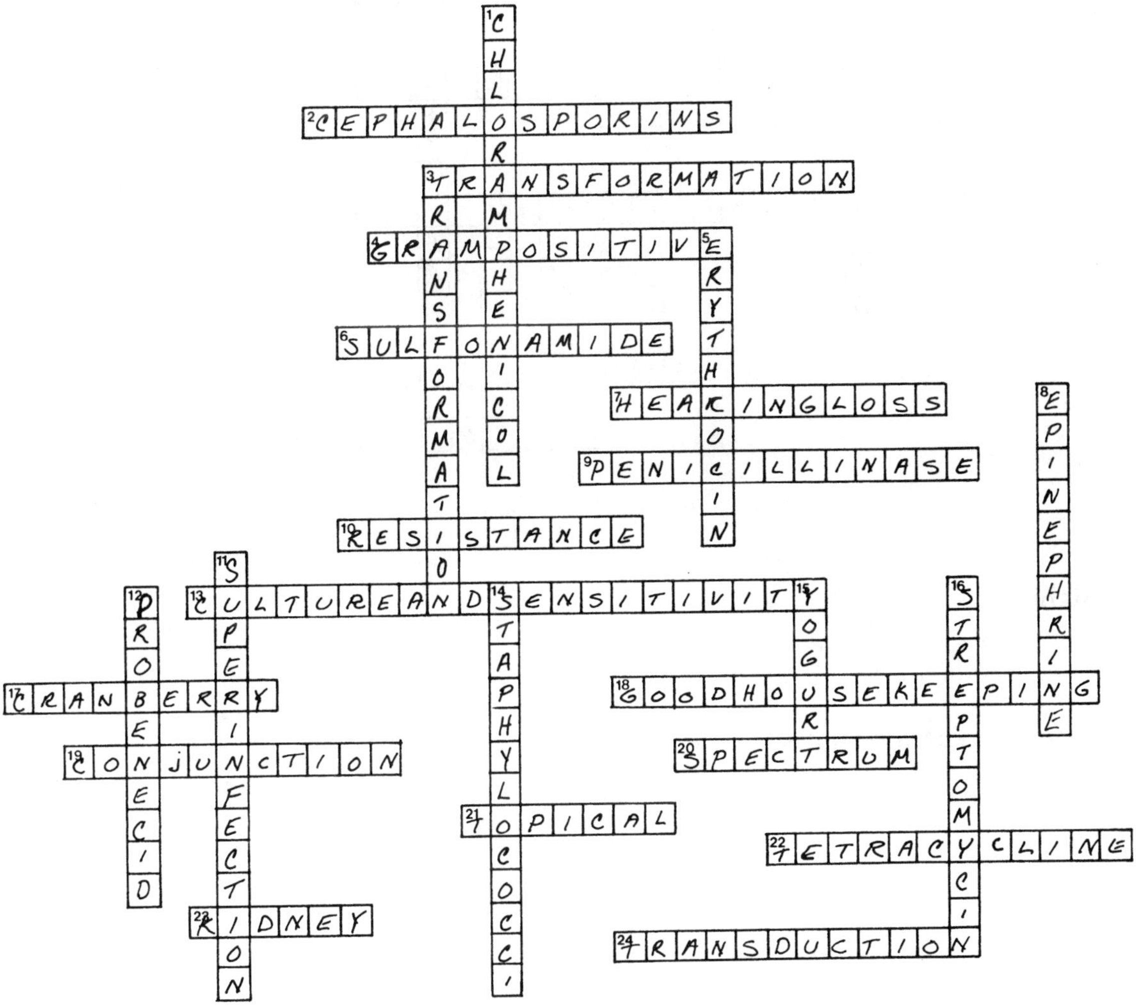

43 ▪ Other antimicrobial drugs

Crossword puzzle

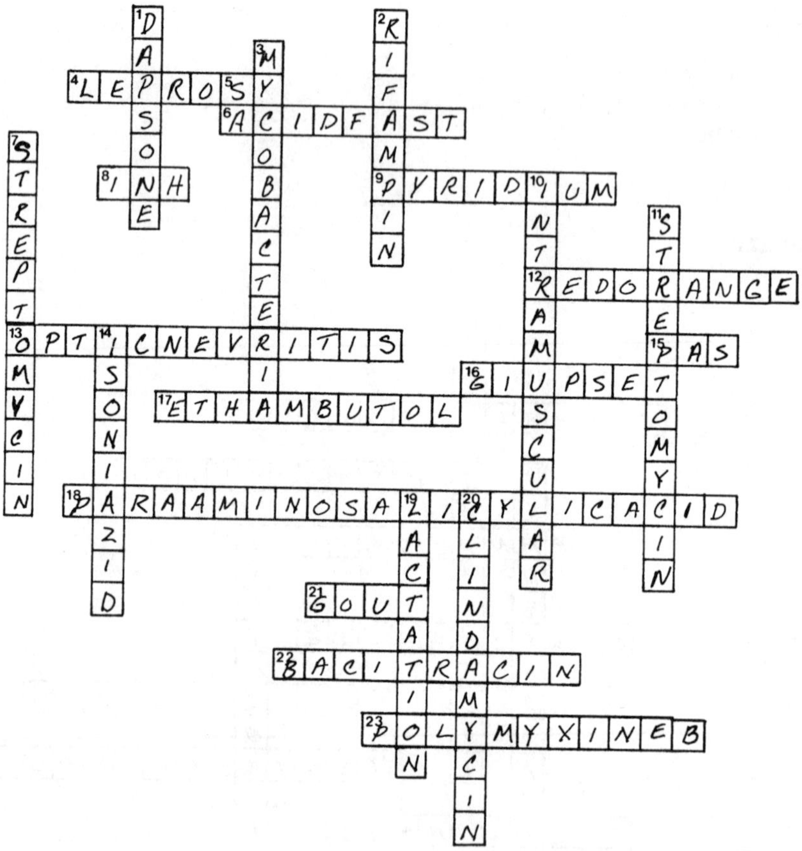

Matching

A. 1. e,f,g 2. d 3. a,c,d,f,h 4. b,c,d 5. a,c,h 6. f,h 7. d, f, g
B. 1. b 2. c 3. d,e 4. a, c

Multiple choice questions

1. a 2. d 3. b 4. d 5. c 6. a 7. b 8. d

Short answer questions

1. Tuberculosis and leprosy
2. Streptomycin
3. Ethambutol, isoniazid, rifampin
4. a. Rifampin
   b. Sweat, urine, feces, saliva, tears, and cerebrospinal fluid tend to become orange-red in color
5. Increase fluid intake, perineal cleanliness from urinary meatus outward, applying and removing perineal pads from front to back, decreasing use of bath salts or bubble baths, decrease fecal contamination of perineum (bowel training programs, prompt cleaning after fecal incontinence), eliminate use of urinary catheters (bladder training)
6. To prevent activation of the drug by stomach acids

44 · *Drugs that treat viral and fungal infections*

Correct the false statement

1. F; preventing contact between virus and host and use of vaccines to stimulate active resistance
2. T
3. F; intravenously, orally, or topically
4. T

Short answer questions

1. The ability to reproduce
2. Tinea pedis (athlete's foot), tinea corporis, tinea capitis (ringworm), tinea cruris (jock itch), candidiasis (thrush/oropharyngeal, diaper rash, vaginal)
3. Promoting ventilation of superficial tissues by using absorbent porous clothing (leather shoes, cotton underwear); avoiding the use of broad-spectrum antibiotics; alternating shoes to allow for thorough drying between wearings

Multiple choice questions

1. c 2. a 3. c 4. d 5. d 6. c

Selection of options

1. a,b,c 2. a,b,c 3. a,b

45 ▪ *Drugs that treat parasitic and helminthic infections*

Matching

1. a 2. d 3. b 4. d 5. b 6. b 7. d 8. d 9. a

Short answer questions

1. Clothing that covers adequately; use of insect repellent containing DEET; planting chrysanthemums; use of insecticides on lawns
2. Rocky Mountain spotted fever (*Rickettsia rickettsii*), epidemic typhus (*Rickettsia prowazekii*), endemic typhus (*Rickettsia typhi*), trench fever (*Rickettsia quintana*), scrub typhus (*Rickettsia tsutsugamushi*)

Correct the false statement

1. T
2. F; whites of Mediterranean origin and blacks
3. T
4. T
5. F; wearing of shoes
6. F; pinworms, caused by Enterobius vermicularis
7. F; toxoplasmosis
8. T

Multiple choice questions

1. c 2. b 3. c 4. c 5. d 6. d 7. a 8. b 9. b 10. a

Selection of options

1. a,b,c 2. a,b,c 3. a,d,e,f,g

46 ▪ Chemotherapeutic drugs: Alkylating agents and antimetabolites

Matching

1. c 2. a 3. b 4. b 5. c 6. b

Short answer questions

1. Triethylenethiophosphoramide, Thio-TEPA; hexamethylmelamine, HMM
2. Carmustine/BCNU, lomustine, CCNU, and streptozocin
3. Ototoxicity means that there are harmful effects on the ears. Symptoms would include hearing loss and possibly tinnitus. Signs would include changes in the whisper and watch tick tests, in the Weber and Rinne tests, and in audiometric testing. An alkylating agent which causes ototoxicity is cisplatin (Platinol).
4. a. A folic acid analogue competitively inhibits dihydrofolate reductase, the enzyme that reduces dihydrofolic acid to tetrahydrofolic acid. Tetrahydrofolic acid is converted to various coenzymes required for several one-carbon transfer reactions. The reaction most sensitive to lack of coenzyme is the conversion of 2-deoxyuridylate (dUMP) to thymidylate (dTMP), an essential component of DNA.
   b. Metabolism of a pyrimidine analog produces fluorodeoxyuridylate (FdUMP). FdUMP inhibits thymidylate synthetase, which catalyzes methylation of dUMP to dTMP. Thus, with this inhibition, a DNA precursor is not available and DNA synthesis is prevented.
   c. The activation of a purine analogue produces a nucleotide, which inhibits purine biosynthesis at its first step and blocks the conversion of inosinic acid to adenylic acid or guanylic acid.
5. It is used to treat premalignant skin keratoses, superficial basal cell carcinomas, and carcinoma *in situ* of the vulva.
6. Avoid spicy and greasy foods; use cold meats rather than hot ones; stress a high-protein breakfast; encourage eggs and cheese; allow foods the client "craves"; use smaller servings, and even use smaller dishes; eat six meals rather than three; make sure the environment is clean, odor free, and free of unsightly items; avoid unpleasant treatments too close to mealtime; be sure the client is positioned properly; provide mouth care; encourage company during mealtime.
7. Be ever mindful of the possibility of infection, and assess for its signs and symptoms; use extremely careful handwashing technique; teach client and family the importance of handwashing; give meticulous care to invasive devices (e.g., urinary and venous catheters, respiratory therapy equipment); consider placing the client in reverse isolation; administer prophylactic antibiotics as ordered by the physician.

Completion exercises

1. a. Adverse reactions are anorexia, nausea, vomiting, alopecia, hyperpigmentation of skin and nails, cardiotoxicity, hemorrhagic colitis, stomatitis, hepatic dysfunction, gonadal suppression, ovarian suppression, pulmonary fibrosis, hypersensitivity reactions, water retention, leukopenia, hemorrhagic and nonhemorrhagic cystitis, nephrotoxicity, renal and bladder tumors.
   b. When the drug is discontinued, your hair will grow in again. Sometimes, however, your new hair may be a different texture or color. Vigorous brushing or teasing of the hair or the use of brush rollers will increase hair loss. You might like to consider using a wig because most women have found a wig satisfactory. If you choose a wig and purchase it now before your hair loss, you might be more satisfied because you could make sure that the wig is a good color match for your own hair.

2. a. Normal saline solution
   b. Juices high in citric acid, rough-textured foods, and hot foods
   c. Nystatin as an oral suspension
3. Mercaptopurine
4. Chlorambucil

Essay questions

1. The concept of synergism is being applied when combination chemotherapy is used. Drugs used in combination chemotherapy would have different sites and mechanisms of action. Using several drugs with different actions may create multiple flaws in the tumor cells, which may prevent rapid repair of the damage, delay regrowth of the tumor, and prevent or delay the development of resistant tumor cells. Differences in toxicity to normal tissues among the several drugs being used in combination may permit full therapeutic dosages of each drug to be given without unacceptable adverse reactions in the client. The rate and duration of remission obtainable with combination therapy is greater than with single drug therapy.
2. Factors that affect whether or not antineoplastic drug therapy is used include the type of malignancy, the client's status, cell growth factors, and pharmacologic considerations.

   Some malignancies respond favorably to drugs in nearly all cases, and other malignancies respond only a small fraction of the time.

   Certain drugs may not be chosen if the client has preexisting heart, liver, or kidney disease. Some drugs are toxic to these specific systems.

   If the client has previously received antineoplastic drug therapy, the choice of drugs is limited because cancer cells develop resistance to drugs by more than one mechanism.

   Tumors in which a large percentage of cells are actively making deoxyribonucleic acid and dividing during a short span are said to have a large growth fraction. These tumors are more susceptible to drug action because a large percentage of cells will be killed by the drug. Tumors in which a small percentage of cells are making deoxyribonucleic acid and dividing have a small growth fraction and will lose a smaller percentage of their cells when exposed to drugs.

   The distribution of a drug within the body may influence drug therapy. Some drugs are excluded from certain areas of the body. For example, tumor cells in the brain are inaccessible to most antineoplastic drugs due to the blood–brain barrier.
3. Phase M: mitosis; prophase, metaphase, anaphase, telophase.

   Phase G_0: resting or dormant phase; normally all genetically assigned functions are performed except reproduction.

   Phase G_1: predeoxyribonucleic acid synthesis phase, ribonucleic acid, and protein synthesis increased, cell growth occurs.

   Phase S: synthesis phase, deoxyribonucleic acid synthesis occurs.

   Phase G_2: premitotic phase, deoxyribonucleic acid synthesis ceases, ribonucleic acid and protein synthesis continues, manufacture of mitotic spindle apparatus
4. In rescue therapy, an agent is given to "rescue" normal cells from the toxic effects of the chemotherapeutic agent. An example is the use of folinic acid in association with methotrexate.

   Certain tumors are treated with doses of methotrexate that are so large that such a dose would ordinarily destroy the client's bone marrow. However, the bone marrow can be protected if the client receives intravenous folinic acid. Folinic acid is a folate coenzyme that does not need reduction by dihydrofolate reductase. When folinic acid is supplied to cells, the methotrexate inhibition of production of tetrahydrofolic acid is bypassed.

47 ▪ *Other anticancer drugs: Natural products, hormones, and antineoplastics*

Matching

A. 1. c 2. c 3. b 4. c 5. d 6. c 7. b 8. a 9. a 10. a
B. 1. d 2. a 3. c,e 4. h 5. a 6. b,f,g 7. a
C. 1. c 2. a 3. e 4. b 5. d
D. 1. e 2. d 3. c 4. a 5. b

Short answer questions

1. Vincristine's adverse reactions involve the central and peripheral nervous systems and the autonomic nervous system. When the central and peripheral nervous systems are affected, the symptoms are paresthesias, loss of deep tendon reflexes, neuritic pain, muscle weakness, footdrop, ataxia, difficulty in walking, slapping gait, sensory loss, cranial nerve manifestations, and headache. Optic atrophy with blindness has occurred. When the autonomic nervous system is involved, severe constipation, abdominal pain, paralytic ileus, and bowel obstruction can occur.
2. The anthracycline antibiotics are inhibitors of topoisomerase II. Topoisomerase II is critical for DNA function and cell survival. These antibiotics bind to DNA and topoisomerase enzymes, resulting in DNA damage (single and double-strand breaks) that interferes with replication and transcription.
3. Two types of kidney damage can occur. One type is an acute renal failure that can be fatal in 3–4 weeks, and the other is a chronic progressive type of damage. The acute form is accompanied by microangiopathic hemolytic anemia, thrombocytopenia, and hypertension. Most of the clients experiencing the acute form had been given mitomycin in combination with fluorouracil, but some had received the mitomycin in combination with other drugs.
4. Hypercalcemia can cause renal calculi and physiologic disturbances because of an increase in the concentration of ionized calcium in the extracellular fluid. It may be so significant as to be life-threatening. Plicamycin is one agent used to lower serum calcium.
5. Clients whose tumors lack estrogen receptors do not respond to hormone administration, but clients with receptor-containing tumors benefit from hormone treatment. Antiestrogens (e.g., tamoxifen) use this concept in their functioning.

Completion exercises

1. a. bone marrow suppression (especially leukopenia), alopecia, stomatitis, diarrhea, nausea, and vomiting.
   b. testicular cancer, small cell lung cancer, non-Hodgkin's lymphoma, and Kaposi's sarcoma
2. Chronic granulocytic leukemia
3. A rapid reduction in the levels of adrenocorticosteroids and their metabolites in blood and urine
4. cross the blood-brain barrier; brain tumors
5. hairy cell leukemia
6. mitotane
7. lowers serum calcium

Essay questions

1. Lungs do not contain bleomycin hydrolase, an enzyme that normally hydrolyzes the bleomycin and inactivates it. The reaction in the lungs usually begins insidiously as a pneumonitis that can progress to fatal pulmonary fibrosis. The process involves most prominently the peripheral areas of the lower lobes of the lungs. Early signs and symptoms are decreased pulmonary function, rales, shortness of breath, and cough.
2. There are two forms of cardiac toxicity: acute and delayed. The acute form occurs 1–3 days after administration and is not considered a contraindication to continued therapy. It is characterized by electrocardiographic abnormalities, including ST-T wave alterations and arrhythmias. The delayed form can produce a life-threatening cardiomyopathy. It is characterized by tachycardia, arrhythmias, dyspnea, hypotension, and congestive heart failure that is unresponsive to digitalis. The mortality rate is over 50 percent. This form appears to be dose-related and the risk is significant if total doses over 550 mg/square meter (in adults) are used.
3. Asparaginase's mechanism of action is quite different from that of other antineoplastic drugs. Most tissues need asparagine and synthesize it. The lymphoblast in acute lymphocytic leukemia does not synthesize asparagine, but it does require it for growth purposes. The enzyme asparaginase catalyzes the hydrolysis of extracellular supplies of asparagine to aspartic acid and ammonia, thereby depleting the supply available to the lymphoblasts and leading to their death.
4. The tissues of the prostate and breast depend on the androgens and estrogens for growth and function. Carcinomas that occur in the prostate and the breast often retain the hormonal requirements of the nonmalignant tissue. It is possible to change the course of the neoplastic process to some degree by changing the hormonal environment of such tumors.

48 ▪ Parenteral supplements

Matching

1. b,d 2. f 3. a,c

Correct the false statement

1. F; total parenteral hyperalimentation solutions
2. F; phthalate (or filters)
3. F; is sometimes administered in the home to clients on long-term therapy
4. F; saline solution

Short answer questions

1. Hyaluronidase (Wydase)
2. They tend to delay it
3. Lipids
4. One with a microscopic filter that removes aggregate particles
5. The client should be placed immediately on the left side to trap the air in the right ventricle.
6. A maximum of 3 weeks (21 days)
7. Typing and cross matching
8. In the refrigerator, away from the coils to prevent freezing
9. 18 years; 65 years

Multiple choice questions

1. c 2. b 3. a 4. e 5. c 6. c 7. b 8. a 9. c 10. b 11. c 12. b 13. a 14. a 15. a 16. b 17. a 18. c 19. e 20. a

Selection of options

1. a,b,d 2. a,b,c,d 3. b,c,d 4. a,b,c,d 5. a,b 6. a,d 7. a,c 8. a,c,e,f,g 9. d only 10. b,c 11. a,b,c,d 12. a,b,d

49 · *Oral nutritional supplements*

PART 1: MINERALS AND VITAMINS

Matching

A. 1. b 2. a 3. h 4. e 5. d 6. h 7. g 8. a
B. 1. f 2. h 3. g 4. e 5. c 6. b 7. d 8. a
C. 1. b,e 2. a 3. d 4. a

Correct the false statement

1. F; ultraviolet light
2. T
3. F; may be cheaper than
4. F; on an empty stomach
5. F; potassium
6. F; magnesium
7. F; potassium
8. F; rickets
9. T

Short answer questions

1. a. An organic chemical found in food that cannot be synthesized by the human body but is essential in small quantities for health and normal growth
   b. Inorganic chemicals used by the body for essential physiologic functions
   c. The minimal intake of a nutrient that is required to prevent the development of deficiency disease in most people
   d. Levels of intake of essential nutrients considered to be adequate to meet the nutritional needs of almost all healthy persons (as defined by the Food and Nutrition Board of the National Research Council)
2. a. Therapeutic strength: vitamin preparations that contain dosages high enough to correct vitamin deficiencies
   b. Maintenance preparations: vitamin preparations designed to prevent deficiencies in people with no existing deficiencies
3. Not usually, because it is not well absorbed when given with food, but it is given with food when necessary to reduce adverse gastrointestinal side effects

Multiple choice questions

1. c 2. b 3. e 4. a 5. b 6. d 7. f 8. f 9. e 10. b 11. a 12. a 13. e 14. a 15. c 16. e 17. d 18. c 19. a 20. d 21. f 22. b 23. c 24. b 25. b 26. d 27. d 28. b 29. b 30. b 31. d 32. f 33. c 34. d 35. d 36. a 37. a 38. a 39. c 40. c 41. d 42. a

Selection of options

1. a,d,e,f 2. a,b,d 3. a only 4. a,b,c,d,g 5. d only 6. b,e 7. b,c 8. a,e,f 9. b,c,d,e 10. b,c,d 11. c,d,e 12. c,d 13. b,d,e 14. a,d,e 15. d only

PART 2: HEALTH FOOD PRODUCTS

Correct the false statement

1. F; are not required to adhere
2. F; seldom recommend
3. F; Health Food Literature
4. T
5. F; sometimes
6. T
7. F; exercise caution because the preparations are not controlled by the Food and Drug Administration

50 ▪ *Diagnostic drugs*

Multiple choice questions

1. a 2. b 3. b 4. b 5. a 6. d 7. c 8. b 9. c 10. d 11. c 12. d 13. b 14. b 15. d 16. b 17. b 18. b 19. d 20. d 21. a 22. e 23. a 24. d 25. b